ARTICLES ON HYPOTHYROIDISM

Recovering from Hypothyroidism series

Covering Hypothyroidism,
Thyroid Treatment, Lab Testing,
Cortisol and Related Issues

PAUL ROBINSON

The information provided in Articles on Hypothyroidism is for educational purposes only. This book is not intended to replace the care by a qualified, licensed and competent medical professional. Care by a medical professional may be necessary to meet the unique needs of an individual patient. The author and publisher are clear that this book does not in <u>any</u> way represent the practice of medicine.

The author, publisher and others involved in the production and publication of this book do <u>not</u> recommend that readers alter their treatment that has been created for them by their own doctor or other health care professionals without individualised and clear guidance from these health care professionals.

Neither the author, publisher, nor any medical or health practitioners or researchers mentioned, nor any other parties involved in the preparation or publication of this book warrant that the information contained in this book is indicated, applicable, effective or safe in any individual case.

The author, publisher and others involved in the preparation or publication of this book disclaims any liability resulting directly or indirectly from the use of the information contained in this book. A qualified doctor should supervise in all matters relevant to physical or mental health.

Every effort has been made to make this book as complete and accurate as possible. However, there may be mistakes, both typographical and in content. Furthermore, this book contains information that is current only up to the date of publishing.

First published by Elephant in the Room Books 2025

ISBN: 978-1-7384579-2-2

To all thyroid patients, who wish to have access to the extensive number of additional articles that I have written over many years on hypothyroidism, important hormone relationships and other significant issues.

Acknowledgements

My grateful thanks to Helen Macdonald who helped me run thyroid forums for over ten years. The website blog posts that form the basis of the articles in this book were often first published on these forums. Without Helen's support I could never have run the forums.

The other person to thank profusely is my wife Fiona. She has supported me through many years, as I continued to try to help thyroid patients as best I could. She is also the best proof reader that I could ever wish for. So, if there are any typos then it is her fault!

Contents

CONTENTS

Chapter 1

Introduction

I am a thyroid patient advocate, with over thirty-five years of personal experience of thyroid hormone issues. I also have over fifteen years of experience of supporting thyroid patients.

Recovering with T3 is still the definitive book on T3-Only therapy. Together with The CT3M Handbook it provides a means for patients to finally resolve their hypothyroidism and low cortisol issues. The Thyroid Patient's Manual is also extremely useful and covers hypothyroidism diagnosis and treatment in a broader way. All the main thyroid treatments are dealt with in pragmatic detail. A host of other issues, from cortisol to low B12 and sex hormones issues, are also covered, but too numerous to list. The feedback on all three books has been excellent.

After completing The Thyroid Patient's Manual, I have continued to state that I would never write a fourth book. Clearly, something must have changed in my thinking.

Why did I decide to write this book?

Over the past several years, I have been wrestling with the thorny issue of what to do about my website after my death. My website was originally created in 2011, but then it underwent a facelift and a new name in 2020 and became https://paulrobinsonthyroid.com

Whether this website still exists at the time of you reading this I cannot say – and this issue is at the heart of why I wrote Articles on Hypothyroidism.

Over the years, I have written many articles which contain additional information above and beyond the content of the books. In some cases, they cover subjects that were not referred to in my books. In other instances, the subject of my article was based on a new piece of research or information that was not available when the books were written. Therefore, the content of these articles is extremely useful to many thyroid patients and needs to be preserved to complement the content of my books.

However, a website takes a lot of work and money to keep it available:

1. You have to pay a yearly hosting charge to the company that owns the servers and gives you the space on the website plus the CPU and memory to run the website.
2. You have to pay to keep the domain (URL), i.e., the name of the website.
3. I have to pay for some specific plug-in software which the site uses.
4. I also pay for the update and backup software.

5. The site has to be backed up and checked for any updates required. Sometimes an update can have a problem and it breaks something making the website unusable. This often means that a previous backup needs reloading.

It is all a manual process. Any errors in 1-5 would cause the website to either crash, or simply vanish.

I originally thought that there must be companies who offer to keep websites running indefinitely, but these do not appear to exist. I suspect that this work it is too specific to an individual website and too much work to make a viable business. This is likely why so many great websites have vanished sometime after the owner has died.

Hopefully, you can now see my motivation for producing this book. You never really know what is around the corner. I am 66 years old as I write this introduction. Although I do not have heart issues, or any impending life-threatening condition, this does not make me immune from some health event. I might never be in a position to preserve all that I have written.

I have been agonising for the past few years on how to keep my work available for patients. I have virtually given up on the idea that my website will be able to continue for very long once my wife and I die. This is why I am working hard on the fourth book.

Putting the articles into a book makes them far easier for my family to continue to keep them available after my death. My books do not require a print run, as they are print on demand. So, the effort to keep them available is relatively minimal. A modest effort on the part of those that come after me will avoid the books going out of print.

Why would I worry about my books going out of print? Well, this is because of the work of two of my thyroid heroes. Dr John C. Lowe wrote the forward to my Recovering with T3 book. His website has vanished now and his books are out of print. He was a pioneer in T3 therapy and is no longer paid attention to. Dr Broda Barnes wrote a book called "The Unsuspected Illness". This book is still in print, even though it was published in 1976. Broda Barnes does not go as far as I do in my books, but we are in line. His ideas are now nearly 50 years old, and endocrinology and thyroid treatment have got worse since then. His book looks like being as relevant in twenty-five to fifty more years as it was when he first wrote it.

So, because of the near-Dickensian treatment of thyroid patients, I need my books to keep being available in some form for a long time – perhaps another one hundred years or even more. The website would definitely not achieve this longevity.

Who is this book aimed at?

This book is meant to help anyone who has read my books and is still looking for additional information and background on hypothyroidism and a wide range of associated issues. In many cases, as always in my written work, I try to back up my content with research references. Where this is not feasible, then my explanations are logically and cogently laid out.

The book includes articles about my books, my videos, general information on hypothyroidism and low cortisol, on the dismal failures of modern treatment, thyroid laboratory testing and how to use it, the contentious issue of low TSH, thyroid hormone dosing and management, cortisol, research studies and other related issues.

Many readers who have not examined my website will find the content extremely useful. Those who have used my website should feel reassured that they will still have access to the articles should the website no longer exist.

Overall layout of the book

After this introduction, I have managed to organise what I consider to be the most useful of my articles into related groupings, each of which appears in its own chapter. There are 9 of these chapters, not including this short introduction, and around 110-120 articles. A huge amount of information is covered.

Special considerations

In the process of preparing this book, I assumed that my own website would no longer exist so I have removed the mention of any of my own website links.

I have worked on the assumption that the websites of others may still be running and have included the links to those articles. However, it is entirely possible that over the course of time some of these links may actually break. I have no control over this.

In the case of published research, I have not only included the link but also the authors, the research paper title and any DOI (digital object number that uniquely identifies the research paper).

The last book

I can safely say that this is my fourth and final book. I had no intention of writing another book after the first three. However, I could see no other solution available in order to preserve nearly 15 years of work that have gone into the writing of the articles contained here. Many of these have been edited, extended, and honed over that time to make them as useful and clear as I could possibly achieve. In doing this editing, I have striven as always to keep my writing as simple as it could be, in order to deliver the information into the hands of thyroid patients.

The current treatment of hypothyroidism is still flawed and limited. Far too many patients are left with symptoms of hypothyroidism. In many cases, this can go on for years and even decades. I do hope that, together, my books continue to provide insights that help you all recover from hypothyroidism. It really should be far more straightforward to recover from this condition, even in complicated cases. As always, I wish you all good health!

Chapter 2

The Books

1. THE BOOKS ARE NOW AVAILABLE IN PAPERBACK, HARDBACK & KINDLE

The first three books in The Recovering from Hypothyroidism series include:

- The Thyroid Patient's Manual – covers the diagnosis of hypothyroidism, various treatments & a huge number of important and related issues.
- Recovering with T3 – covers the safe & effective use of the T3 thyroid hormone.
- The CT3M Handbook – covers how to correct low cortisol levels using T3.

With Articles on Hypothyroidism the series is now four books and is complete. At the time of writing this book, I am only planning on a paperback version.

The books are some of the best and most practical books written about the diagnosis and treatment of hypothyroidism. They are now available in multiple formats – paperbacks, hardbacks and Kindle (an E-Book which can only be purchased from Amazon).

The hardback and paperback versions are available via most online bookstores, e.g., Amazon. If you cannot find one of the books on your usual online bookstore, then do try another online retailer in your country. On Amazon, the Kindle option is also available.

All of the books have undergone extensive revision over the years since they were first published. Often, I have not communicated these changes as they have not significantly affected the core of the books. Nevertheless, a great many changes have been made and all the up-to-date text is now in the currently available hardback, paperback and Kindle formats. The hardbacks are in the same format size as the paperbacks.

More information about each book can be found in the other articles in this chapter.

I hope that you find one or more of the books suitable for you.

2. THE THYROID PATIENT'S MANUAL BOOK – IS IT THE BEST THYROID BOOK FOR ME?

The Thyroid Patient's Manual is a practical, easy-to-read book, which provides an excellent resource for people who are trying to understand hypothyroidism and how to recover from it. It is a great book to read for those trying to recover from hypothyroidism as fast as possible.

It is also the ideal first book to read in the Recovering from Hypothyroidism series of books by Paul Robinson.

The book covers the following topics:
- Information on how the thyroid and thyroid hormones fit into a larger system. In particular, it explains how TSH, the T4 thyroid hormone, the T3 thyroid hormone and cortisol all interact.
- How to tell if someone has hypothyroidism. The book discusses thyroid laboratory testing and lab test results in detail. It refers to recent research findings and points out some of the flaws in current diagnosis and treatment. Most importantly it highlights the main symptoms and signs that might suggest that someone has hypothyroidism. Symptoms and signs are often far more telling than laboratory test results.
- For those about to start thyroid treatment, or those already on thyroid medication but are still unwell, the book suggests some other important laboratory tests to do to ensure treatment has a chance of success. Sometimes, other issues get in the way of successful thyroid treatment and the book will help you to identify and resolve them.
- A large core of the book is focused on the use of the main thyroid treatments: Levothyroxine (T4), Natural Desiccated Thyroid (NDT), T3-Only and T4/T3 Combination Therapy. Each of these has a detailed chapter that explains how to introduce the medication type and then manage dosage changes.
- Less common problems are discussed including sex hormones and other issues that might affect some thyroid patients.
- Throughout the book, suggestions are made to overcome common pitfalls that thyroid patients may face along the road to recovery.

The Thyroid Patient's Manual is presented in a very practical and logical way. It helps thyroid patients to move systematically from the current place in their own health journey and recover from hypothyroidism as quickly as possible.

The book is aimed at several different patient groups. These include:
- Those who suspect they have hypothyroidism but have not yet been diagnosed.
- Patients who have just been diagnosed with hypothyroidism, and need to understand enough about their condition to assess if their treatment is the right one.
- Those who are on thyroid medication but remain unwell, and want to know what might be preventing their recovery.
- Thyroid patients who want to know exactly what laboratory tests they should do and how to interpret the results.

- Those who believe that they may be on the wrong medication for them, and want to know what the other options are and how to use them.
- Thyroid patients who wish to understand the best way to use the thyroid medications (T4, NDT, T3-Only and T4/T3). For those thyroid patients who decide that T3-Only is definitely their best option, they should also read Recovering with T3.
- Thyroidectomy patients, or thyroid patients, who believe that they may have lost significant T4 to T3 conversion capability.
- Overall, it is the foundation of the Recovering from Hypothyroidism series and ideally should be read prior to reading any of the other books.
- The Thyroid Patient's Manual may also be of value to many doctors who are out of date with recent research findings, and their implications for the diagnosis and treatment of hypothyroidism.

The Thyroid Patient's Manual book is a practical manual written to help thyroid patients recover as fast as possible. Amazon also uses Look Inside so you can view sample pages of the book there.

3. RECOVERING WITH T3 – IS IT THE BEST THYROID BOOK FOR ME?

Recovering with T3 is still the most helpful and practical book to read about using the T3 (Liothyronine) thyroid hormone.

Recovering with T3 is part of the Recovering from Hypothyroidism series of books. It is usually best to read The Thyroid Patient's Manual first before progressing to Recovering with T3.

Everyone who is on T3, whether in a small dosage or a large dosage would benefit from reading Recovering with T3.

Recovering with T3 contains the full protocol for the safe and effective use of the T3 thyroid hormone. It also describes an additional protocol for correcting cortisol balance, called the Circadian T3 Method (CT3M). There is an additional book focused just on CT3M, called The CT3M Handbook, but it is important to read Recovering with T3 first. The CT3M Handbook is a companion book and is only needed by some patients, who feel that they need more information on CT3M.

The Recovering with T3 book covers the following topics:
- The background on how Paul Robinson became ill and did not recover from hypothyroidism on Levothyroxine (T4 medication), Natural Desiccated Thyroid (NDT) or T4/T3 combination therapy. It explains how Paul eventually recovered his

health through the use of Liothyronine (T3). This background story will likely resonate with many thyroid patients who find they are struggling to recover from hypothyroidism with standard thyroid treatment.

- with many thyroid patients who find they are struggling to recover from hypothyroidism with standard thyroid treatment.
- Information on how the thyroid and thyroid hormones, the adrenal glands and cortisol work together. Sometimes correcting cortisol can be of equal importance to correcting thyroid hormone function. This was true in the author's case.
- Essential background information on the T3 thyroid hormone, how it works, why it is so crucially important and how it affects other hormones.
- The most important laboratory testing for a thyroid patient to have done prior to starting T3 treatment.
- Many practical pieces of advice on how to go about using T3 therapy safely and effectively. There is a lot to know about using T3, if treatment is to progress smoothly and safely – the book covers all of this.
- The book explains the problems of trying to manage T3 therapy using the standard laboratory ranges for thyroid hormones, and what to do instead.
- Some of the most important chapters of the book provide the detailed protocol on how to safely begin using T3 therapy and how to adjust the T3 dosage. This protocol is described in a step-by-step manner, with guidance on how to assess the efficacy of T3 doses and how to safely adjust them.
- The Recovering with T3 book also describes the Circadian T3 Method (or CT3M). This is an approach created by Paul Robinson, based on research findings. CT3M allowed Paul to correct his own very low cortisol, and he continues to use it himself today. CT3M has proven over the years to be very effective in helping many other thyroid patients to correct their own low cortisol, thus enabling the T3 thyroid hormone to work effectively.
- The book also discusses why some people might never be able to correct their hypothyroidism without the use of T3.

The book is aimed at several different groups of people. These include:
- Those thyroid patients who have been unable to get well on Levothyroxine (T4), NDT or T4/T3 combinations and wish to try an approach that is based on using T3-Only.
- Those thyroid patients who remain symptomatic, with low FT3 levels on any dosage of conventional thyroid treatment. These patients might also have high reverse T3 levels even on NDT or T4/T3 combination therapy.
- Thyroid patients who have been sick and symptomatic for a very long time and want to get well as soon as possible. In these cases, using T3-Only can be very effective. Some T4 based medication could be added later, if so desired.

- Those thyroid patients who wish to use mostly T3 (with a small amount of T4).
- Those thyroid patients for whom any amount of T4 medication appears to be problematic and need to use T3-Only with no T4 medication.
- Thyroid patients who are already on T3-Only therapy but have not been able to find a dosage that eliminates their symptoms.
- Physicians who wish to learn a safe and effective protocol for using the T3 thyroid hormone in anything other than tiny amounts.

Recovering with T3 remains the go-to book for those patients who need to use T3 in order to get well.

Amazon also uses Look Inside so you can view sample pages of the book there.

4. THE CT3M HANDBOOK – IS IT THE BEST THYROID BOOK FOR ME?

The CT3M Handbook was written about two years after the Recovering with T3 book was released. Recovering with T3 covers both a protocol for using the T3 thyroid hormone safely and effectively and an optional protocol to help those with low cortisol. This optional protocol is called the Circadian T3 Method, or CT3M.

Paul Robinson wrote The CT3M Handbook because he had received lots of questions from patients about certain aspects of using CT3M. The CT3M Handbook was written as a companion book to Recovering with T3, in order to cover those things that patients felt needed more explanation.

Many thyroid patients will find the Recovering with T3 book perfectly adequate on its own. Recovering with T3 explains why CT3M can be very helpful and exactly how to use it if required. However, for those that really depend on using the CT3M protocol, and find they have additional questions, The CT3M Handbook is an excellent companion book, as it discusses CT3M in more detail.

The CT3M Handbook was written assuming the reader would read Recovering with T3 first (as Recovering with T3 provides the overall protocol for using T3).

The CT3M Handbook covers the following topics:
- Information on the circadian rhythm of thyroid hormones and cortisol and how the CT3M actually works.
- How to assess if CT3M is relevant to you.
- Practical considerations of using CT3M including what thyroid medications can be used, how adrenal hormone supplements fit in, and many other things.
- Discussion on any issues that can be a problem and prevent CT3M from working effectively.

- How CT3M can be used to allow a thyroid patient to reduce and eventually stop being dependent on adrenal steroids like hydrocortisone (HC). This is only going to be feasible if there is no fundamental adrenal damage (Addison's disease) or hypopituitarism.
- Details of the CT3M protocol are explained in a step-by-step manner.

The CT3M Handbook is relatively short, only numbering some 162 pages, but it does address most of the questions regarding CT3M that have been asked by patients.

The CT3M Handbook is aimed at several different patient groups. These include:
- Those who continue to be plagued with low cortisol issues even though their thyroid treatment appears well adjusted.
- Those who have low cortisol but have been shown to not have Addison's disease or Hypopituitarism, i.e., there is no known reason for the low cortisol levels.
- Thyroid patients who are on effective thyroid treatment, but who are also on adrenal steroids, like hydrocortisone (HC), and do not want to continue to take these. HC and other steroids are sometimes essential but some thyroid patients do not feel well on them and are sometimes given these drugs far too quickly, before other approaches like CT3M are attempted.
- Those thyroid patients who are left with some questions about CT3M, even after they have read the Recovering with T3 book.

Amazon also uses Look Inside so you can view sample pages of the book there.

Chapter 3

General Topics

1. THE ELEPHANT IN THE ROOM

He has never told me his first name. I just have to call him by the name that fits him best! I call him 'The Elephant in the Room'. How do I describe him to you?

Many endocrinologists and doctors have the belief that synthetic T4 (Levothyroxine / Synthroid) is always an effective treatment for hypothyroidism. During my years on Levothyroxine, I continued to feel very ill. I knew the treatment I was being given was utterly failing. My doctors thought that Levothyroxine always worked and my thyroid lab test results were normal. There was a gulf between my view and the view of my doctors. I wanted to find a description for the flawed beliefs that the doctors and endocrinologists had. I ended up calling this 'The Elephant in the Room'. It made it easier for me to describe it to myself and others that I spoke with about it.

Thyroid patients who feel desperately ill on T4 replacement therapy often appear to be the only group of people who know that synthetic T4 is not working for them. These patients can see the elephant.

Many thyroid patients go along to visit their doctor and they sit down in the doctor's waiting room and nervously rehearse what they are going to say, in order to try to get better treatment. Patients often find that this preparation and the appointments themselves are hugely stressful,

Thyroid patients know that their thyroid blood test results are not showing the whole story. For many of these patients, the elephant in the room is clearly visible. The large grey beast may be sitting in one of the waiting room chairs, in heavy disguise. It may be wearing an extra-large pair of shoes, a nice suit and a large hat and be reading a newspaper. The elephant's trunk may be tucked behind the newspaper!

However, some thyroid patients are able to see the elephant very clearly, even though every attempt has been made to not draw attention to it.

The doctor's office staff and nurses do not appear to have a clue that there is an elephant in the room. They do not think there is a false belief, a bad assumption, a flawed paradigm or anything incorrect at all about the idea that Levothyroxine always works for all patients!

If the patient were to ask the doctor, or one of his staff, about the elephant directly, a range of reactions might be elicited, from total denial through to irritation for describing one of the doctor's most valuable assistants as some sort of beast. The patient may even be 'diagnosed' as having a psychological problem and be offered anti-depressants!

However, make no mistake, the elephant is there! Once a patient has recognised the elephant in the room, it is very easy to spot from that point onwards!

I got to the point when I expected to see the elephant. I often heard an endocrinologist speak the inevitable sentences indicating that my thyroid hormones were normal, and I could actually see the elephant sitting in the endo's office – grinning at me!

The above simple analogy is very relevant.

So, many thyroid patients feel that they understand what is happening to them and yet no doctors or nurses appear to recognise it. The doctors and staff simply ignore the very obvious hypothyroid symptoms that have not been eliminated and just keep talking about thyroid lab test results being in range, or about Levothyroxine always working, or that the patient's symptoms must be connected to depression or some other condition. For many thyroid patients, the elephant is very clearly visible!

Recovering with T3 and The Thyroid Patient's Manual will explain why some patients can see the elephant, and why many doctors cannot. These books are written to help thyroid patients to recover from hypothyroidism, and not have to worry about the elephant in the room again.

2. SYMPTOMS OF HYPOTHYROIDISM

I thought this article would go a long way to explain why people with hypothyroidism have such a large range of symptoms and why people often experience hypothyroidism differently.

The thyroid gland is a small, butterfly-shaped gland that sits in your neck. It is part of your endocrine system.

The simplest definition of hypothyroidism is that the thyroid gland is not able to produce enough thyroid hormones. It is also sometimes called underactive thyroid or simply low thyroid.

The main purpose of thyroid hormone is to keep your metabolism running at a healthy rate. So, it should be no surprise to learn that people with this condition will have symptoms associated with a slow metabolism.

Hypothyroidism is more common than you would believe, and millions of people are hypothyroid and are often not aware of it.

Common causes of hypothyroidism.

Hypothyroidism can result for many reasons.

One cause is due to inflammation of the thyroid gland, which leaves a large amount of the thyroid damaged (or dead) and incapable of producing sufficient hormone. This is often as a result of autoimmune attack (also called Hashimoto's thyroiditis).

It is also quite common for middle aged and elderly people (often women), to have lower thyroid hormone production and require some thyroid hormone treatment.

Some thyroid patients require the partial or total surgical removal of the thyroid gland (thyroidectomy). These types of procedures are sometimes needed due to thyroid cancer, nodules, or Graves' disease (hyperthyroidism). Surgical intervention may remove differing amounts of thyroid gland tissue. If there is some thyroid gland left, it may or may not be sufficient to produce enough thyroid hormone.

Goitres and some other thyroid conditions can be treated with radioactive iodine therapy (RAI). The aim of the RAI is to destroy a portion of the thyroid to prevent goitres from growing larger or producing too much hormone (hyperthyroidism). Sometimes RAI can leave a patient without enough thyroid gland and this also results in hypothyroidism.

There are other causes of hypothyroidism beyond the basics above.

Medical categories of hypothyroidism.

Hypothyroidism has been classified historically by the medical profession into several categories:

- Primary hypothyroidism – this is where the thyroid gland fails to produce enough T4 and T3. It is the most common type of hypothyroidism and the patient is said to have an under-active thyroid. It is usually diagnosed through finding high Thyroid Stimulating Hormone (TSH) and low Free T4 (FT4) and low Free T3 (FT3). If this is caused by Hashimoto's thyroiditis, the thyroid peroxidase autoantibodies (TPOAb) and/or thyroglobulin autoantibodies (TGAb) may be raised.
- Secondary hypothyroidism – this is less common and occurs if the pituitary gland fails to produce enough TSH.
- Tertiary hypothyroidism – occurs due to a fault within the hypothalamus gland, which in turn fails to stimulate the pituitary gland, resulting in low TSH and low thyroid hormones.
- Secondary and tertiary hypothyroidism may be collectively referred to as central hypothyroidism.
- Sub-clinical hypothyroidism – is defined by raised TSH above the top of the reference range but with in-range FT4 and FT3. However, we now know from research that simply having an FT4 and FT3 somewhere in the reference range does not mean you are well (see The Thyroid Patient's Manual book for more details).

My definition of hypothyroidism.

The two main thyroid hormones produced by the thyroid gland are Thyroxine (T4) and Triiodothyronine (T3). It is a scientific fact that T4 only has very weak effects, whilst it is the biologically active T3 that makes our cells work correctly. T4's main function is to be converted into the active hormone T3. Therefore, T4 is often referred to as a pro-hormone, i.e., something that is not really an active hormone unless the body is able to convert it into T3.

If for any reason the action of the thyroid hormone T3 is inadequate to regulate metabolism, this is still hypothyroidism (this broadens the definition to include syndromes like thyroid hormone resistance).

So, therefore, if for any reason an individual does not have sufficient T3 hormone converted from T4, or there are any issues within the cells making T3 hormone less effective, this will still result in symptoms of hypothyroidism.

So, my definition of hypothyroidism is 'the sub-optimal effect of the biologically active T3 within some or all of the cells'. In some cases, this is due to too few thyroid hormones, but in every case, it is down to too little effect from T3 within the cells. Many things can cause this. Some examples are:

- Low cortisol, or more properly, hypocortisolism, as cortisol and T3 work together.
- Total thyroidectomy or Hashimoto's thyroiditis (causing thyroid gland damage) – both result in too little T3 (including the loss of T3 converted from T4 by the thyroid gland).
- Poor conversion of T4 to T3.
- Some form of thyroid hormone resistance.
- Central hypothyroidism, resulting in insufficient TSH, and therefore, low T4 and T3.
- Reduced thyroid gland production of hormones or atrophy.
- Any other reason that can result in the sub-optimal effect of T3 within some or all of the tissues that cause the symptoms associated with hypothyroidism.

So, when I use the term hypothyroidism, I mean the sub-optimal effect of T3 thyroid hormone within some or all of the cells of the body.

This definition includes everything that stops T3 from working well within the cells. It is a more precise definition, and is far less ambiguous than just low thyroid hormones, because sometimes the thyroid hormones may not appear to be low – they just are not working correctly.

Note: some of the issues that result in hypothyroidism may not be visible on any current medical test. This can be the case, even though the individual clearly appears to have many of the main symptoms of hypothyroidism. Thyroid lab test results may still be in range.

Why is there such a wide range of symptoms in hypothyroidism?

This is because the active thyroid hormone T3 needs to be at good levels inside all of our cells in order to make them work to their full potential. When T3 is not working optimally in the body, each collection of cells that form glands, organs or tissues may not work at the right metabolic rate and this is when symptoms begin to show up.

Let me provide some examples:

- If the brain has low or ineffective T3, the person experiencing this may have memory problems, brain fog, fuzzy thinking or poor concentration.
- If T3 is not sufficient or effective in the gut, the individual may have digestive symptom issues like poor absorption of vitamins and minerals, bloating or indigestion. They may be more likely to develop leaky gut syndrome or be susceptible to infections, candida, bacterial overgrowth or other imbalances.
- If T3 is low in the body, the liver can be less effective at managing a person's cholesterol and high cholesterol can be a result.
- The heart and cardiovascular system also need good levels of T3 thyroid hormone. A variety of cardiovascular problems including high heart rate, low heart rate, heart palpitations, atrial fibrillation, and heart disease may all result if FT3 is not at the level needed for the individual. The variation of the heart rate often depends on how low FT3 is. If extremely low, then heart rate is usually very low. If just a little low then the heart rate can rise.
- Low T3 can also cause bone loss and lead to osteoporosis if the hypothyroidism is not addressed.
- I could cite many more examples.

In general, the metabolism of an individual person is likely to be low when active thyroid hormone, T3, is too low within their cells. Therefore, it is not going to be a surprise at all to see that the list of possible symptoms of hypothyroidism is vast.

Symptoms of hypothyroidism (this may not be complete):

- Abnormal or painful menstrual cycles.
- Acne and skin infections.
- Allergies.
- Anaemia.
- Anxiety, tension and low stress tolerance.
- Appetite low.
- Blood pressure high.
- Blood pressure low.
- Blood sugar low (hypoglycaemia) – can cause dizziness, hunger.
- Bone loss (osteoporosis, osteopenia).
- Brain fog (see Cognitive Impairment).
- Changes in voice (slower, rougher).
- Cholesterol high.
- Cognitive impairment (brain fog, not thinking clearly).
- Cold hands or feet.
- Concentration poor.

- Constipation.
- Decreased libido.
- Depression.
- Digestive system issues, e.g., absorption of nutrients, bloating, IBS.
- Dry eyes (due to reduced tear production, which may lead to the eyes becoming dry).
- Eyebrows – loss of outer eyebrows.
- Fatigue, tiredness- can be severe and can be the cause of chronic fatigue.
- Feeling cold, cold intolerance.
- Feeling hot, heat intolerance.
- Fibromyalgia (widespread pain and tiredness).
- Fingernails – thin, brittle or cracked.
- Fuzzy-headed feeling.
- Hair – dry or coarse.
- Hair loss – body, head, legs etc.
- Headaches or migraines.
- Heart disease.
- Heart palpitations.
- Heart rate high.
- Heart rate low.
- Insomnia – difficulty sleeping.
- Irritability, mood swings.
- Joint pain or muscle pain or fibromyalgia.
- Memory poor.
- Miscarriages (and difficulty in becoming pregnant).
- Muscles weak or cramping.
- Myxoedema (swollen skin especially on the face, eyelids, upper arms and hands) – see note below.
- Pain – or aches, in muscles, joints, fibromyalgia.
- Reflex responses poor.
- Relaxing is difficult.
- Shortness of breath, laboured breathing.
- Skin dry, rough or pale, cracked, itchy.
- Sleeping a lot. Falling asleep even when you do not want to.
- Slow movement.
- Sore throat.
- Swallowing problems.
- Sweating reduced.
- Temperature low.
- Tinnitus.
- Tongue swollen.
- Vertigo.
- Voice slower or rougher.

- Water retention.
- Weight gain
- … and I expect some of you will know of other symptoms.

Note: Myxoedema is common in severely hypothyroid patients. It is caused by mucin, a glue-like substance that fills parts of the skin. If myxoedema is present, it is often difficult to slightly lift up areas of the skin, using the thumb and forefinger. The presence of this particular clinical feature, combined with low body temperature and any of the other more common symptoms listed above, used to be the main method of diagnosing hypothyroidism prior to the advent of thyroid blood tests.

If extreme iodine deficiency is a cause of the hypothyroidism, the thyroid can become very large and is then called a goitre. This problem used to be less common, as people used to buy iodized salt. However, the use of less salt or sea salt (which usually does not have added iodine) has resulted in a higher level of iodine deficiency.

Potential dangers of having improperly treated hypothyroidism.

Undiagnosed, untreated or improperly treated hypothyroidism is highly detrimental to your health. In some cases, this can leave the individual with on-going debilitating symptoms that make work or home life very difficult. In the worst cases, it can lead to other health conditions like heart disease, high cholesterol, heart failure, osteoporosis or severe depression. Severe untreated hypothyroidism can even result in coma and death in extreme circumstances.

In many cases, if hypothyroidism is not properly treated the poor patient can continue to struggle with their health for months, years or even decades. It can make having a career or job almost impossible. It can impact relationships and home life. I have worked with so many thyroid patients over the years and the collateral damage that improperly treated hypothyroidism can cause is heart-breaking. This is especially sad because hypothyroidism is such a treatable condition.

Note: In this section, I am carefully using the term 'improperly treated' because there are a large number of thyroid patients who have been given the most common form of treatment with T4 medication (Levothyroxine/Synthroid) and for various reasons, they are still severely symptomatic and struggle with their health.

A few comments on the diagnosis and treatment of hypothyroidism.

Hypothyroidism can often be diagnosed with a simple blood test of all the important hormones including:

- TSH – the signal from the pituitary gland to request the thyroid gland to make hormones.

- FT4 – the inactive form of thyroid hormone that in healthy people is converted subsequently to T3.
- FT3 – the active form of thyroid hormone and one of the most important tests to run. Note: testing Total T3 is not sufficient. The bio-available form of T3 needs to be measured – Free T3 (FT3).
- RT3 (Reverse T3) – can also add some useful insights.

In some people, diagnosis of a thyroid problem by blood tests alone is not clear-cut and more account needs to be taken of clinical history. It might even require a trial of thyroid hormone as the ultimate diagnostic test. However, my book, The Thyroid Patient's Manual, provides a lot of insight into how best to interpret the above laboratory tests.

Hypothyroidism is completely treatable in most patients. However, this is a simplified statement, and it is not always easy. There are several types of thyroid hormone preparations and one type of medicine will not be the best therapy for all patients. In particular, the standard treatment with T4 (Levothyroxine/Synthroid) can leave some patients with on-goings symptoms of hypothyroidism. In which case, one of the other treatments should be considered, e.g., T4/T3, Natural Desiccated Thyroid (NDT) or T3-Only. Unfortunately, in some countries, it is getting more difficult to find doctors willing to explore the use of other thyroid medications.

Many factors must be considered in establishing a sound plan for the treatment of hypothyroidism and it has to be different for every patient. Again, many health systems appear to be moving in the direction of trying to assume that every patient is the same. This latter trend usually means focus on thyroid laboratory test results as the primary means of assessing whether a thyroid patient is correctly treated or not. Recent research findings have shown the flaws in this latter approach. Research has also shown that the symptoms and signs of the patient ought to be the most important means of assessing treatment success.

Final comments on the symptoms of hypothyroidism.

Each individual patient may have any number of the symptoms of hypothyroidism, and they will vary with the severity of the thyroid hormone deficiency and the length of time the body has been deprived of the proper amount of hormone.

You may have one of these symptoms as your main complaint, while someone else will not have that problem at all and will be suffering from an entirely different symptom.

Most people will have a combination of some of these symptoms.

Very occasionally, some patients with hypothyroidism have no symptoms at all, or they are just so subtle that they go unnoticed.

If you have some of these symptoms, you need to discuss them with your doctor.

I do recommend getting enough knowledge so that you can tell if the diagnosis and treatment you are being given appears to be correct for you.

The Thyroid Patient's Manual as a resource.

The Thyroid Patient's Manual is an excellent resource for any thyroid patient learning about hypothyroidism and how to recover from it. It is aimed at patients who suspect they have hypothyroidism, those who have just been diagnosed and are beginning treatment, and those who are on thyroid treatment already but are still feeling ill.

The Thyroid Patient's Manual provides a solid foundation of knowledge about hypothyroidism and treatment. The book includes information on thyroid and adrenal hormones, diagnosis of hypothyroidism and selecting the right treatment. It covers treatment with medications like T4, T4/T3, NDT and T3-Only. It also covers many other problems that might get in the way of your treatment working successfully, and how to deal with them.

Everyone deserves good health!

3. SYMPTOMS OF LOW & HIGH CORTISOL AND ISSUES WITH ALDOSTERONE

This article is based on a few extracts from Chapter 5 of my book, The Thyroid Patient's Manual. Please see the book for a more complete description of the adrenal glands, adrenal hormones, and issues that can arise in connection with these.

I am not going to discuss treatment options for low cortisol in this article. I do discuss this in my book The Thyroid Patient's Manual. I also describe how to tackle low cortisol in my other two books, Recovering with T3 and The CT3M Handbook.

Low cortisol often goes hand in hand with thyroid problems, as it is often induced by hypothyroidism, or incorrectly treated hypothyroidism, which leaves the thyroid patient with low FT3, or a poor combination of FT3 and rT3.

This article will focus on the symptoms that can be caused by severe, moderate, or mild levels of low cortisol.

It will also briefly cover the symptoms of high cortisol and both low and high aldosterone. Please be aware that people vary in the number of these symptoms that they experience, and the severity of the symptoms.

Let me first cover the most severe type of low cortisol caused by adrenal gland failure - Addison's disease.

Addison's disease is a life-threatening condition. Proceeding with thyroid treatment without diagnosing and treating Addison's disease could risk an Addisonian crisis and death. In Addison's disease, the adrenal cortices are destroyed. This is usually caused by an autoimmune attack. In this case, adrenocorticotropic hormone (ACTH) from the pituitary is not effective in producing sufficient cortisol.

Sufficient cortisol is required to maintain health and quality of life. In states of physiological stress, particularly caused by infection or physical exertion, the body produces significantly more cortisol – sometimes even by a factor of 10. Consequently, in Addison's disease, the body cannot meet the demand for higher cortisol, and an Addisonian crisis can result.

Sufficient aldosterone is required to maintain blood pressure and sodium/potassium balance. Many deaths from Addisonian crisis, or adrenal crisis, are caused by the nearly complete absence of aldosterone. With low aldosterone, potassium levels become very high and can cause cardiac arrhythmias.

Note: in central adrenal insufficiency (in which there is little or no ACTH stimulation), the cortices will continue to produce sufficient aldosterone in most individuals. They will also produce a little cortisol – even with no ACTH secretion at all.

Addison's disease is extremely serious and must be ruled out before proceeding with thyroid treatment. To begin thyroid treatment in the presence of undiagnosed Addison's would risk causing an Addisonian crisis. Addison's disease symptoms usually develop slowly over many months.

The symptoms of Addison's disease include:

- Extreme fatigue.
- Weight loss and decreased appetite.
- Darkening of your skin (hyperpigmentation).
- Low blood pressure, fainting, worse on standing.
- Salt craving.
- Low blood sugar (hypoglycaemia).
- Nausea, diarrhoea or vomiting.
- Abdominal pain.
- Muscle or joint pains.
- Irritability.
- Low mood, mild depression.
- Body hair loss or sexual dysfunction.
- Frequent urination.
- Drowsiness.
- Increased thirst.
- Dehydration.

If some or all of these symptoms are not responded to, the situation can worsen over time. These symptoms typically worsen when even a mild illness like a cold occurs.

Acute adrenal failure/Addisonian crisis symptoms:

- Pain in your lower back, abdomen or legs.
- Severe vomiting/diarrhoea.
- Low blood pressure, worse when standing up.
- Severe drowsiness or loss of consciousness.
- High potassium and low sodium.
- Muscle cramps.
- Severe dehydration.
- Pale, cold and clammy skin.
- Sweating.
- Rapid, shallow breathing.
- Severe muscle weakness.
- Headache.

If the above is not promptly attended to, the risk of an Addisonian crisis is significantly higher.

Addison's disease needs to be diagnosed and treated by an endocrinologist, as it can be life-threatening as I have said many times now. Extremely low cortisol in Addison's disease is treated with hydrocortisone (HC), which is bio-identical cortisol.

Once on HC treatment, the individual needs to be aware that there are situations where a higher HC dosage needs to be used. The reason for this is that the HC an Addison's patient requires will suppress any remaining ability to make cortisol. So, in the event of higher physiological stress, the body cannot respond to it by making more cortisol. The need has to be met by using more HC medication.

If your doctor suspects severe hypocortisolism, or adrenal gland damage or low aldosterone you need to be referred to an endocrinologist for further investigation.

Severe hypocortisolism may also prompt the doctor to consider low aldosterone as a possible problem, as this is often also present in Addison's disease.

What about less severe low cortisol that is not caused by Addison's disease?

Many thyroid patients experience milder levels of low cortisol, sometimes known as partial adrenal insufficiency, or adrenal fatigue. Both of these terms are misleading, as I will discuss soon.

Some of the symptoms of hypothyroidism may be confused with some of the symptoms of low cortisol since both can lower metabolic rate. Low cortisol may interfere with the conversion of T4 to T3 and result in lower FT3 and elevated rT3. Low cortisol also reduces T3-effect in the cells. When cortisol is low, blood sugar may also be low. Insufficient blood sugar will slow down the mitochondria – thus slowing down metabolism.

31

The mechanism that most frequently causes low cortisol is hypothalamic-pituitary (HP) dysfunction. This means that for some reason the HP system is not controlling one or more endocrine glands correctly, even though there may be no damage or disease in either the hypothalamus or pituitary.

Contrary to what many alternative medicine practitioners claim, the adrenal glands do not become 'fatigued' or 'tired'. They can continue to make and secrete cortisol in large amounts as long as they are stimulated to do so by sufficient ACTH from the pituitary gland. For instance, cortisol levels remain very high indefinitely in Cushing's disease – when a pituitary tumour produces excessive ACTH. So, even in the state of constant and prolonged excessive cortisol production, the adrenals just keep making cortisol. The adrenals can continue to make all the steroid hormones, as long as there is sufficient cholesterol in the blood.

The rate-limiting step in cortisol production is the amount of ACTH-stimulation of the adrenal cortices. Hence, the terms 'adrenal fatigue' or 'tired adrenals' are misleading. The term 'partial adrenal insufficiency' tends to imply that the adrenals are 'partially insufficient'. It is a vague term, but it is misleading too, as the adrenals themselves are usually not the issue.

The cause of most cases of low cortisol is inadequate secretion of ACTH by the HP system. It is a dysfunctional state, not a 'disease' state, i.e., there is usually nothing at all wrong with the adrenal glands themselves.

Often the cause of this HP dysfunction is unknown, although many studies have shown that it can result from extreme or prolonged stress. The net effect of this is that cortisol and DHEA eventually fall. Dysfunction of the hypothalamic-pituitary-adrenal axis (HPA axis) is thought by some doctors to be the number one cause of low cortisol problems.

Genetic mutations can also cause adrenal cortex dysfunction. Mutations can reduce the function of the enzymes needed to make cortisol, resulting in a condition known as congenital adrenal hyperplasia (CAH). Milder versions of this disorder occur in adults – where it is known as non-classical CAH. In CAH, DHEAS levels are high as more ACTH is secreted to super-stimulate the cortices to make enough cortisol.

Mild to moderate low cortisol problems are far more common than the severe cortisol insufficiency of Addison's disease. Unfortunately, most doctors do not test, recognise, or treat moderate to mild low cortisol.

I prefer to use the term 'hypocortisolism' versus 'low cortisol'. Low cortisol is better defined as the sub-optimal effect of cortisol within some or all of the cells. This definition includes all the possible causes, e.g., HP dysfunction, adrenal gland disease, and even cortisol resistance. It includes everything that stops cortisol from optimally operating within the cells. Consequently, I use the terms hypocortisolism and low aldosterone – which are far more specific.

Some of the main symptoms of hypocortisolism include:
- Low blood sugar – dizziness, unwell, hunger.

- Severe fatigue, tiredness.
- Dizziness (even when sitting down).
- Low blood pressure.
- Intolerance to even low dose thyroid medication.
- Poor response to thyroid treatment or dose raises.
- Anxiety or inability to cope with stress.
- Irritability or anger or panic feelings.
- Feeling cold.
- Low body temperature as thyroid hormone is not as effective.
- Fluctuating body temperature.
- Aches and pains.
- Pale skin or slight darkening of the skin.
- Skin appears thinner.
- Digestive upsets – may include diarrhoea.
- Nausea.
- Weight loss if cortisol very low.
- Worsening allergies.
- Trembling, shakiness or jittery/hyper feeling.
- Rapid heartbeat especially after thyroid meds.
- Insomnia - difficulty sleeping.
- Flu-like symptoms.
- Dark rings under the eyes.
- Low back pain (where adrenal glands are).
- Hair loss.
- Worsening symptoms in presence of stress.
- Clumsiness.
- Fatigue in the morning but better in the evening.

Some of the main symptoms of low aldosterone include:

- Low blood pressure.
- Postural hypotension (lower BP on standing).
- Craving for salty foods.
- Thirst.
- Light headedness on standing.
- Frequent urination (esp. during the night).
- Excessive sweating.
- Slightly higher body temperature than usual.
- High heart rate/palpitations.
- Cognitive fuzziness.

- Dizziness or fainting.
- Low sodium and high potassium.

Note: low aldosterone can occur with or without Addison's disease. It can also occur with or without hypocortisolism. So, your doctor should be aware of this and be on the lookout for any indications of it, even if you do not have Addison's disease.

Low levels of thyroid hormone can cause several symptoms of hypocortisolism.

This can obviously make recognising hypocortisolism a bit of a challenge. If someone has been hypothyroid for a considerable time before diagnosis and treatment, it is possible that there will be hypocortisolism present. Therefore, hypocortisolism is something that a family doctor or endocrinologist should either check for, or at the very least, be on the lookout for.

Let me now briefly discuss high cortisol.
These are some of the clues when high cortisol is present:

- High blood pressure.
- Vasoconstriction causing pain in the chest, similar to angina.
- The latter can also cause arrhythmia – changes in heart rate, missing beats, extra beats.
- Heart rate variations including pounding heart, high heart rate - see the previous point.
- Bruising easily.
- Fluid retention.
- Weight gain, obesity, or moon-shaped face.
- Increased belly fat, fat on the back of the neck.
- Fatigue.
- Weak muscles and muscle loss.
- Facial flushing.
- Bile acid indigestion – burning in stomach.
- Excess stomach acidity – this can be severe.
- Mood swings – anxiety, depression, irritability.
- Increased anxiety is particularly common in high cortisol.
- Note: gut issues including diarrhoea are usually linked with low cortisol. But the effect of the stress hormone cortisol within the brain can cause it to send signals to the large intestine and cause mild diarrhoea (getting the body ready for flight or fight). Also, chemicals released due to stress/anxiety/possible depression etc. can cause the chemicals released by this to disrupt the gut flora and also cause gut symptoms.
- Hair loss.

- Reduced TSH.
- Reduced FT3, increased rT3.

These are some of the clues when high aldosterone is present:

- High blood pressure.
- Low potassium (weakness/muscle spasms).
- Numbness or tingling in the extremities.
- Frequent urination.

If you suspect low or excess adrenal hormones then please ask your doctor to run lab tests for cortisol, aldosterone, renin, potassium and sodium, in order to get a more complete picture.

For a fuller description of the adrenal glands, adrenal hormones, disease states, and treatment options, please see The Thyroid Patient's Manual.

4. PAUL ROBINSON'S STORY

This is the story of how Paul Robinson recovered from hypothyroidism, became a thyroid patient advocate and wrote his books

I have had Hashimoto's thyroiditis for over thirty years. I am now well into in my sixties.

During the first seven years of my illness, I was on Levothyroxine (T4, Synthroid) only and my symptoms hardly changed at all, i.e., I still felt chronically hypothyroid with most of the same symptoms I had prior to diagnosis apart from the myxedema.

I saw five or six endocrinologists during the first six to seven years and received the same response: I was told my TSH, FT4 and FT3 were all normal and that my symptoms could not be due to the thyroid treatment – which was apparently fine. The fact that my health was perfect before Hashimoto's thyroiditis and was dreadful since the 'treatment' with T4 seemed to elude the specialists I saw. It was obvious to me that I still had hypothyroidism symptoms.

I felt that this really very simple logic was totally lost on them – it was very frustrating!

I was offered anti-depressants because they thought that my distraught pleadings with them to get to the bottom of my problem was just depression. I was offered a place in an ME patients' support group because I was clearly going to have to live with my symptoms and accept that I had ME as well as thyroid disease. For any USA-based reader, 'ME' is what we often call chronic fatigue syndrome (CFS) in the UK.

I was offered a lot of things but no solution and no real explanation (that I believed).

The so-called specialists that I went to see (some private ones), said very unhelpful and I thought stupid things to me:

"Your lab test results are in range, so there is nothing wrong with your thyroid hormones."

"You are on the correct treatment, so your symptoms are due to something else."

"It is chronic fatigue syndrome or ME, so you are just going to have to learn to live with it."

"No, you don't need extra T3 to get your level higher – it is already in range."

"FT3 in the lower part of the reference range is still fine."

The Internet was in its infancy at that time. So, I began buying endocrinology books, using the library and borrowing books on endocrinology and the thyroid. I began educating myself. I had to. My health had deteriorated by this point because the T4 medication was not working. I had severe fatigue and weakness. My career, which I loved, was close to ending, as I was more often not able to go to work due to my worsening health.

Things got even worse. I was not able to walk far and spent most days laying on my sofa or in bed. I could barely get up the staircase at home. I had to go to sleep for at least four hours in the middle of each day in order to cope. I felt so ill and dizzy with low blood pressure that I used to blackout regularly (most days). I had digestive system issues. I was weak. I had lost over 30% of my body weight due to low cortisol. My bones were sticking out. My doctor and the doctor at work both had concerns about how my health might deteriorate further. No doctor could understand what was going on or how to help me.

I began to believe that I was actually dying and that it would be only a few years at most before this happened. I was forced to put plans in place, so that when I died, my family would be looked after as well as possible. This was when I was about 36 or 37 years old! I did lose my job and my career. Everything was black.

My life at home was also a train wreck. I was married and I had two young children. I felt too exhausted and too ill to be a good parent, and as a consequence, I lacked the patience and the ability to provide my children with the care and attention that they needed. It was an extremely bad time for all concerned. There have been terrible long-term consequences of this.

I had to find out how to get myself well because the medical profession had failed to help me.

The gradual increase in knowledge paid off because I began to develop an understanding of what I thought might be happening. I began to use the burgeoning Internet to see what relevant research might have been published.

I realised that something had fundamentally changed within my body after the advent of Hashimoto's thyroiditis. The change had altered the way my body is able to process and utilise thyroxine (T4).

I knew that I needed to confirm this with a trial of liothyronine (T3). In fact, I knew that a trial of T3-Only was the ONLY way to confirm what I thought was happening, as there was no test for it.

After a lot of my own investigation, I managed to find a doctor who was prepared to offer a series of trials of alternative thyroid hormones.

Trials with natural desiccated thyroid (NDT), and with synthetic T4 + T3, and some adrenal support all failed dismally. So, I began to use T3-Only.

Within two weeks of getting on a moderate dose of just T3 (and no T4), I began to see some small improvements.

There was almost no useful information on using T3 available at that time. So, it took me nearly three years to finally arrive at a T3 dosage that made me feel really well again. I only managed to do this, because I kept believing that I could get well. I also learned very quickly that I had to be very organised, collect data and not make rapid changes. I began to learn that I would make mistakes along the way, but I could rectify these. In working through this, I developed the basis of the protocol that is now described in The Recovering with T3 book.

During those years, my knowledge of T3, and all issues surrounding its use, grew exponentially. I gained information from numerous sources including my own personal experience with T3.

I obviously went back to see my endocrinologists and doctors, when I first began to respond to T3. I knew the T3 on its own was what I had needed. However, I was met with scepticism and anger.

They did not believe me. One of the endocrinologists actually said I should not be on T3 at all, that it was not needed. He said my symptoms had been caused by some other condition! The fact that they had gone completely on the T3-Only therapy did not shake his view! I found this type of thinking difficult to understand, as it just is not logical. I never saw him again and I did not go back to T4.

I have been on T3-Only treatment for over 30 years. After the first 3 years of working out a safe and effective protocol for its use, I began my real road to recovery.

I take 60 micrograms per day of T3 and no adrenal medication, as I have corrected my cortisol level using the optional part of my T3 protocol (CT3M).

I have no FT4 in my blood test results and my TSH is suppressed to near zero. My FT3 levels are over the top of the population reference range, but I am neither hyperthyroid nor thyrotoxic.

Blood tests – well, I could say a LOT about them. As soon as I was on only T3 and no T4, it became apparent to me and my new family doctor, and a new endocrinologist, that the conventional method of managing dosage via TSH, FT3 and FT4 was not going to work. The fluctuating levels of T3 in the bloodstream from the individual T3 doses and the effect that this has on TSH, make using TSH or even FT3 too unreliable and unhelpful. I use a different method. This is covered in the Recovering with T3 book, and other articles.

Oh! The other interesting thing is that if I take any T4 now it just interferes with T3 treatment and I go hypothyroid very quickly.

One thing is very clear though that this is not a unique problem. I have spoken to thousands of thyroid patients all over the world with this type of problem. Many have bought my Recovering with T3 book and have made their own recovery using T3-Only or T3/T4 combinations. I have now seen very large numbers of thyroid patients make full recoveries on T3 without any T4.

One of the most horrifying things is that NONE of my hypothyroidism problems were highlighted through countless thyroid BLOOD TESTS. Even full thyroid panels which included TSH, FT4 and FT3 revealed nothing. They just elicited the response from doctors that my thyroid hormone levels were 'normal'.

All the problems were going on inside my cells and were never visible through the use of any laboratory blood tests.

I was not depressed.

I was not psychologically disturbed.

I did not have ME, chronic fatigue syndrome (CFS) or Fibromyalgia.

I did not have to accept my ill health and just live with it!

All of the above 'diagnoses' that were given to me were just plain wrong and if I had accepted them, then I would still be ill now, or more probably dead! They were more than 'wrong' – they were bad science and bad diagnostic work.

I had a problem with thyroid hormones that simply could not be seen through blood tests.

I personally lost what could have been my very best years. These were the years during which I could have developed a really successful and satisfying career. Instead, I lost my career.

More importantly, my young children were born and grew up during that time. I was not the father I wanted to be. There have been consequences to this that have been hard to deal with. My marriage suffered also and eventually ended as a result.

I will never, ever be able to consider thyroid disease without also thinking about the collateral damage it can do to the person involved, their career, their family and others around them.

I will not ever get over the damage that was done to me. It occurred because of a lack of timely and correct treatment.

Very little appears to have changed in the intervening years. In fact, from talking to other patients, I would say it is now harder to get believed and get the right treatment than it was back then.

It is a disgrace that so few people get adequately treated if T4 does not work. Yes, many people do get better on the standard T4 treatment, but so many, in terms of pure numbers, are cast aside and have ruined lives as a result.

All the various thyroid treatments do need to be available.

However, due to a variety of reasons, most endocrinologists and family doctors still refuse to use all the available treatments at their disposal.

Recovering with T3, The CT3M Handbook and The Thyroid Patient's Manual, together with this collection of articles are a part of my continued effort to communicate better ways to treat thyroid patients.

5. WHY PAUL NEEDED T3-ONLY THYROID MEDICATION

This is an update on the reasons why I could not get well using T4, T4/T3 or NDT medication. I needed T3-Only medication in order to recover my health.

Firstly, I have defective DIO1 and DIO2 genes that are responsible for producing the D1 and D2 deiodinase enzymes correctly.

I have tested the DIO2 gene defect and the two DIO1 gene defects. See Article 2 in Chapter 5 for more information on both DIO2 and DIO1 gene defects and how to test them.

I have discovered that I have the homozygous variant of both the DIO1 and DIO2 gene defects. Homozygous means that I inherited both copies of the defects (one from each of my parents). Given I have both copies of all the defects then I am more likely to be a poor converter of T4 to T3.

The D2 deiodinase enzyme is used by the brain, pituitary, thyroid gland, heart, and muscles. D2 is far more efficient in converting T4 to T3 than D1.

See the Watts Study for more information on the DIO2 deiodinase gene defect. This is referenced in Article 2 in Chapter 5.

The D1 deiodinase enzyme is produced by the cells of the liver and kidneys. D1 is less efficient in converting T4 to T3. However, in the liver D1 is very important, as it is used to clear rT3, i.e., to convert rT3 to T2, T1 and then T0 before removing it from the body within 24 hours. So, a DIO1 defect can cause higher rT3, because the rT3 will not be cleared as fast. We know that high rT3 also tends to lower the number of D2 deiodinase enzymes, thus making the conversion of T4 to T3 even worse.

There are two DIO1 gene defects. I am homozygous for both of these, and got both copies of each defect. So, I have all the defective mutations for the DIO1 and DIO2 gene defects. I was always likely to have T4 to T3 conversion problems.

Secondly, Hashimoto's Thyroiditis destroyed my thyroid gland. This is another reason that so many with Hashimoto's, or thyroidectomy patients, need additional T3, as it causes a significant loss of conversion ability from T4 to T3.

The thyroid is the biggest converter of T4 to T3 in the body. The contribution of the thyroid gland to conversion is far more important than the liver, or kidneys or peripheral tissues. The blood flowing through the thyroid gland carries FT4, and the thyroid converts some of this FT4 to FT3. The conversion contribution of the thyroid gland is more significant than any T3 produced by the thyroid itself in normal circumstances. The thyroid is responsible for 25% of our total circulating T3 (through T3 production and mostly through T4 to T3 conversion capability). So, when you lose thyroid tissue, you also lose this T3 and the important T4 to T3 conversion capability. It is gone – permanently!

Thirdly, my thyroid gland is now completely atrophied and barely there. Hashimoto's does not do this. However, Atrophic Thyroiditis (AT) does do this. I cover AT in Article 1 in Chapter 10, so I will not go into details here. However, it is worth noting that someone with AT often finds it difficult to tolerate T4 medication and convert it to T3. In addition, AT can cause rapid atrophy of the thyroid gland – resulting in the loss of significant T4 to T3 conversion ability.

Fourthly, I was also driven to T3 medication use, because I had extremely low cortisol levels when on T4-based medication.

The pituitary uses the D2 deiodinase enzyme to convert 80% of the T4 that passes through its cells. It keeps this converted T3 within its own tissues, i.e., the pituitary gland NEEDS high levels of FT3 in order to function. With worsening conversion through the DIO2 gene defect and the loss of thyroid conversion, on T4-based medication, I would have had lower T3 levels in the pituitary. This can induce dysfunction in the pituitary, and lower the output of ACTH and TSH. T3-Only is known to stimulate the hypothalamic-pituitary system and the mitochondria far more than T4 or T4/T3.

My cortisol levels were so poor, that my blood pressure was horribly low and as a result, I used to pass out quite often. Only when I managed to rectify my hypocortisolism (low cortisol) through the use of T3 and the Circadian T3 Method (CT3M), did my full recovery begin.

Note: Anything that lowers T3 levels, including lower conversion through any mechanism, can affect the pituitary, and the way it is supposed to work. It is not surprising that so many thyroid patients also have low cortisol issues.

The above combined to be a perfect storm for me and T4 would not work.

I believe the above points may be relevant to a large number of thyroid patients.

I was driven to need T3 in order to compensate for the active effects of the DIO1 and DIO2 gene defects, plus the loss of conversion capability due to Hashimoto's and AT. On top of all of this, when someone takes T3, it tends to suppress TSH more effectively than T4 medication. A low TSH reduces T4 to T3 conversion, (see my books and more information on this in Article 14 in Chapter 7).

The combination of everything above would have made it very difficult for me to recover with a T4 or T4/T3 combination.

I cannot cope with T4 medication, even in small amounts. T4 in any quantity brings back my hypothyroid symptoms.

As I write this, I am healthy and an active sixty-six-year-old man. I remain symptom-free on T3 replacement therapy. So, when I hear views like, "Everyone needs some T4", I would like to be able to respond, "Why would I wish to be ill once again, just to appease your incorrect view!" These types of views are stated from time to time, usually by doctors, but also, sometimes by thyroid patients. Unsurprisingly, the patients concerned that make these statements are usually on some form of T4, T4/T3 or NDT medication. They think everyone else should be taking it too. They have sometimes found a not especially compelling piece of research that shows that T4 has some minor effect on some systems in the body, and they extrapolate from there that everyone needs T4. This is not the case. One of the big flaws in that type of argument is that people who are living well on T3 alone have not been studied for the compensatory adjustments that the body makes when using T3 on its own. The other big flaw is that small pieces of research are often found to be inadequate or incomplete when further research comes along.

I have used T3 replacement for over thirty years. I know many thyroid patients, who have recovered their health using T3-Only and have been using it for a very long time. There are well-understood reasons that explain why I could not get well on more conventional T4-based (T4/T3 or NDT) thyroid treatment.

For many thyroid patients, T4 monotherapy works well, for others a T4/T3 combination is what they need to eliminate all their symptoms. However, for those thyroid patients that require it, T3-Only replacement therapy can be a very effective, safe, long-term thyroid hormone treatment. There are too many thyroid patients like me who are well on T3-Only to doubt its value as a useful thyroid treatment for those who cannot get well with any T4-based therapy (NDT and T4/T3 included).

T3 replacement therapy also provides people with sufficient T2 thyroid hormone. T2 only has minor effects but some people do not understand that as long as someone has sufficient T3 they will also produce sufficient T2.

This is a quote from the late Dr John C. Lowe who wrote the foreword for my Recovering with T3 book:

"Studies indicate that T4 is of no use to anyone except, figuratively, as a storage unit for the metabolically-active thyroid hormones T3, T2 and possibly T1. When T4 ends its long ride through the circulating blood, it enters cells. There, enzymes convert it to T3 and, after a while, other enzymes convert T3 to T2. The T2 becomes T1 and eventually, T1 becomes T0 (T-zero). T0 is just the amino acid backbone (called "tyrosine") with no iodine atoms attached. Because it has no attached iodine atoms, T0 is no more a hormone than T4.

Rather than being a hormone, T4 is a pro-hormone. That means that enzymes have to convert T4 to T3 before T4 benefits us. T4 is no more a hormone than beans in an unopened can are a food. For all practical purposes, canned beans become food only when a can opener frees them, so you can eat them. Hence, T4, like canned beans, only potentially benefits us, but actually does so only after being freed from its metabolically unusable form.

Your endocrinologist may say that T4 is a gentler way to get T3 into your body. This to me, however, is a specious argument. When taken properly, T3 can affect one as gently as T3 derived from T4."

More research will prove me right. The current prevailing attitude of negativity to T4/T3 and T3-Only therapy will eventually be blown away, when the research that is already known is accepted and when more studies are done, that focus on people who are very healthy on some form of T3 treatment.

6. TEN IMPORTANT LESSONS I LEARNED ON MY JOURNEY WITH THYROID DISEASE

I was diagnosed with hypothyroidism (Hashimoto's) when I was about 30 years of age, but symptoms had been developing since I was 28. Over the following 7 years, I went from one doctor to another and from one endocrinologist to another. I was put on Levothyroxine (Synthroid) at various doses. I was given natural desiccated thyroid (NDT) at various doses, then T4/T3 combinations. I was even given some of these medications with hydrocortisone, as I had also developed severe low cortisol. In all cases, I was pronounced 'correctly treated' because my lab tests were apparently normal. However, all my original symptoms persisted.

I went gluten-free, grain-free, and dairy-free for several years but this did not alleviate the whole range of symptoms, which included debilitating fatigue, terrible gut and digestive system issues, low blood pressure, and a general inability to cope with life. I could not function as I had done previously.

It got to a point where the doctors were no longer interested and they even had the rudeness to say that something else was now causing all the same symptoms but it was no longer hypothyroidism! By this stage, the disease had wreaked havoc on my body. The low cortisol alone had caused me to lose about 35% of my body weight. I was so exhausted I was virtually an invalid. I also lost the career that I loved. Sadly, various relationships were also damaged.

I took matters into my own hands after about 7 years. The Internet was only just starting, so I bought endocrinology books – a lot of them! I taught myself. My background is in science, so I did not find it difficult. I learned that it was still hypothyroidism that was causing my symptoms. Something had altered in my body and I felt sure that I needed more T3 and less T4, so as not to rely on the conversion of the T4 into the active form (T3).

The bottom line is that after about 10 years had elapsed, I was on T3-only treatment with no T4 medication. I had also found a novel way to regulate cortisol using the T3 and it worked. I began to recover. I no longer needed to be on a restrictive diet because all my digestive issues cleared up once I was on enough T3 thyroid medication. I had been so ill for so long that full recovery took a few more years as I had to build myself up and get fit again.

Once on enough T3 medication, I had almost no FT4 in my blood test results and low TSH. I have never missed the FT4 – it is not a real thyroid hormone. I now know that T4 does not connect to the thyroid receptors in the cell nuclei. It is mainly present as a means of producing T3 through conversion – but so often this does not work well enough. Plus, sometimes, the thyroid patient needs T3-Only therapy in order to recover.

As a result of all of this, I have written 3 books that cover many aspects of thyroid diagnosis and treatment: Recovering with T3, The CT3M Handbook, and The Thyroid Patient's Manual. I fully understand what had happened to me and why I did not respond to any of the other thyroid medications.

I am now into my late 60s and have been living well on T3-only for over thirty years. I am fit and healthy, with no signs of either hypothyroidism or hyperthyroidism.

These are some of the main lessons that I learned through my own journey:

1. Do not believe all you are told by doctors OR other patients. This includes diagnosis, thyroid laboratory test interpretation, vitamin and mineral levels, and whether they are okay or not. Yes, take it on board, but always check things out if there is the slightest doubt OR it is easy to verify. There are so many thyroid forums that exist these days. It is possible to get bad advice on these too. Use my books! Take all views on board but do not just believe everything you are told.

2. Always get copies of your test results – with the actual result numbers, the reference ranges, and the units they are measured in. Frequently, you need to check if what you are being told about these results is actually correct or not. Insist on getting the actual results – not a statement that they were okay. They are often helpful later on when you are trying to work out what happened at what point in your illness. Try to stick to the same laboratory each time, as different labs can produce slightly different results. Results often vary a lot depending on what treatment you are on at the time of the lab test, so this will become part of the chronological history of your diagnosis and treatment progression. Because of this, always make a note of the exact thyroid medication you were on, including doses, at the time of the test. Note the timing of your thyroid medication as this can influence the test results at the time of the blood draw. Note down any other supplements or medication you were taking at the time. This information can end up being invaluable to you and your doctor at a later time.

3. Do your own research. Read books. Use my books and other peoples' resources as references.

4. Knowledge is critical – so gain it as FAST as you can. Knowledge allows you to gain some control of the situation vs feeling like you are on a raft, adrift on a stormy sea. Gaining more control gives you the ability to make better decisions and to ask better questions of your doctor(s). Getting knowledge FAST means you have a better chance to get well FAST. Getting well quickly is the best way to avoid the kind of damage and havoc that this disease can cause when it is not properly treated. A speedy recovery is the best way to prevent career damage, relationship damage, and other related health issues from developing.

5. Do not stay with a doctor who is not supporting you. That is a recipe for staying sick. There are usually solutions. You really need to have a good working relationship with your doctor, so that you know they are actually listening to you and understand how you are feeling. You also need to feel that they are doing their very best for you. It is hard enough to recover from hypothyroidism without feeling like your doctor is letting you down. In particular, if a doctor is managing your health based on keeping TSH in range and FT4 in range and is not concerned with your low FT3 (even if it is in the reference range), then that doctor is likely to be keeping you sick. FT3 is the most important lab test result and usually, it needs to be high enough for you as an individual for you to feel well. This needs to be done without very high Reverse T3. Sometimes this requires less T4 medication and more T3 medication. Sometimes it needs to be done with low TSH – contrary to the opinion of many doctors.

6. Never just turn your health over to someone else. You need to remain in the driver's seat. It is your body and you need to own it and look after it during your return to good health. If you are not happy with the opinions or treatment you are receiving from your doctor, do not simply accept this situation. Start looking for a more supportive doctor and seek input from others regarding this, so that you have some evidence that the new doctor will be more helpful.

7. Never, ever, give up!

8. Never, ever, give up! I cannot say this often enough. It is so important. Sometimes it can be a huge struggle to get well, given the relatively poor diagnosis and treatment policies that seem to exist for thyroid patients these days.

    The next two are suggestions rather than lessons:

9. Read: The Thyroid Patient's Manual. I wrote it to help people gain knowledge quickly and to enable them to see the entire picture of the thyroid hormones in the context of other systems in the body. I wanted to give all the key information related to diagnosis and treatment, especially since so much new research has been done over recent years. The goal of the book is to help people recover FAST – before too much damage occurs in their lives.

10. Read Recovering with T3 and The CT3M Handbook if you need to use more than a small amount of T3. Having the knowledge to correctly use T3 is critical if you are one of the few who has to go down this route. Sadly, many doctors simply do not know how to use T3 safely and effectively – but they may think that they do. They often believe that adding a little T3 will actually result in higher FT3 but this is often not true. Frequently, the person ends up with some improvement for a short time and then FT3 sinks back to the previous level. My books explain why this is and how to fix it.

I hope these lessons help you avoid having your thyroid issues being poorly treated. Getting well fast should be your goal!

7. A COLLECTION OF SOME OF PAUL'S YOUTUBE VIDEOS & VIDEO INTERVIEWS

This is just a simple list of my favourite videos & video interviews:

- A YouTube Video about Paul Robinson's own journey in recovering from thyroid disease: https://youtu.be/oOHHmO7WNiE

- A follow up YouTube video which adds more information and is a bit less emotional: https://youtu.be/ZcDb9Cm7Zj0

- The Thyroid System - What you need to know (and what your doctor might not know): https://www.youtube.com/watch?v=ani654TROnc

- The Thyroid Treatment Mess: https://www.youtube.com/watch?v=gqBqqDtQpmw&t=0s

- Dr Westin Childs interviews Paul Robinson: https://www.youtube.com/watch?v=Lgo0hnnEDkE&t=0s

- Dr Amie Hornaman interviews Paul Robinson: https://www.youtube.com/watch?v=QP_1788AOUU&t=0s

- Karen Martel interviews Paul Robinson: https://youtu.be/L0GxGjIYcp4?list=PLr4GYKvjP-lBta_pfgyngkA58kdjtM4W6

- Chemaine Linnie interviews Paul Robinson: https://youtu.be/FuGgTvBQRYQ

- This is a very old video I made which describes CT3M: https://youtu.be/gGs6po4D-YI

Note: I am working on the assumption that my own YouTube channel still exists and that those channels of the other individuals are also still available.

8. MUSINGS AT AGE SIXTY-SIX

I hardly recognise myself at age 66 compared to the person I was when aged thirty.

By the time I was thirty years of age, I was married and had two children. My career was enjoyable, satisfying and paying me a lot of money because I was good at it. The future looked bright.

Thyroid problems came and turned everything upside down.

The many endocrinologists and doctors that I saw during the first seven years of my thyroid problems, were completely incapable. They had a belief system that made them unable to help me. I have written about the broken paradigm and dogmatic beliefs inherent in thyroid treatment so many times. Levothyroxine does not always work. It does not always convert to enough T3. Laboratory test results that are in range, do not mean that the person is correctly treated, and the patient can still be horrendously symptomatic. That is what happened to me.

It took me many years of hard work, research, reading endocrinology text books, and persuading doctors to prescribe what I knew I needed, to get well. I had to create a protocol for using the rarely prescribed thyroid medication, T3. Many aspects of that protocol were highly inventive.

As a result of my experience, I have written three books and am working on this fourth one. My books are widely read and used by thyroid patients in order to recover from hypothyroidism. The books are also increasingly used by doctors around the world.

It was never my intention to write any books, let alone do all the work that I have done subsequently. It has been an incredibly strange journey for me, and it was a road that I would definitely not have chosen for myself.

My life changed dramatically due to my thyroid condition, which was untreatable by the endocrinologists and doctors that I saw. The end result was the loss of my career, the end of my marriage. Eventually, as a result of all the damage, I lost contact with my children through their estrangement of me.

One of my main concerns now, is how to enable my books to continue to be available. Dr Broda Barnes wrote 'The Unsuspected Illness' in 1976. His book is more relevant now, nearly fifty years later, than it was when he first wrote it. Liothyronine (T3 thyroid hormone), is now more needed by those patients who cannot process enough Levothyroxine (T4) into enough T3. Doctors do not want to prescribe T3, and they do not understand thyroid treatment, or T3, well enough. Thyroid treatment is actually worse now than when I was first diagnosed. It is more mechanical, less flexible and less focused on the individual patient.

I am still trying to work out how to keep my books available for another one hundred years and maybe even longer than that – I think they will be needed for at least that length of time.

As a result of my journey, I am a very different person now than I was when I was young. Am I glad that I took this road? Well, I had little choice at the start of it. But I could have just got well and then got on with my life. What I have managed to do has made a contribution. However, it has been a very, very hard road. I hope that my choice to do this work has made, and will continue to make, a difference.

Here are two quotes from poems that I really like and also seem to sum things up for me:
Firstly, from The Road Not Taken - Robert Frost:
"I took the one less travelled by, and that has made all the difference."

Secondly, from Stopping by Woods On A Snowy Evening - Robert Frost:
"But I have promises to keep, And miles to go before I sleep, And miles to go before I sleep."

Chapter 4

Failures of Current Treatment

1. HISTORY OF THYROID TREATMENT AND WHY THE CURRENT PARADIGM IS BROKEN

The history of thyroid treatment is interesting as it makes it so clear why we are in the mess that we currently are in with lab test driven treatment, and having so much difficulty getting T3 prescribed when it is required

Some History Prior to the 1970s.

Synthetic T4 (Synthroid, Levothyroxine) was first introduced in the 1950s. Current thyroid lab tests (TSH, and the other thyroid labs) were invented in the 1970s.

Before these events, all doctors had available was good clinical judgement, based on the symptoms and signs (body temperature etc. and possibly basal metabolic rate), of the patient, and the option to use natural desiccated thyroid (NDT). NDT contains both T4 and T3 thyroid hormones! It seemed a reasonable way to replace thyroid hormones, as we make both T4 and T3 within the thyroid. A healthy thyroid gland converts a significant amount of T4 to T3. So, prior to the 1970s, it seemed sensible to replace low thyroid hormones with a mixture of T4 and T3 hormones in the form of NDT.

When doctors worked with a patient, they would assess many things and try to reach a judgement over whether the patient might have a thyroid problem or not. If low thyroid hormones were suspected, a trial of NDT would be started. If there were improvements in symptoms and signs, the NDT would be adjusted (titrated) to a higher or lower dose if needed. This titration process would continue based on the presenting symptoms and signs of the patient. This meant that the doctor would have to work with the patient and listen to what they were saying about how they were feeling in response to treatment. There were no laboratory tests to get in the way between the doctor and the patient in front of them.

This approach worked pretty well a lot of the time. It ought to have moved forward from there, taking advantage of modern lab testing (but not being a slave to it), and having all the other thyroid medications available.

What Happened from the 1970s Onwards.

In the 1970s, the TSH test became the standard way to assess whether thyroid treatment was working. Levothyroxine/Synthroid/T4 became the standard medication for treatment. Both of these required almost no effort on the part of the doctor or endocrinologist compared to what happened in the past. It vastly reduced the work of the physician. The reliance on the TSH test and the use of T4 medication also virtually guaranteed that no patient would ever be over-medicated.

This sea-change was the beginning of conveyor-belt thyroid treatment, optimised for the doctor and far less likely to result in over-medication of the patient. However, it was much more likely to result in the under-medication of the patient!

Unfortunately, it is a method that frequently results in improperly treated hypothyroidism. It is a broken paradigm.

I have written about this in many other articles, but here is a summary:

- TSH can be totally suppressed in some cases when the person is on thyroid treatment, i.e., near zero. This is fine and it does not mean the patient is hyperthyroid if they show no symptoms or signs of hyperthyroidism. Keeping someone to an in-range TSH may leave them under-medicated!
- TSH does not track symptom improvement. So, a doctor cannot see a change in T4 medication and a lowering of TSH and assume that the patient is doing better.
- FT4 does not track symptom improvement either. A higher level of FT4 does not mean that the patient will be feeling better.
- Free T3 does track symptom improvement. However, FT3 is not the measure that most doctors focus on.
- The reference ranges for FT4 and FT3 are population ranges. These are far too wide to conclude anything about whether a patient is well-treated or not. Real individual reference ranges (which cannot be known before treatment) are less than half as wide as the wide population ranges for FT4 and FT3. These individual optimal ranges within the reference range are closer to one third the width of the reference range, and can be positioned much further up the reference range for some patients.
- Reverse T3 (rT3) may or may not be an issue, and there is no ideal FT3/rT3 ratio for all patients. Just as the lab ranges are wide population ranges, people all have their own individual requirements for their labs. No ratio or reference range can be applied to all people. Very high rT3 is usually an issue but that is about all you can say about it in isolation. Symptoms and signs of the patient say more.
- T4 does not work for all patients. Some patients cannot get well using T4 medication.
- We also know that the thyroid gland itself is responsible for around 25% of our T3, mostly through conversion, so tissue damage through Hashimoto's, or through the removal of the thyroid, loses a huge amount of ability to convert from T4 to T3. This can often not be compensated for with T4 alone.

- We also know from research that some people have genetic defects that reduce the capability to convert from T4 to T3 (DIO1 and DIO2 gene defects).
- Research has shown that the loss of the thyroid gland and of conversion capability makes it difficult to achieve a balance of thyroid hormones. T3 often has to be added to treatment.

Moreover, we know from the experience of thyroid patients that many of them need different medications to get well: T4, NDT, T4/T3, or in some cases T3-Only.

Logic and patient experience also suggest that once a thyroid patient is on a combination of T4 & T3 treatments the laboratory reference ranges can break down. The ranges are based on people with no thyroid issues or those on T4 treatment. They are not based on those on combined T4/T3 or T3-Only. It is not reasonable to lower a thyroid patient's T3 medication level, in order to satisfy the need to keep FT3 within the range, or to keep FT4 in range, or TSH in range, if the patient has no indication at all of being over-medicated or is feeling under-medicated.

So, the current paradigm of thyroid treatment is broken, and the research has shown this.

The Consequences of the Broken Paradigm.

This is the really sad aspect of all of this. Thyroid patients are being left improperly treated in many, many cases. They are either on the wrong medication for them, or they are being left under-medicated.

Patients actually got better treatment prior to the invention of Levothyroxine/Synthroid and the new laboratory tests.

Thyroid treatment ought to have got better!

2. WHY SO MANY THYROID PATIENTS FAIL TO RECOVER ON LEVOTHYROXINE (T4)

This is article is from a fellow thyroid patient advocate. The post clearly spells out the reason why so many thyroid patients who are taking Levothyroxine continue to feel unwell. Levothyroxine is the synthetic version of the T4 thyroid hormone (also known as Synthroid in the USA).

Levothyroxine simply does not provide the same amount of T3 that healthy people have. On Levothyroxine, the thyroid patient often has higher T4 and far lower T3 levels than healthy people. T3 is the biologically active thyroid hormone, so being deficient in T3 compared to healthy people is a real issue, and is why so many on T4 medication remain symptomatic.

The research paper that her blog post on was actually published in 2011. So, this information has been with endocrinologists and doctors for a long time! However, treatment practices did not change because of the research!

The article fits totally with what thyroid patients already know and what so many doctors and endocrinologists refuse to believe: Levothyroxine frequently leaves some thyroid patients with remaining symptoms.

To make things worse, in far too many cases FT3 is not the primary thyroid hormone test that is being used alongside the patient's symptoms and signs to assess the efficacy of treatment.

Something really needs to change with thyroid treatment. The current approach is based on false assumptions. It is a failed treatment paradigm.

The article is well worth a read:
https://thyroidpatients.ca/2020/11/12/gullo-lt4-thyroid-loss-inverts-ft3-ft4/

3. CURRENT DIAGNOSIS AND TREATMENT OF HYPOTHYROIDISM ARE FLAWED

I have recently been given a new paper written by Professor Rudolf Hoermann, Mel Rowe and Peter Warmingham. The three authors have joined forces to try and improve patients' knowledge of effective diagnosis and treatment of hypothyroidism.

The title of their paper is, "A Patient's Guide to the Diagnosis and Treatment of Hypothyroidism". I will provide a link to it at the end.

When I was sent the paper by one of the authors, I read it and responded immediately with:
'It is a brief, simply-explained, to-the-point and altogether excellent paper".

The paper is extremely worth reading and may help many thyroid patients in discussions with doctors or endocrinologists. Of course, sometimes, the doctor you speak with may be very certain of their point of view. They may not even realise that what they have been taught was only introduced post-1985 when the TSH assay was created. These post-1985 views, that are currently being used by most doctors and endocrinologists, have now been shown to be very flawed, and this new paper by the three authors points this out very clearly.

The paper points out several major FLAWS in current diagnosis and treatment. I will pick out the major ones listed in the paper, all of which have now been refuted by extensive scientific evidence.

The flawed views are:

1. A subnormal assessment of free T4 (FT4) serves to establish a diagnosis of hypothyroidism. Also, TSH is exquisitely sensitive to minor changes in FT4, leading to the

adoption of TSH as "the single best screening test for primary thyroid dysfunction for the vast majority of outpatient clinical situations."

2. T4 is converted to T3 as needed, leading to treatment being changed to levothyroxine (T4) only.

3. TSH within its reference range represents euthyroidism (normal), leading to the treatment dosage of T4 being adjusted to return TSH within its normal range.

All three of the above assumptions are fundamental to current guidelines for doctors and endocrinologists. They need to be replaced with new guidelines that fit the science and help far more thyroid patients fully recover.

We know TSH does NOT correlate to symptomatic improvement and that low TSH does not mean someone is overtly hyperthyroid.

TSH should not be the predominant means of determining whether a patient is hypothyroid or not, especially when TSH is not overtly high. Both FT3 and FT4 need to be used in the determination of whether a patient is hypothyroid or not.

We now know that improvement in serum FT3 concentrations correlates to symptomatic improvement. We also know that conversion from T4 to T3 does not always work well. Only the T3 hormone provides genomic effect in the cells of the body.

We also know that the clinical presentation of the patient and symptom improvement should be at the forefront of treatment and that any lab assessment of thyroid hormones must include FT3 as well as TSH, FT4 and possibly Reverse T3.

The paper supports all of the statements with research references.

The authors recommend what ought to be done instead of the current practices. These recommendations include the focus on patients' symptoms, what testing really needs to be done and which labs are the ones to see improvement in. This is what needs to happen and it is what my books and website have been saying for many years. Eventually, this will happen – but it may take a long time.

I highly recommend reading the paper. Many thanks to all three authors!

Here is the URL link to the new paper:

https://thyroiduk.org/further-reading/a-patients-guide-to-the-diagnosis-and-treatment-of-hypothyroidism/

4. WE NEED A NEW PARADIGM OF THYROID TREATMENT

It is desperately clear to thyroid patient support groups and to many well-informed thyroid patients that there is an urgent need for a new paradigm for the treatment of hypothyroidism.

The Cambridge English Dictionary defines 'paradigm' as: "A model of something, or a very clear and typical example of something".

We need a new, effective, and very clear model of how doctors should be using thyroid laboratory test results, together with symptoms & signs, to treat thyroid patients. This new paradigm has to include all thyroid treatments, including T4, T4/T3, NDT and T3-Only.

This new model of treatment has to take into account the individuality of each patient. We are not robots that have come off the end of a production line. We do not have identical requirements for thyroid hormone replacement. Each of us needs to have the right level of thyroid hormones for us. The variation between thyroid patients of required FT4 and FT3 levels for good health is too large to attempt to treat everyone using the same approach (as happens today).

We need a new paradigm for thyroid treatment!

Why do I assert this so firmly?

The answer to that comes from several sources of information. I will discuss each of these and will try to divide the points into several categories. I will number the points within each category to make them easier to refer to. I also include many of the relevant research articles below. Hopefully, this will be of use to thyroid patients as they try to persuade their own physicians to provide the treatment that they require in order to get well.

Research regarding the current use of thyroid laboratory tests:

1. TSH is not a measure that can be used to assess whether a thyroid patient is properly treated or not. The TSH laboratory test result does not track symptom improvement, as medication is adjusted. It provides little or no guide as to whether the thyroid dosage is correct. See references 1, 2, 3, 4, 16, 18, and 19 at the end of this article.

2. TSH can be suppressed (at or near zero) when a patient is on thyroid treatment. This does not mean the patient is hyperthyroid at all. It simply means that the TSH from the pituitary is suppressed. Endocrinologists and doctors are mistakenly applying the reasoning that suppressed TSH means hyperthyroidism, based on people who are on no thyroid medication at all! An individual suffering from hyperthyroidism, who is on no thyroid medication, will have a suppressed TSH and typically high FT3 and high FT4, due to excess thyroid hormone production.

However, the concern over suppressed TSH for hypothyroid patients already on thyroid treatment is misplaced. If this flawed reasoning is applied to thyroid patients on treatment, it may well stop some of them from getting enough thyroid medication and keep them symptomatic. See references 2, 5, 6 and 15 at the end of this article.

3. FT4 & FT3 lab ranges are wide population ranges. A thyroid patient's personal FT4 and FT3 ranges are less than half as wide as the lab ranges. So, when a doctor is assessing a patient's lab results against the lab ranges, he has no idea if the results are in the right place for that individual patient. This makes reliance on thyroid lab results as the prime decider of correct treatment dubious at best. Thyroid patients on treatment with T4 medication have also been shown to have lower FT3 levels than healthy people. Since the test results for these people are included, when laboratories construct the reference ranges, this will influence the bottom and the top end of the FT3 lab range, making them both lower than they ought to be for healthy people. See reference 7 at the end of this article.

4. FT4 does not track symptom improvement as the patient's medication is adjusted. Just like TSH, the level of FT4 provides little or no guide as to whether a thyroid patient's dosage is correct. See reference 5 at the end of this article.

5. FT3 laboratory test results DO track symptom improvement during the adjustment of thyroid medication. It is the only lab that goes up as symptoms improve. This should be no surprise at all to those thyroid patients who now realise that it is the T3 thyroid hormone that is biologically active and does all the good things for us within our cells. The big problem is that FT3 is the one lab test that many doctors do not test! Madness!

    FT3 should be the most important lab test to do. Of course, if doctors do not test FT3, they will not see the issue and they can carry on looking at nice, in-range TSH and FT4 results. They can keep telling thyroid patients that they are correctly treated, even though they are still very ill! See references 5 and 17 at the end of this article.

Levothyroxine (T4 medication) leaves some patients ill and symptomatic:

6. Previous clinical trials comparing T4 to T4/T3 treatment were flawed. They were subject to amalgamation problems (Simpson's paradox). They were not designed correctly and were always liable to conclude that T4/T3 offered no benefit.

    Unfortunately, clinical trials are not the best way to assess medications as they lack the subtlety that occurs when a doctor is working with a patient to titrate medication correctly. For example, the Federal Drugs Administration (FDA) places actual experience of drugs in the hands of physicians as more important than the proof of effectiveness under clinical trials because clinical trials can be fraught with issues. See reference 8 at the end of this article.

7. Research already exists that shows that some people will never recover using T4 medication alone. There are some good reasons for this. See references 9 and 10 at the end of this article.

8. There are good reasons for adding T3 to therapy.

We know that the thyroid gland is typically responsible for around 25% of our T3, and can be far higher in some individuals. This T3 is produced by a healthy thyroid, primarily through the conversion of the T4 in the blood flowing through it. Consequently, any thyroid tissue damage through Hashimoto's, or through the removal of all or part of the gland, will lose significant ability to convert from T4 to T3. T4 treatment may struggle to provide sufficient T3 to overcome symptoms.

Research has shown that athyreotic (thyroid-less) patients usually require sufficient T4 medication to completely suppress TSH before they ever get a high enough FT3 level to resolve their symptoms. In other cases, T4 alone is not enough to raise FT3 and additional T3 medication is needed. In many cases, TSH may need to be very low or suppressed.

The loss of thyroid gland tissue not only loses a large amount of conversion capability but importantly, it loses the ability of the thyroid to act as a control system in managing thyroid hormone conversion and balance. This loss can occur through any form of thyroid tissue damage, e.g., thyroidectomy or Hashimoto's. Losing some or all of a healthy thyroid gland has a profound impact on T3 levels that often cannot be compensated for by the conversion of Levothyroxine (T4) medication into T3.

Moreover, we know from research that some people have genetic defects that can also reduce the capability to convert from T4 to T3 (DIO1 and DIO2 gene defects).

If TSH, FT4, FT3 and Reverse T3 (rT3) were routinely tested, then the ability of the individual to produce enough FT3 for them without excess rT3 could be assessed. We know from research that with high rT3 the effect of any FT3 is reduced – rT3 is effectively a 'T3 blocker'. See references 4, 9, 12, 13, 17 and 20 at the end of this article.

9. Many doctors and endocrinologists all over the world have treated patients successfully using mixtures of T4/T3 and even with T3-Only. The evidence is already there for the use of many different types of thyroid medications: T4, T4/T3, NDT, T3-Only, and Slow Release T3.

   The proof for the inclusion of T3 in treatment for some patients is already out there! This comes from both research findings and clinical experience with T3 in combination therapy (T4/T3 and NDT) and on its own. See references 1, 6, 11, 14 and 17.

Symptoms & signs should be paramount:

10. Clinical presentation is more important than laboratory test results. If we are going to have thyroid treatment that leaves fewer patients dissatisfied, doctors need to begin by focusing far more on the patient in front of them using symptoms and signs, with laboratory test results in a supporting role. See references 1 and 11.

11. Endocrinologists and doctors are trying to force every thyroid patient into a little standard box.

    This box contains T4 medication, the TSH and FT4 lab tests and very little else. It contains very little compassion for the suffering of the patients. Symptoms and signs are not at the forefront of the doctors' minds when assessing the treatment. These are often dismissed as being caused by something else, e.g., depression, not exercising enough, chronic fatigue syndrome etc.

    This flawed treatment paradigm is simple and fast to use for the endocrinologists and doctors who have adopted it. They can get their patients in and out of their offices very quickly, without having to consider whether the medication is high enough, or contains the right blend of thyroid meds. This flawed paradigm is a 'blessing' in terms of time management for the doctors concerned. However, it is harming thyroid patients all over the world!

Patient experience is clear – T3 & T4 medications are both needed:

12. We know from an immense body of thyroid patients that many of them need different medications to get well: T4, NDT, T4/T3, or in some cases T3-Only. Thyroid patient experience is clear and we should not need to keep shouting this. It is so obvious to us.

Lab reference ranges are based on healthy people or thyroid patients on T4:

13. For those taking T3-Mostly or T3-Only, the lab ranges for FT4 and FT3 become unfit for purpose. The current laboratory ranges are designed for healthy people on no thyroid medication or for those on T4 monotherapy. The lab ranges are not designed for patients on T3-Only or T3-Mostly therapy. So why would anyone in their right mind attempt to apply the lab ranges in this case?! T4/T3 combination therapy is subject to the same problem but to a less significant extent.

It makes no scientific or logical sense to attempt to apply the ranges developed for healthy or T4-medicated patients to those patients who are on T3-Only or T3-Mostly.

If there was a need to have lab ranges for those on T3-Only or T3-Mostly thyroid medication, then this population of people on T3 therapy would have to be studied and ranges would need to be developed specifically for this usage of thyroid medication. Force fitting the current labs for use with T3-Only or T3-Mostly patients cannot work and is likely to leave the majority of them under-medicated. The FT3 range for those on T3-Only, needs to have a higher bottom and top end of the range, and the FT4 range needs a lower bottom and top end of the range.

For T3-Only and T3-Mostly therapy, none of the current lab ranges are useful in assessing whether the T3 dosage is too high, too low or just right – not TSH, not FT4 and not even FT3. These lab results are only useful by observing how they change as the T3 is being adjusted. The changes in TSH, FT4 and FT3 show trends during T3 dosage adjustment. They cannot be used to assess the adequacy, inadequacy or excess of the T3 medication. The absolute values of the thyroid lab results cannot answer the question of whether the patient is on the right T3 dose or not.

The same argument applies to more standard T4/T3 combination therapy. Currently, many doctors are satisfied if the patient's labs are sat somewhere in the range. In many cases, the patient is left undermedicated as they need much higher FT3 and lower FT4 (to avoid high rT3).

We know from research, that many patients on T4 have lower FT3 than healthy people. The current FT3 lab range is lower for both top and bottom of the range, due to thyroid patients on T4 therapy contributing to the construction of the FT3 range.

The other thing that happens is that the patient on T3-Only has less ongoing T4 to T3 conversion within the cells (because they have less T4). This means that they need extra T3 medication to replace this missing converted T3. The converted T3 within the cells cannot be seen on a blood test BUT the extra T3 medication can. So, the more T3 in the T3/T4 combination that the patient has, the more the top of the FT3 range will become an unfair constraint.

I believe that the top of the FT3 range is too low for those on T4/T3 and definitely too low for those on T3-Only. I know many people on T3-Only medication who often have had FT3 results slightly above the top of the FT3 reference range, and they are healthy and definitely not hyperthyroid. I am one of these people.

It is not reasonable to hold a thyroid patient's T3 medication level down in order to satisfy the need to keep FT3 within the range if the patient has no indication at all of being over-medicated. On T3-Only in particular, the patient often has to have FT3 at or above the top of the range before they feel well (for good reasons I have explained in my books and in other articles in this book).

Summary of the above.

The current paradigm of thyroid treatment is well and truly broken. Scientific research, patient experience, and the experience of some physicians are evidence of this. Logic is screaming that the current approach is flawed in many ways.

The consequence of the current broken treatment approach is the really sad aspect of all of this. Thyroid patients are being left improperly treated in a large number of cases. I know. I talk to many of these thyroid patients every day. They are either on the wrong medication for them, or they are being left under-medicated – often both. Often, they are not even having the right thyroid tests done and FT3 is not being monitored.

Many patients have severe symptoms and are often left with them for many years. This broken paradigm is harming patients all over the world!

We need a new paradigm for the treatment of hypothyroidism. I describe this new paradigm very clearly in my latest book, 'The Thyroid Patient's Manual'. Here are the key points:

- TSH can be totally suppressed when on thyroid treatment, i.e., near zero. This is fine and it does not mean the patient is hyperthyroid. So, not increasing thyroid medication in order to maintain an in-range TSH, may leave the patient under-medicated.
- TSH does not track symptom improvement. So, a doctor cannot see a change in T4 medication and a lowering of TSH and assume that the patient is doing better.
- FT4 does not track symptom improvement either. A higher level of FT4 does not mean that the patient will be feeling better.

- FT3 does track symptom improvement but this is not the measure that most doctors focus on. This needs to become the most important of the lab tests performed.
- The reference ranges for FT4 and FT3 are wide population ranges. Real individual reference ranges (which cannot be known before treatment) are less than half as wide as the wide population ranges for FT4 and FT3. Doctors cannot conclude, just because a patient has FT4 and FT3 numbers in the range, that they are now correctly treated.
- Reverse T3 (rT3) may or may not be an issue, and there is definitely no ideal FT3/rT3 ratio for all patients. Just as the lab ranges are wide population ranges, people all have their own individual requirements for their labs. No ratio or reference range can be applied to all people. However, very high rT3 is usually an issue. It can impact T4 to T3 conversion and may be a flag that the D3 deiodinase enzyme is high (which may block T3 action) but that is all you can say about it. Symptoms and signs of the patient say more.
- T4 does not work for all patients. Some patients cannot get well using T4 medication. This is clear. Doctors need to realise this and be prepared to use the full range of thyroid medications. Even if this means they need to spend more time with individual thyroid patients and not just whisk them out of their office in five minutes!
- We also know that the thyroid gland itself is typically responsible for around 25% of our T3 (more in some people), mostly through conversion, so tissue damage through Hashimoto's, or through the removal of the thyroid, loses a huge amount of ability to convert from T4 to T3. This cannot always be compensated for with T4 alone. Doctors must expect to push up the dosage of thyroid medication or consider adding T3 treatment in these situations.
- We know from research that some people have genetic defects that reduce the capability to convert from T4 to T3 (DIO1 and DIO2 gene defects). This needs to be taken into account.
- We know from an immense body of thyroid patients that many of them need different medications to get well: T4, NDT, T4/T3, or in some cases T3-Only. All thyroid medications must be on the table. If one fails to work, another must be offered. Doctors and thyroid patients need to start working in partnership with thyroid treatment. It seems that this can be more of an adversarial relationship compared with other health issues. Time for a change!
- Once a thyroid patient is on a combination of T4 & T3 treatments, the laboratory reference ranges can break down. The ranges are based on people with no thyroid issues or those on T4 treatment. They are not based on those on combined T4/T3 or T3-Only. It is not reasonable to hold a thyroid patient's T3 medication level down in order to satisfy the need to keep FT3 within the range if the patient has no indication at all of being over-medicated. On T3-Only in particular, the patient often has to have FT3 above the top of the range before they feel well.

Doctors need to stop treating us as if we are all the same. We are not identical robots. We have individual needs which the current broken process does not account for.

It is absolutely necessary at this time to move to a new paradigm of thyroid treatment!

References.

Reference 1:

"Time for a reassessment of the treatment of hypothyroidism"
John E. M. Midgley, Anthony D. Toft, Rolf Larisch, Johannes W. Dietrich & Rudolf Hoermann.
BMC Endocrine Disorders volume 19, Article number: 37 (2019)
https://bmcendocrdisord.biomedcentral.com/articles/10.1186/s12902-019-0365-4

Reference 2:

"Homeostatic Control of the Thyroid-Pituitary Axis: Perspectives for Diagnosis and Treatment."
Hoermann, Midgley, Larisch, Dietrich.
Front Endocrinol 2015 Nov 20;6:177. doi: 10.3389/fendo.2015.00177.
Abstract: http://www.ncbi.nlm.nih.gov/pubmed/26635726
Full article: https://www.frontiersin.org/articles/10.3389/fendo.2015.00177/full

Reference 3:

"TSH Measurement and Its Implications for Personalised Clinical Decision-Making"
Rudolf Hoermann and John E. M. Midgley
Volume 2012 Article ID 438037 https://doi.org/10.1155/2012/438037
http://www.hindawi.com/journals/jtr/2012/438037/

Reference 4:

"Recent Advances in Thyroid Hormone Regulation: Toward a New Paradigm for Optimal Diagnosis and Treatment"
Rudolf Hoermann, John E. M. Midgley, Rolf Larisch and Johannes W. Dietrich
Front. Endocrinol., 22 December 2017 https://doi.org/10.3389/fendo.2017.00364
https://www.frontiersin.org/articles/10.3389/fendo.2017.00364/full

Reference 5:

"Symptomatic Relief is Related to Serum Free Triiodothyronine Concentrations during Follow-up in Levothyroxine-Treated Patients with Differentiated Thyroid Cancer"
Rolf Larisch, John E M Midgley, Johannes W Dietrich, Rudolf Hoermann

Exp Clin Endocrinol Diabetes 2018; 126(09): 546-552
DOI: 10.1055/s-0043-125064
https://www.thieme-connect.de/DOI/DOI?10.1055/s-0043-125064

Reference 6:
"Thyroid hormone replacement – a counterblast to guidelines"
J R Coll Physicians Edinb 2017; 47: 307–9 | doi: 10.4997/JRCPE.2017.401
http://www.rcpe.ac.uk/sites/default/files/jrcpe_47_4_toft.pdf

Reference 7:
"Narrow Individual Variations in Serum T4 and T3 in Normal Subjects: A Clue to the Understanding of Subclinical Thyroid Disease"
Stig Andersen, Klaus Michael Pedersen, Niels Henrik Bruun, Peter Laurberg
The Journal of Clinical Endocrinology & Metabolism, Volume 87, Issue 3, 1 March 2002, Pages 1068–1072,
https://doi.org/10.1210/jcem.87.3.8165
https://academic.oup.com/jcem/article/87/3/1068/2846746

Reference 8:
"Lessons from Randomised Clinical Trials for Triiodothyronine Treatment of Hypothyroidism: Have They Achieved Their Objectives?"
Journal of Thyroid Research. Volume 2018 Article
ID 3239197 https://doi.org/10.1155/2018/3239197
Rudolf Hoermann, John E. M. Midgley, Rolf Larisch, and Johannes W. Dietrich.
https://www.hindawi.com/journals/jtr/2018/3239197/

Reference 9:
"Differences in hypothalamic type 2 deiodinase ubiquitination explain localized sensitivity to thyroxine"
Joao Pedro Werneck de Castro, Tatiana L. Fonseca, Cintia B. Ueta, Elizabeth A. McAninch, Sherine Abdalla, Gabor Wittmann, Ronald M. Lechan, Balazs Gereben, and Antonio C. Bianco
Journal of Clinical Investigation 10.1172/JCI77588
http://www.jci.org/articles/view/77588

Reference 10:
"Homeostatic equilibria between free thyroid hormones and pituitary thyrotropin are modulated by various influences including age, body mass index and treatment"

Rudolf Hoermann, John E.M. Midgley, Adrienne Giacobino, Walter A. Eckl, Hans Günther Wahl, Johannes W. Dietrich, and Rolf Larisch
https://doi.org/10.1111/cen.12527
See: Clin Endocrinol (Oxf) (2014) 81:907–915. doi:10.1111/cen.12527
URL: https://www.researchgate.net/publication/263321383_Homeostatic_Equilibria_Between_Free_Thyroid_Hormones_and_Pituitary_Thyrotropin_Are_Modulated_By_Various_Influences_Including_Age_Body_Mass_Index_and_Treatment
and
http://www.thyroiduk.org.uk/tuk/TUK_PDFs/Homeostatic-equilibria-cen-final-080714.pdf

Reference 11:
"Individualised requirements for optimum treatment of hypothyroidism: complex needs, limited options"
Hoermann, Midgley, Larisch and Dietrich.
Drugs in Context
DOI 10.7573/dic.212597
https://www.drugsincontext.com/individualised-requirements-for-optimum-treatment-of-hypothyroidism:-complex-needs,-limited-options/

Reference 12:
"Dual control of pituitary thyroid stimulating hormone secretion by thyroxine and triiodothyronine in athyreotic patients"
Hoermann R, Midgley JEM, Dietrich JW, Larisch R.
See: The Adv Endocrinol Metab (2017) 8:83–95.
doi:10.1177/204201881771640112.
https://www.ncbi.nlm.nih.gov/pmc/articles/PMC5524252/

Reference 13:
"Relational stability of thyroid hormones in euthyroid subjects and patients with autoimmune thyroid disease"
Hoermann R, Midgley JEM, Larisch R, Dietrich JW.
See: Eur Thyroid J (2016) 5:171–179.
doi:10.1159/000447967
https://www.ncbi.nlm.nih.gov/pmc/articles/PMC5091265/

Reference 14:
"Effects of Long-Term Combination LT4 and LT3 Therapy for Improving Hypothyroidism and Overall Quality of Life"
Anam Tariq, Yijin Wert, Pramil Cheriyath, and Renu Joshi.
South Med J. 2018 Jun; 111(6): 363–369.

Published online 2018 Jun 1. doi: 10.14423/SMJ.0000000000000823
https://www.ncbi.nlm.nih.gov/pmc/articles/PMC5965938/

Reference 15

"Biochemical markers reflecting thyroid function in athyreotic patients on levothyroxine monotherapy"
Ito M, Miyauchi A, Hisakado M, Yoshioka W, Ide A, Kudo T, Nishihara E, Kihara M, Ito Y, Kobayashi K, Miya A, Fukata S, Nishikawa M, Nakamura H, Amino N.
Thyroid. 2017;27:484-490. doi:10.1089/thy.2016.0426
https://www.ncbi.nlm.nih.gov/pmc/articles/PMC5385443/

Reference 16:

"Is a Normal TSH Synonymous With "Euthyroidism" in Levothyroxine Monotherapy?"
Sarah J. Peterson, Elizabeth A. McAninch, Antonio C. Bianco
The Journal of Clinical Endocrinology & Metabolism, Volume 101, Issue 12, 1 December 2016, Pages 4964–4973,
https://doi.org/10.1210/jc.2016-2660
https://academic.oup.com/jcem/article/101/12/4964/2765082
and
https://www.ncbi.nlm.nih.gov/pubmed/27700539

Reference 17:

"Defending plasma T3 is a biological priority"
Sherine M. Abdalla and Antonio C. Bianco
Clin Endocrinol (Oxf). 2014 Nov; 81(5): 633–641.
Published online 2014 Aug 7. doi: 10.1111/cen.12538
PMCID: PMC4699302
https://www.ncbi.nlm.nih.gov/pmc/articles/PMC4699302/

Reference 18:

"Does TSH Reliably Detect Hypothyroid Patients?"
Ling C1, Sun Q1, Khang J1, Felipa Lastarria M1, Strong J1, Stolze B1, Yu X1, Parikh TP1, Waldman MA1, Welsh K1, Jonklaas J2, Masika L3, Soldin SJ1,2.
Ann Thyroid Res. 2018;4(1):122-125. Epub 2018 Feb 20.
https://www.researchgate.net/publication/323809727_Does_TSH_Reliably_Detect_Hypothyroid_Patients

Reference 19:

"TSH Should not be used as a Single Marker of Thyroid Function"

S. Soldin, Qian Sun, Brian Stoize
DOI: 10.26420/annalsthyroidres.2018.1038
https://www.researchgate.net/publication/328881749_TSH_Should_not_be_used_as_a_Single_Marker_of_Thyroid_Function

Reference 20 (shows that a high rT3 implies a blocking effect on T3 within the cells):
"Qualitative and quantitative differences in the pathways of extrathyroidal triiodothyronine generation between euthyroid and hypothyroid rats."
J E Silva, M B Gordon, F R Crantz, J L Leonard, and P R Larsen
10.1172/JCI111313
https://www.jci.org/articles/view/111313

More recent understanding of the blocking effects on T3 suggests that it is actually D3 enzymes that block T3 binding to receptors. D3 converts T4 to rT3. So, it may not actually be rT3 itself, but rT3 is a marker of this and as such is still useful to test. RT3 also has a small effect on reducing the rate of T4 to T3 conversion, i.e., it reduces the number of D2 enzymes being produced in cells.

5. HOW SUCCESS IN TREATING THYROID PATIENTS SHOULD BE MEASURED

I wrote about this in 2011, in Chapter 30 of the Recovering with T3 book. I have always thought that it was critically important that doctors should be primarily measuring their own success on something more important than getting TSH or other thyroid labs into the 'right' range. Now, it is even more important, as we seem to have moved further away from a patient-focused approach.

This article is about how doctors and endocrinologists measure their own success when treating thyroid patients, and how they are assessed by their peers and managers.

Currently, family doctors and endocrinologists appear to be satisfied that they have successfully treated the hypothyroid patient when thyroid blood test results conform to certain ranges. This appears to be the main way in which doctors assess whether they have treated the patient adequately.

They do not like to see a suppressed TSH, even though there is research that clearly shows a suppressed TSH is not an issue for a patient on T4/Levothyroxine therapy, as long as the patient has no evidence of being hyperthyroid and FT3 is not over the top of the reference range.

They are also perfectly happy if FT3 and FT4 sit somewhere in the reference range.

In fact, TSH is often the only thing that is measured. Sometimes TSH and FT4 are measured.

But increasingly, FT3 is not tested at all, even though research has shown that it is the only thyroid lab that rises as symptoms improve, i.e., symptom improvement is linked to getting FT3 higher. FT3 is the only thyroid lab test result that is linked to symptom improvement but this is increasingly ignored by medical professionals.

We know from research that TSH and FT4 do not correlate to symptom improvement, yet they are usually the only ones tested.

Thyroid laboratory tests appear to be the prime focus of most family doctors and endocrinologists and they often pronounce the patient adequately treated even if the poor patient is still very symptomatic.

As long as the above situation continues, no substantial change for the better will occur. In particular, it should no longer be acceptable to believe that thyroid replacement treatment has been a success just because thyroid blood test results are 'normal', i.e., sit somewhere within a reference range. The level of dissatisfaction with thyroid treatment should motivate those that manage the process of thyroid treatment to consider a change for the better.

People in other professions re-orient themselves and work differently depending on the measures that are used to determine whether they are successful or not.

In my previous professional life, I was measured using various criteria that included whether a certain new technology worked according to its design specification, and also whether it was produced in time for a customer to use. Doing one of these on its own, but not the other would have been deemed a failure.

Lawyers are ultimately assessed on whether they get good levels of acquittals or convictions.

Heart surgeons are judged on their % of successful surgeries and survival rates.

Teachers have yearly assessments and schools are assessed on their actual examination results.

In all the above cases, trying to ensure the customer was satisfied with the work is of paramount importance and is relevant to how the professionals are judged.

Why are the people involved in treating hypothyroidism not measured in the same way? Why should the quality of health care of a thyroid patient not be tracked properly? What would it mean to track the success of the health care of a thyroid patient? Should not the satisfaction of the thyroid patient with their health be as important in assessing the performance of the doctor or endocrinologist? Surely our health is as important as education, law, and engineering? Why cannot the health of thyroid patients be taken as seriously as the 'customers' of other professionals?

At present, a doctor can feel satisfied if thyroid blood test results are normalised according to certain criteria. However, we know that thyroid blood test results are not sufficient on their own. The normalisation of TSH or any other thyroid lab may have nothing at all to do with whether the patient recovers their health.

Doctors need to begin to measure the progress of the treatment mostly in terms of improvements in symptoms and other useful signs that actually reflect how the patient feels. If the patient does not feel better, the treatment is not working well enough, regardless of thyroid labs. Thyroid labs should not be the most important focus. Symptom improvement is not the paramount focus for most doctors treating thyroid patients – this urgently needs to change. The satisfaction of the patients with their therapy needs to be taken into account.

If the thyroid patient's lab test values are brought into the reference ranges, any remaining symptoms are frequently written off as, "It must be some other condition now!", "You have chronic fatigue syndrome!", or in medical-speak, there is some other co-morbidity (other conditions causing the symptoms). Often these 'other conditions' are not investigated to show if they exist or not. Sometimes, the poor thyroid patient may simply be told that they are getting older or need to exercise more!

The current approach that focuses almost entirely on laboratory test results is simply NOT GOOD ENOUGH.

Doctors and endocrinologists need to measure their success in treating a patient by how the patient's symptoms improve. If the patient genuinely feels they are better, this is what counts.

Changing how the success of thyroid hormone replacement is measured, to explicitly include what a thyroid patient most cares about, i.e., how well they feel, is a profoundly important change. It would alter the process of thyroid treatment, and the relationship between doctor and patient – for the BETTER!

I honestly believe that this needs to be incorporated into medical training of doctors involved in treating thyroid problems. I also believe that, over time, it would improve the quality of care and treatments offered to thyroid patients.

If T4 (Levothyroxine/Synthroid) replacement therapy fails, a focus on symptoms and signs would enable the patient and the doctor to have a common understanding that this has occurred.

The doctor would feel at a deeper level that the treatment has not been successful and would be more likely to continue to explore how to fix this.

These measures should become part of how the doctor assesses his or her own ability to treat patients. A focus on symptoms and signs would be a potent tool.

This assessment of the success of thyroid treatment could be more formalised. Just look at the school system as an example. In the UK, schools and individual teachers are rated in various ways. Most schools have a system where each teacher is rated/assessed each year based on exam results of classes they have taught and through observation. Schools and individual teachers are assessed even more formally every four or five years by external assessors. Education is obviously critically important.

Why is not health also critically important? I honestly think the paramount measure of success of thyroid treatment is symptom relief for the patient. This could be tracked quite easily and it has to be assessed with the patient being the primary judge of whether the symptoms are still present, better, worse, or completely gone. This is possible.

Thyroid patients need a new assessment scheme (other than thyroid labs) that properly represents how they feel and are responding to treatment. Doctors/Endocrinologists need to be looking at how a patient actually improves (or does not) in terms of symptoms. Thyroid labs are not enough. Pointing at the possibilities of other co-morbidities (other contributing conditions) without identifying them explicitly and putting treatments in place for them, is not good enough.

Being labelled as chronic fatigue, or ME, or just old, is not sufficient. Symptom improvement is the most important thing when treating thyroid patients. Specialists who are treating heart or cancer patients are viewed on their success rate with getting their patients well or extending their life. They are not measured simply on laboratory test results.

This is not rocket-science. It is just common sense. If there is to be an improvement in the quality of care of thyroid patients, I believe that placing patient symptom relief at the forefront of the focus of the medical professionals is an essential step.

I am sure a simple scheme focusing on a minimum set of the most common hypothyroid symptoms and rating them could be developed. The score could then be tracked and progress could be measured. This assessment could be graphed in the patient's medical records. It is feasible.

This change needs to be a central part of the new paradigm for thyroid treatment for all thyroid patients. If the change happened, a great many doctors would soon realise that they need access to all the thyroid treatments (T4, T4/T3, NDT, and T3-Only), in order to make their patients recover – it would be a game-changer! They would not be measured as successful with some patients if they only had access to T4 medication. They would also need to keep up to date with important research findings and adapt their approach accordingly. Treatment would improve. More thyroid patients would get better and live healthier and happier lives!

6. WHY DO I STILL HAVE ALL THE SYMPTOMS OF HYPOTHYROIDISM?

Doctors & the Current Treatment Approach are Keeping Many Patients Sick.

There are many reasons why some thyroid patients cannot get well. However, some thyroid patients are not allowed to get well. They are being kept sick.

In this article, I will discuss a few of the significant issues holding back the recovery of some patients and leaving them with ongoing symptoms of hypothyroidism.

The T3 thyroid hormone is not the main thyroid hormone being focused on.

T3 thyroid hormone does almost all of the work for us within our cells. T3 binds at the thyroid receptors in the cell nuclei. It is T3 that makes our cells run at the right rate. So, FT3 is the most important laboratory test to do. We know from research findings that it is ONLY when FT3 increases that symptoms improve.

Endocrinologists and doctors are not usually focused on the FT3 level of their patients in a way that helps their patients get well. This is a massive issue. Currently, just being in range with TSH, and FT4 is all that is required for most doctors to think that their patients are well-treated. Even an FT3 result that is just inside the bottom of the reference range, or mid-range, is thought by many doctors to be a good result. However, some thyroid patients need their FT3 level to be a lot higher. This is not a focus for most doctors. Hence it is stopping the recovery of many thyroid patients.

T3 is the most important thyroid hormone, but this fact is often overlooked.

Thyroidectomy patients lose some T4 to T3 conversion ability.

Thyroidectomy patients often lose about 25% of their T3 production (and it can be more in some patients). Most of this loss comes from the T4 to T3 conversion that occurs within the thyroid. The thyroid gland is the most important converter of T4 to T3 in the body (more important than the liver). The thyroid gland uses both D1 and D2 deiodinase enzymes in order to convert the T4 flowing in the bloodstream to T3. It is like a 'little machine' in the blood flow that converts T4 to the active hormone T3. So, the loss of the thyroid gland means the permanent loss of that important ability to convert T4 to T3. It can never be replaced with 'additional conversion' from other organs in the body. You cannot make T4 convert better than the body is doing it. So, the loss of the thyroid in cases of thyroidectomy causes a serious loss of T4 to T3 conversion capability.

Hashimoto's thyroiditis patients may also have conversion issues.

Hashimoto's thyroiditis patients also lose thyroid tissue. Over time, unless the autoimmune response can be halted, the same thing will happen to them as in thyroidectomy patients! They are just on a sliding scale with respect to T4 to T3 conversion loss from the thyroid gland vs. a total loss with thyroidectomy. After many years, a Hashimoto patient is also likely to become thyroid-less. So, Hashimoto's thyroiditis patients also risk a serious loss of conversion capability.

Note: this exact same situation occurs whenever the thyroid gland atrophies, e.g., in Atrophic Thyroiditis (see Article 1 in Chapter 10).

Genetic reasons can play a part in poor T4 to T3 conversion.

The DIO1 and DIO2 gene defects affect the ability of our cells to make good, effective D1 and D2 deiodinase enzymes. There are two copies of each gene – one from each parent. If someone has only one bad copy (gene defect) and one good copy, they are said to be heterozygous for the gene defect. If they have both bad copies, they are homozygous. This applies to both the DIO1 and DIO2 genes. The gene defects often do not manifest until someone is in their late twenties or early thirties. If these gene defects do appear to be causing issues, the homozygous situation (both copies of each gene defect) is usually more serious. DIO2 is also more serious, as the D2 enzyme converts T4 to T3 more efficiently than D1. Having both D1 and D2 defects is also worse of course. So, these gene defects can seriously affect the ability of someone to recover, if only given T4 medication. See Article 2 in Chapter 5 for more information on DIO1 and DIO2 gene defects.

Laboratory test ranges are being used poorly by doctors.

Lab ranges are the side of a barn door! I have discussed this before. The lab ranges are wide population ranges and have little resemblance to the range an individual's FT4 and FT3 need to be in for them to feel well. Lab ranges are not 'normal' ranges. The way lab test results and lab reference ranges are being used today is leaving many thyroid patients inadequately treated. We do not know where an individual's own personal ranges are. So, the wide population ranges are not useful for fine-tuning a thyroid patient's medication. We know from medical research that an individual's ranges are far less than half as wide as the population ranges used for thyroid testing. The laboratory reference ranges are simply a guide and it is still essential to look at the clinical presentation of the patient.

This situation gets even worse when a thyroid patient is on thyroid medication that includes T3, e.g., T4/T3, NDT or even T3-Only. Laboratory reference ranges are created based on healthy people with no thyroid problems, or those patients on T4-Only medication. To even attempt to use the standard laboratory ranges for those on T3, laboratories would need to take a population of thyroid patients who are healthy on T3 and develop different ranges for these people. Shoehorning all thyroid patients to fit within the standard population ranges is extremely bad logic. It keeps a lot of thyroid patients who are on T3 sick!

TSH is being relied on far too much as an insight into thyroid hormones.

TSH itself is also no measure of thyroid hormone action. It is profoundly misleading and research has proven that the movement of TSH under thyroid treatment does not track the patient's symptoms at all.

Losing thyroid function leaves the thyroid patient deficient in T3.

In addition to the above, we know that when someone becomes ill with hypothyroidism, their entire thyroid system balance (homeostasis) is changed. The system does not work as well as it did in the past. The thyroid gland no longer steps in and keeps the level of Free T3 up to the level that is in a healthy person. On thyroid treatment, it is critical to ensure that the thyroid patient has enough T3 to correct their symptoms. Sadly, this usually does not happen.

Other issues are frequently not looked at thoroughly.

Often other lab tests are either not done, or the results are said to be Ok when they are clearly too low, e.g., cortisol, ferritin, vitamin D, B12 etc. Other issues are thus not diagnosed or ignored.

Symptoms and signs are rarely at the forefront of doctors' focus. Thyroid labs are just too easy to use instead!

Symptoms and signs need to be centre-stage – they do indicate how thyroid treatment is working. Symptoms might include energy level/fatigue, feeling cold/warm etc. Signs might include body temperature, and heart rate.

Symptoms and signs show the actual response of the body, whereas blood test results just show what is in the blood. The latter is made worse by comparing the individual's results to a wide population range.

Unfortunately, symptoms and signs are looked at as less important than TSH and other thyroid lab tests (if others are even done).

T4 monotherapy often fails to work but most doctors are not aware of this.

We are also in a seriously messed up situation where most endocrinologists and doctors believe that T4 monotherapy works well for all thyroid patients. However, T4-Only cannot work well for the many patients who have lost T4 to T3 conversion capability.

Here is a summary of the reasons why so many thyroid patients remain sick:

- T4 to T3 conversion issues can affect a lot of thyroid patients to varying degrees. These have multiple possible causes.
- The flawed application and interpretation of lab tests.

- The flawed belief by most endocrinologists and doctors that the TSH-centric, lab-test-centric, and T4 monotherapy paradigm actually works.
- The lack of focus on improvement in symptoms and signs as the main guide on whether the thyroid treatment is working
- The near-total disbelief that T3 in combination with T4, or NDT, or in a few cases T3-Only, is needed at all. In many parts of the world, T3 is not being prescribed at all, as it is thought to be unnecessary. Lunacy.

All of the above issues (and others) are keeping many thyroid patients from recovering. These issues are even keeping some thyroid patients desperately ill.

Patients are not being allowed to get well due to current treatment practices!

Far too often the thyroid patient is left deficient in the active hormone FT3. When this happens a host of hypothyroid symptoms remain. Frequently, the thyroid patient has high blood pressure and high heart rate and their doctor even cites these as reasons for not increasing the thyroid medication or adding T3 to therapy. This is a mistake in so many cases because low FT3 causes cardiovascular stress and this can manifest as one or both of high blood pressure and high heart rate. I see this over and over again when I talk to thyroid patients and look at their lab test results.

It is time to accept the new research findings and embrace a new treatment paradigm (approach) that will actually work.

The research findings are already out there to show how treatment needs to change. Past clinical trials are flawed but randomised clinical trials (RCTs) are not the best way to prove treatment anyway.

There is plenty of clinical evidence for the need for all the treatments to be available already. T4 monotherapy will not make everyone well!

We need to have all the thyroid treatments available and we need a sound approach to the use of clinical presentation and thyroid labs during treatment.

It is absolutely necessary at this time to renew the paradigm and move forward!

Without a new paradigm of thyroid treatment, thyroid patients will continue to ask the question, "Why do I still have all the symptoms of hypothyroidism?"

7. USING TSH TO MANAGE TREATMENT IS A HOUSE OF CARDS WAITING TO FALL

In Article 3 in Chapter 6, there is a research paper that makes it clear that a suppressed TSH whilst on thyroid treatment does not mean that the patient is hyperthyroid. I am keeping the articles on Suppressed TSH together, all in Chapter 6.

The research paper shows that thyroidless (athyreotic) thyroid patients require sufficient T4 (Levothyroxine, Synthroid) medication to get their FT3 levels up high enough to feel well. When this happens, TSH is suppressed but as already stated, the research shows that TSH suppression on thyroid treatment does not mean the patient is hyperthyroid. This argument can be extended to those with some thyroid function left as long as they have no hyperthyroid symptoms or signs and their FT3 is not high.

A person not on any thyroid treatment who has suppressed TSH could easily be hyperthyroid (unless they have a pituitary issue, e.g., hypopituitarism which results in low TSH). But the genuinely hyperthyroid person on no thyroid medication, with low TSH, is a totally different case. However, this assumption of low TSH always implying hyperthyroidism, is routinely being used with thyroid patients on thyroid treatment. It is keeping many of them under-medicated.

Being thyroid-less is just at one end of the spectrum of thyroid patients. Many thyroid patients who are on thyroid hormone treatment have some thyroid gland function and with this, some T4 to T3 conversion ability. Some of these people may also need very low TSH in order to get well.

However, IF you accept that TSH can be suppressed in a thyroid patient on treatment (which you have to because the research is compelling), then the consequences of this are significant.

It means that on thyroid treatment, TSH could be anywhere from just inside the top of the lab range right down to near zero. Thyroid treatment might even need to be increased when TSH is suppressed in order to get a therapeutic response i.e., to eradicate a thyroid patient's symptoms. This does not mean that the patient is hyperthyroid. It simply acknowledges that the person needs more T3 in order to feel well, i.e., enough of the actual active thyroid hormone.

Currently, TSH is being interpreted in the same way as it is for an individual not on any thyroid treatment (and who may be genuinely hyperthyroid). This is incorrect and is likely to keep many thyroid patients under-medicated.

Ok, so where does that leave us in terms of knowing if a thyroid patient is properly treated?

The answer is "Nowhere" if TSH is the only measure!

TSH tells us very little about whether the thyroid medication dosage the patient is on, is correct for them. It may not provide a clue as to whether the right type of thyroid medication is being used. If TSH does change, as the thyroid dosage is increased or lowered, then it might be safe to assume that the pituitary gland is at least working. However, being low in the range on TSH does not mean the patient is correctly treated with the right amount of thyroid medication, or even the right type of thyroid medication!

The use of TSH to determine the correct treatment and dosage level is flawed!

Doctors and endocrinologists are ultimately going to have to face up to the science and begin to ignore their sacred TSH. It is not the beacon of light onto the correct treatment level at all.

The logic of using TSH comes crashing down!

The house of cards collapses!

This has to happen at some point.

Research findings and science cannot be ignored forever!

8. LAB TEST AND REFERENCE RANGE THYROID TREATMENT IS FAILING PATIENTS

Doctors who are focusing primarily on the laboratory testing of TSH, FT4 and FT3, and who are satisfied when each lab test result falls somewhere within its reference range, are often failing thyroid patients.

All of this information (and a lot more besides) is in my book The Thyroid Patient's Manual.

There are two important points that I need to make.

The first point is that thyroid laboratory tests do not take account of the individual needs of thyroid patients.

Thyroid lab tests all suffer from a 'low index of individuality'. The range of variance in the population is much wider than the range of variance in the individual (this is also known as non-ergodicity). We know from research that the actual individual person ranges for levels like FT3 and FT4, are far less than half as wide as the population ranges that doctors are using to assess our thyroid lab test results. When you make generalisations based on the population and try to apply them to the individual, you have problems. Basically, the lab reference ranges do not help much when assessing whether FT3 or FT4 is at the right level for the individual thyroid patient. We do NOT know what each thyroid patient's actual reference range is!

The following research study shows that the FT4 and FT3 reference range for each individual is less than half as wide as the population reference ranges for FT4 and FT3:
"Narrow individual variations in serum T(4) and T(3) in normal subjects: a clue to the understanding of subclinical thyroid disease." Stig Andersen, Klaus Michael Pedersen, Niels Henrik Bruun, Peter Laurberg
The Journal of Clinical Endocrinology & Metabolism, Volume 87, Issue 3, 1 March 2002,

Pages 1068–1072. https://doi.org/10.1210/jcem.87.3.8165 and
https://academic.oup.com/jcem/article/87/3/1068/2846746

The use of TSH in monitoring thyroid hormone therapy is highly unsatisfactory and should be replaced by triple FT4/FT3/TSH measurement. The presentation of symptoms of the patient should be the primary focus, above lab-test results, but supported by them. Unthinking, automatic, biochemical definition of treatment success, independent of the patient must cease. Individuality should be the decision-maker for optimum therapeutic outcomes:

"Time for a reassessment of the treatment of hypothyroidism." John E. M. Midgley, Anthony D. Toft, Rolf Larisch, Johannes W. Dietrich & Rudolf Hoermann.
BMC Endocrine Disorders volume 19, Article number: 37 (2019)
https://bmcendocrdisord.biomedcentral.com/articles/10.1186/s12902-019-0365-4

This research article shows that the current protocols for managing thyroid hormone issues are very wrong. The way TSH is currently used is wrong. The way people are treated as if they are all the same is wrong. Simply being 'in range' on levothyroxine monotherapy is not going to guarantee a good outcome. We are all individuals. Many of us require either some T3 with T4 or T3-Only in a few cases. We also know that we cannot be managed by simplistic measures like TSH. This is a complex article but well worth the read:

"Recent Advances in Thyroid Hormone Regulation: Toward a New Paradigm for Optimal Diagnosis and Treatment." Hoermann, Midgley, Larisch, Dietrich.
https://www.frontiersin.org/articles/10.3389/fendo.2017.00364/full.

The top and bottom of the FT4 and FT3 lab test ranges are limiting treatment.

The second point is that we also know that some laboratories include data from thyroid patients with in-range TSH levels. However, thyroid patients under treatment with T4 medication, tend to have higher FT4 and lower FT3, than non-thyroid patients.

This is because the T4-Only medication does not result in as much FT3 as a healthy person has from the conversion of T4, plus there is often a loss of T3 from the thyroid gland itself.

The net effect of this is that the bottom and the top of the reference ranges for FT4 and FT3 are influenced by the inclusion of the thyroid patient data. The top and bottom of the FT4 ranges are likely to be higher than for healthy people. The top and bottom of the FT3 ranges are likely to be lower than in healthy people.

As a result of this practice, you may be more likely to be considered healthy with higher inactive pro-hormone FT4 and lower biologically active FT3.

Current treatment focusing mainly on lab test results is failing patients.

It is currently impossible to assess what the unique individual person ranges are, other than through the treatment of a thyroid patient. In many instances, doctors are satisfied if the patient's thyroid labs sit within the population reference ranges – virtually anywhere within them! Even though the patient may need much higher FT3 and lower FT4 (and the rT3 that comes from this) in order to feel well.

Moreover, thyroid blood tests cannot measure the FT3, FT4 and rT3 levels within the cells. They only measure the blood portion and as such are an approximation to what might be present and active within the cells. Since conversion occurs within the cells, we cannot know specific information about FT3, FT4, and rT3 inside the cells. So, focusing on the clinical presentation of the patient through their symptoms and signs is critical.

The bottom line is, there is not as much value to the thyroid laboratory test results and reference ranges as is being assumed and relied upon, by most doctors and endocrinologists at the present time.

Simply having results that fit inside each lab test reference range is no guarantee of symptom relief. What is important, is finding a treatment regime that relieves symptoms, and allows the thyroid patient to live a healthy life.

The response to treatment and the changing relationships between TSH, FT4, FT3, and rT3 should be what guides dosing decisions. Sticking mechanically to the existing reference ranges without using good clinical judgement is a desperately flawed approach.

We need to have ALL the thyroid treatments available to thyroid patients, in order to ensure every individual has the right level of FT3 and FT4 for them.

The thyroid treatments using T4, T4/T3, NDT and T3-Only (when needed) all have to be available, as options from our doctors.

Current thyroid treatment is failing patients – it does not take into account the research that clearly contradicts current practices.

9. WHY THYROID PATIENTS NEED TO GET BETTER FASTER

I have described hypothyroidism to a lot of people as being the illness that is the 'death of a thousand cuts.'

Hypothyroidism is often a slow process that gradually wears the sufferer down. Sometimes the symptoms just slowly creep up on the person. To begin with they may not even notice the symptoms. Issues, like gaining weight, feeling tired, getting depressed, difficulty in thinking straight and feeling cold, can be so general that the individual may think that they are just working too hard, or have too much stress etc. Months or years can go by as the symptoms worsen and new ones appear before they eventually might get a diagnosis of hypothyroidism.

Even when a proper diagnosis has been made, it is common for poor treatment to leave the thyroid patient with many or all of the original symptoms. The quality of care may be quite good for those patients that respond well to Levothyroxine (T4 only). But for the large numbers of patients that find T4-Only does not alleviate their symptoms the quality of care can be dreadful. The life that the patient used to have before hypothyroidism can be lost. Precious time simply vanishes after more and more visits back to the doctor or endocrinologist. Eventually, many patients look back with sadness at multiple years or even decades during which they have suffered debilitating symptoms.

During this time, the thyroid patient often has more thyroid blood tests done by their doctor or endocrinologist (frequently not including FT3 and reverse T3). Sometimes, increases in Levothyroxine (T4) are made and sometimes, the dose is lowered. Usually, any improvement is very short-lived. The T4 dosage often ends up being cycled up and down many times over years, with little or no benefit to the thyroid patient. Over time, it is common for the thyroid patient to get more ill. This frequently stops the thyroid patient from enjoying their life and living it to the full. It can leave the patient severely debilitated (it did this to me and I know it does to many others). In this way, more of the person's precious life is lost.

Worse still can be the collateral damage that hypothyroidism frequently causes. This damage can be to the thyroid patient's career or job, or to their relationships with friends or family members (partner, children etc.). This type of collateral damage only occurs if the hypothyroidism has not been successfully and quickly treated. Sadly, this happens all too often.

Recovering from hypothyroidism as fast as possible is the only effective way to avoid the 'death of a thousand cuts.'

This requires a correct and early diagnosis. Critically it has to be followed by really effective treatment that focuses on the clinical presentation of the thyroid patient (symptoms and signs), as well as comprehensive thyroid laboratory tests (not just TSH and FT4, but also FT3 and reverse T3). Other factors also need to be examined and corrected, like vitamin and mineral levels.

It ought to be straightforward, but all too often it is not.

The current approach that most doctors and endocrinologists use during thyroid treatment is a broken paradigm. Most of them believe that TSH alone can be used to assess the right dosage – WRONG! Low or suppressed TSH when on thyroid treatment is also believed to represent hyperthyroidism in all thyroid patients – also WRONG! This latter prevents many thyroid patients from ever being given a large enough dosage of thyroid medication to effectively treat them and eradicate symptoms. Many doctors think that TSH and FT4 are definitely enough to assess treatment – WRONG! A lot of them do not believe that laboratory testing of FT3 (the active hormone) is essential – VERY WRONG! Most of them believe that T4 medication always converts well and works – WRONG AGAIN! The focus on TSH and FT4, without attention to FT3, can leave many patients either un-treated, or inadequately treated. I see this time and time again. I have spoken to thyroid patients who have developed other serious health issues as a result of this, e.g., coronary heart disease, or diabetes.

The current broken paradigm assumes we are all robots that work identically and always convert T4 medication perfectly. The current treatment approach is keeping many thyroid patients sick! Some thyroid patients are aware of these issues and even know what they require – they simply cannot persuade their doctor or endocrinologist to test them properly or treat them with the correct medication. However, the vast majority of patients do not even realise that they are being treated poorly. These patients often just believe what they are told. This might be that they are just unfit, or getting older, or have chronic fatigue syndrome, or are depressed. So many different excuses are used to avoid the obvious answer – that the treatment is not working.

The thyroid patients that suffer most are those that do not do well on Levothyroxine (T4). This is extremely common. One common reason for this is that doctors often never raise the Levothyroxine to a high enough level because they fear a low TSH means that the patient is hyperthyroid. Research has shown that low TSH is not a concern if the patient's FT3 is over-range, and the patient has no hyperthyroid signs or symptoms. Another major problem with Levothyroxine treatment is that many thyroid patients do not convert T4 to sufficient amounts of the active T3 hormone. Only T3 does any real work in the body and the thyroid patient needs enough T3 for them as an individual. Simply having FT3 in the reference range is not sufficient. FT3 needs to be in the right part of the reference range for the person. Sometimes, even an okay looking FT3 may not be sufficient because the individual patient needs a higher FT3 level in order to feel completely well.

Sometimes the thyroid patient needs a T4/T3 combination that is tuned with the right amount of T4 and T3 for them as an individual. Occasionally, the thyroid patient needs mostly T3 and only a little T4 medication. It is also possible that someone can only get well if they are given T3-Only medication and no T4 at all – this was my own situation and I know that many other thyroid patients have found this to be the case for them too.

I wrote The Thyroid Patient's Manual because I wanted to provide a very practical, easy to use manual to help patients understand whether they have hypothyroidism and to provide a very practical guide on how to recover as fast as possible. In the book, I try to encourage the thyroid patient to 'get in the driver's seat of their own health' and not completely hand their health over to their doctor. This does not exclude having a good working relationship with their doctor. However, it definitely does mean gaining enough understanding of hypothyroidism and how to treat it effectively, so that the thyroid patient can be an active partner in any discussions about changes in treatment. The book will give the reader enough information to understand their situation and to assess what their next steps ought to be.

In my own case, I lost at least ten years of my life from age 30 to 40 through hypothyroidism. I lost my career and my marriage. Worse still was the damage to the relationship with my children. My own 'death of a thousand cuts' has spanned from the start of the disease when I was about 30 and has continued due to the collateral fallout. I still see and feel the damage in my own life due to being incorrectly treated for so long by so many doctors and endocrinologists. Many years ago, I blazed with anger about this bad treatment. This anger helped me to write the Recovering with T3 book. These days, I just feel sadness at what happened to me. I am also very disappointed that the knowledge that I gained and expressed within my books has not been taken up and used by many doctors or endocrinologists. However, I find some consolation in the way that so many patients manage to reclaim their health using my work.

The above is why I am so passionate about the need for a new paradigm of thyroid treatment that provides the fastest possible route for patients to get diagnosed and get correctly treated as unique individuals. Only by getting well fast can the 'death of a thousand cuts' be avoided.

The Thyroid Patient's Manual is effectively Book 1 in the Recovering from Hypothyroidism series. The Thyroid Patient's Manual was written specifically to help thyroid patients recover quickly. The other two books in the series (Recovering with T3 and The CT3M Handbook) are mainly aimed at those patients who need to use T3-Only or T3-Mostly therapy or who need to deal with low cortisol issues. Articles on Hypothyroidism adds a lot of information to the series that I have developed and acquired over many years.

The Recovering from Hypothyroidism series should help more thyroid patients get 'better, faster', and avoid 'the death of a thousand cuts.'

Chapter 5

Lab Testing: What To Do & What To Avoid

1. ASSESSING YOUR FT4 TO FT3 CONVERSION ABILITY

There is a blog post on the Thyroid Patients Canada website about assessing conversion ability from T4 to T3 in late 2018. It is extremely useful and I think it might help some thyroid patients to understand why they are having problems.

The article is entitled: "Are you a poor T4 converter? How low is your Free T3?"
Here is the link to the article on The Thyroid Patients Canada website:
https://thyroidpatients.ca/2018/09/06/how-low-is-your-t3/

The article refers to this research paper:
> Variation in the biochemical response to l-thyroxine therapy and relationship with peripheral thyroid hormone conversion efficiency. Endocrine Connections, 4(4), 196–205.
> Midgley, J. E. M., Larisch, R., Dietrich, J. W., & Hoermann, R. (2015).
> Here is a link to the research paper:
> https://ec.bioscientifica.com/view/journals/ec/4/4/196.xml

The article highlights one particular finding in the research study; that it is possible to assess the T4 to T3 conversion capability in those people on no thyroid medication and in thyroid patients on Levothyroxine only (T4 only thyroid medication).

You can read both the original research paper by Hoermann, Midgely et. al. and Dr Smith's paper for the details.

However, based on both the above, there is a relatively simple way that may help many of you to assess how well you process your T4 thyroid hormone and how efficiently it is being converted to T3.

Note: this method only works for people on no thyroid meds at all or those patients on T4-Only treatment. In addition, both the FT4 and FT3 results need to be from the same laboratory and converted into the same units (below FT4 and FT3 are in pmol/L, but the important thing is that they are in the same units). It is also important to realise that this is also not the same as conversion ratio or what proportion of FT4 is being converted into FT3. It is just a way of categorising how effective the person converts from T4 into T3.

Simple Method of Assessing Conversion Capability:

Metabolic Category	FT3 in pmol/L Divided by FT4 in pmol/L
Poor Converters on T4 Monotherapy	<0.25
Intermediate Converters on T4 Mono	0.25-0.31
Good Converters on T4 Mono	>0.31

I hope you found this information useful.

2. DIO1 AND DIO2 GENE DEFECTS AND TESTING THEM

The D1 and D2 deiodinase enzymes are produced inside our cells to enable the conversion of FT4 to FT3 to occur there.

Both D1 and D2 enzymes are seleno-proteins, i.e., they have selenium as part of their structure. Hence, if someone has low levels of selenium this can hamper conversion. Many thyroid patients take 100 or 200 mcg of selenium per day to ensure they have sufficient.

The higher the number of these enzymes produced, the higher the conversion rate. TSH also has an impact. If TSH goes up, the D1 and D2 enzymes are up-regulated, i.e., more are produced in each cell, and the conversion rate of T4 to T3 rises. If TSH goes down, the D1 and D2 enzymes are down-regulated, i.e., fewer are produced and the conversion rate lowers (but there is still some conversion occurring).

However, some thyroid patients have gene defects that can mean the quality of the D1 or D2 (or both) enzymes are impaired. The genes involved in producing the D1 and D2 enzymes are referred to as DIO1 and DIO2. It is possible to have mutations in the genetic material that make up these genes. If you received a good copy of the genetic material from one parent and a mutation from the other parent, you would be heterozygous for the gene defect. If you had a bad copy from both parents, you would be homozygous for the gene defect – which is more serious as the quality of the deiodinase enzyme is liable to be worse.

Note: I have heard from one patient whose endocrinologist told her that there is no point in testing these, as if she had them, she would not convert T4 to T3 at all (she is very unwell on T4 medication). This is obviously rubbish. The gene defects, even if present with both copies of each DIO1 and DIO2 mutation, impair the quality of the D1 and D2 enzymes but do not stop them from working totally. It just makes conversion worse – it does not totally stop it.

The DIO1 and DIO2 mutations do not always cause obvious conversion problems either. Some people are better at compensating for the defects than others. Geneticists do not fully understand this yet. However, it is this compensation that tends to make the mutations not affect people until their late twenties/early thirties. Perhaps, a higher TSH might help compensate, as more deiodinase enzymes would be produced – but I am speculating. One thing is true though; if you have a mutation, it is genetically there in your make-up. It cannot be turned off or removed. It will in some way affect the ability of your cells to make good D1 and D2 enzymes. Over the next ten years, more on all of this will no doubt be discovered.

The bottom line is that those people with one or more of these genetic defects may have impaired ability to convert from T4 to T3. This means they may have little or no impaired conversion, some impaired conversion or very severely impaired conversion. Even in the most severe cases, there is still an ability to convert some T4 to T3, but it might be that too little T3 is produced and too much reverse T3 is created as a result.

Genetic testing will provide additional information that can back up a suspicion that conversion from T4 to T3 is an issue. Often this testing only gets done when the individual thyroid patient already suspects conversion issues. In some people with the gene defects, there appear to be no conversion problems. In others, there appears to be severe conversion issues.

The most important indicator of T4 to T3 conversion issues in a thyroid patient is how that individual responds to treatment. This involves assessing how well they are, in term of symptoms and signs, as well as full thyroid labs that include FT3, FT4, and TSH. It may be necessary to switch the thyroid patient from Levothyroxine (T4) medication to T4/T3 medication and perhaps eventually to T3 medication, if they do not respond well enough to treatment. Response to treatment is always going to be the most valuable assessment of T4 to T3 conversion.

Having said the above, the DIO1 and DIO2 genetic mutation tests are very useful to do, even if you have to do them privately. Knowing that you have one or both mutations, will inform you of the potential risk of conversion issues. Both mutations can reduce T4 to T3 conversion, lowering FT3 and raising rT3, thus increasing the chances of on-going hypothyroidism.

A DIO1 mutation may affect conversion by the thyroid, liver, and kidneys.

A DIO2 mutation may affect conversion by the brain, pituitary, central nervous system, thyroid, heart, and peripheral tissues (skeletal muscle). Thus, the DIO2 mutation can also cause hypocortisolism, through the impact on the pituitary, i.e., due to HP dysfunction leading to lower adrenocorticotropic hormone (ACTH). ACTH from the pituitary gland, is the control hormone that tells the adrenal glands how much cortisol to produce. Note: once you have totally cleared T4 and are reliant on T3, this conversion issue becomes unimportant, unless it has caused HP dysfunction that is slow to correct.

Both D1 and D2 enzymes are important in the conversion of T4 to T3. More focus has been on the D2 enzymes and DIO2 polymorphisms over recent years. However, DIO1 polymorphisms are still important and have a bearing on T4 to T3 conversion.

The Watts Study by Panicker, Dayan et al study of DIO1 in 2008 showed that this polymorphism affected FT3, FT4, and RT3 concentrations even in people with healthy thyroids! See: Panicker, V., Saravanan, P., Vaidya, B., Evans, J., Hattersley, A.T., Frayling, T.M., Dayan, C.M.: Common Variation in the DIO2 Gene Predicts Baseline Psychological Well-Being and Response to Combination Thyroxine Plus Triiodothyronine Therapy in Hypothyroid Patients. J. of Clin. Endocrinol. and Metab., Vol. 94, No. 5:1623-1629, 2009. See abstract: https://pubmed.ncbi.nlm.nih.gov/19190113/

The D1 deiodinase enzyme is also important in the liver as it is involved in the clearance of rT3.

The bottom line is that both DIO1 and DIO2 gene defects are useful to check. I am also confident that significantly more will be learned about the deiodinase enzymes and their potential gene defects (polymorphisms) over the coming years.

If you do a full genome mapping, please make sure the company offers both DIO1 and DIO2 in their raw data.

Note on SNPs: some genes have places in the genetic material that can have a mutation that is known to cause problems with the function of the gene. These locations in the genetic material of a gene that can have these defects are referred to as Single Nucleotide Polymorphisms or SNPs. These SNPs are like 'hotspots' in the genetic material of genes where known mutations have been observed to occur and can prevent the genes from doing their proper job. These SNPs are given unique codes. Some genes may have more than one SNP that can cause problems. In the case of the DIO1 and DIO2 genes, if the SNPs have mutations, it is possible for any D1 or D2 enzymes produced to be compromised in their quality, resulting in lower conversion capability from T4 to T3. Researchers are continuing to look at the DIO1 and DIO2 genes and their polymorphisms. We can expect new information over time (some of which might contradict our current understanding).

How to Interpret the Results.

If you have used a company that performs separate DIO1 and DIO2 tests, the results will be obvious in their report.

You have three options to interpret your results, depending on the company you have used for testing your genome:

1. Just use the raw data – it is very simple to do and in my opinion, the best option.

The company may have a raw data browser, or you can look/search through the raw data text file if needed. This latter option requires downloading the raw data from the genome mapping company. Then you can open the raw data file using a TEXT EDITOR (like TextEdit on a Mac, or Notepad on Windows). Do not attempt to use a word processor, as the special characters in the raw data will confuse a word processor. After that, it is simply a matter of doing searches for the particular SNP associated with the gene defect. These SNPs have unique codes (rs numbers) that can be searched for in the raw data. The rs number being searched for, can be typed into the Find or Search area in the text editor and it should take you straight to that particular SNP in the raw data.

DIO1 has two known SNPs that can have mutations and cause problems. These are referred to as "rs2235544" and "rs11206244":
- For the DIO1 "rs2235544" SNP: the 'C' (or 'G') allele can boost the expression of DIO1 and can be associated with higher T3 levels. The 'T' (or 'A') allele is the risk allele; it can reduce T4 to T3 conversion and raise rT3 when active.
- For the DIO1 "rs11206244" SNP: the normal allele (normal, no defect) is 'C' (or 'G'). The 'T' (or 'A') allele is the risk allele; it can reduce T4 to T3 conversion and raise rT3 when active.

DIO2 has one known SNP that can have mutations and cause problems. This is referred to as "rs225014" (and also as the "Thr92Ala-DIO2 polymorphism"), The normal/wild-type allele (no defect) is 'T' (or 'A'). The 'C' (or 'G') allele is the mutation (risk allele); it can reduce T4 to T3 conversion and raise rT3 when active. See Note A below regarding Regenerus Labs.

Important Notes A and B:

A. At least one company (Regenerus Labs) is choosing to use a different notation for the DIO2 mutation – 'A' rather than 'C'. This is their argument, "T92A (this is Threonine is changed at position 92 of the protein into Alanine) you also could write this Thr92Ala. If you look at base level in the DNA (genetic code) the C (=Cytosine) codes for the amino acid Alanine) see below. "A" is not Adenosine but the amino acid alanine in this report. So, Ala = "C" in the genetic code (a Cytosine pyrimidine base). So, the Ala/Ala or AA type corresponds to the CC genotype. The Thr/Thr or TT type corresponds to the TT (Thymine base, NOT THREONINE, in the DNA)." Their argument may be that there is an amino acid code: https://en.wikipedia.org/wiki/DNA_codon_table where Alanine is 'Ala' but also 'A'. So, an 'A' result for DIO2 from Regenerus labs is the mutation, then it is equivalent to what most of the companies are labelling as 'C' for the mutation. I wish they were all consistent.

B. In other genes, the notation for normal vs. abnormal is reversed. This has to do with conventions in designating the change from one base amino acid to another. If looking at other genes, one needs to check each one individually against the main databases. Also, you need to bear in mind that for some other genes, an abnormality may confer health advantages better than the normal un-mutated gene.

As briefly mentioned earlier, the results of testing show both copies of the gene – one from the person's mother and one from the person's father. If both alleles show no defect, there is no mutation at all. If one of them is a mutation, the person is said to be heterozygous for the defect, i.e., they have one copy. This is likely to impair the quality of the deiodinase enzymes (but not definitely). If both alleles have the mutation, the person is said to be homozygous for the defect and the chance of the deiodinase enzymes being impaired is higher and the consequence can be more severe.

So, for instance, if you were looking for DIO2, you would search for 'rs225014' then look at the results there. 'TT' would mean you had no defect inherited from either parent. 'TC' or 'CT' would mean one parent gave you the defect and one did not (you are heterozygous for the defect). 'CC' would mean that you have both defective genes (you are homozygous, but as mentioned some labs may use 'A' instead of 'C').

For DIO1 you would search for "rs11206244". 'CC' implies there are no inherited defects. 'CT' or 'TC' means you are heterozygous for DIO1. 'TT' means you are homozygous for the DIO1 mutation (you have both copies).

2. Use a special filtering program.

Companies like 'Genetic Lifehacks' and 'Genetic Genie' offer software that read your genome mapping raw data and give you a simpler analysis of it.

Personally, I think the raw data is easy enough to look through.

3. Laboratories that do the testing.

Note: it is advisable to always check with the company you are considering using that they still have the DIO1 and DIO2 results in their data, as both these gene defects are important to be aware of. Some companies have removed DIO2 (possibly due to some kind of political pressure).

Ancestry (.com and .co.uk) have both DIO1 and DIO2 in the raw data. All you have to do is to download the raw data file and then load it into a text editor and search for the SNPs outlined above.

Regenerus Labs in the UK also offer the DIO2 test – but please check their website, as at one point they had removed the test from the offerings on their website: https://regeneruslabs.com/

MTHFR Genetics in the UK offer comprehensive genetics testing that includes the SNPs mentioned above: MTHFR-Genetics.co.uk

Blue Horizon Medicals in the UK have a genetic profile test that as of May 2020 includes the DIO1 and DIO2 SNP rs numbers and allele results: https://bluehorizonbloodtests.co.uk/collections/a-z-test-catalog/products/dna-blue-thyroid-genetics

23andMe only offers DIO1 in its raw data now. They do not test DIO2.

Nutrition Genome in the USA had both DIO1 and DIO2 in their raw data in August 2018. But this site only appears to work if you are in the USA.

Fulgent Genetics in the USA also provide DIO1 and DIO2 test results: https://www.fulgentgenetics.com/products/disease/genomictesting.html

Also see SNPedia, a source of information on genes, gene defects etc. You can enter SNPs in the search bar and get information on them: https://www.snpedia.com/index.php/SNPedia

I hope you found this useful. I do believe that the DIO1 and DIO2 tests are useful to do, especially if you can see in your thyroid lab results that you are having poor conversion issues. The presence of one or both of these mutations would at least provide a concrete explanation for why this might be and hopefully persuade your physician to switch the balance of your thyroid medication to more T3 and less T4. However, please remember that the loss of thyroid tissue also lowers the conversion rate – so this can be another reason for issues. I discuss all of these types of problems in my book, The Thyroid Patient's Manual.

I am sure that over time, more gene-related issues will be discovered that affect thyroid hormone action within our cells, the binding to thyroid receptors and much, much more.

3. CHASING 'IDEAL' LAB TEST RESULTS IS THE ROAD TO NOWHERE

During the 1970s, the shift to a lab-test-centric model began. This involved the increasing focus by doctors on laboratory test results, rather than symptom improvement in their patients. This was the start of conveyor-belt thyroid treatment using Levothyroxine (T4) medication. It was much easier and faster for doctors treating thyroid patients. Endocrinologists and doctors could get their thyroid patients in and out of their consulting rooms in record time. However, this approach, which is the default approach today, leaves many patients under-medicated or improperly treated.

Both doctors and patients are now highly focused on lab test results. In many cases, both groups (patients and doctors) are operating under the mistaken belief that by focusing mostly on trying to achieve some 'ideal' lab test results, the patients will fully recover.

This article points out the huge flaws in this approach.

Note: the focus of this article is on lab testing during thyroid treatment. Lab test results are extremely valuable during the diagnosis stage, prior to a patient being given any thyroid hormone – there is no question of this.

What Usually Happens During Thyroid Treatment?

Most doctors use the TSH test to assess their patients' thyroid medication dosage. The standard thyroid medication is Levothyroxine/Synthroid/T4. Some doctors also test Free T4 (FT4) and a few also test Free T3 (FT3).

Most of these doctors are content that their patient is well treated on T4 medication, if the patient's TSH is in the reference range. Some prefer to see TSH low in the reference range.

However, most doctors get concerned if TSH is near zero. TSH has become the de facto way of assessing the T4 medication dosage. T4 has become the de facto treatment. Even if a patient is lucky enough to have a doctor who prescribes a mixture of T4 and T3, the doctor often wants to get the FT4 level in range, even if the patient responds poorly to T4, and has awful conversion ability from T4 to T3.

As for patients, they too are interested in their thyroid lab test results. Some well-informed patients are hoping for an FT3 level that is between the middle and the top of the FT3 laboratory range. Some seem to be trying to achieve some ratio of Free T3 to Reverse T3 (FT3/rT3 ratio), that is if they can get rT3 tested. Most of the well-informed patients are still using T4 medication, or natural desiccated thyroid medication (if they can get it). Some of these patients still want TSH, FT4 and FT3 to be in range and this in itself can be an issue for some of them who convert T4 to T3 poorly.

Some History Prior to the 1970s.

Synthetic T4 (Synthroid, Levothyroxine) was first introduced in the 1950s. Current thyroid lab tests (TSH, and the other thyroid labs) were invented in the 1970s.

Before these events, all doctors had available was good clinical judgement, based on the symptoms and signs (body temperature, etc. and possibly basal metabolic rate) of the patient, and the option to use natural desiccated thyroid (NDT). NDT was based on thyroid tissue extracted from pigs. This had all the normal ratios of T4 and T3 that would have been present in porcine thyroid tissue (which has a slightly higher ratio of T3 to T4 than human beings produce in their thyroid glands) and was therefore a T4/T3 treatment.

When doctors worked with a patient, they would assess many things and try to reach a judgement over whether the patient might have a thyroid problem or not. If low thyroid hormones were suspected, a trial of NDT would be started. If there were improvements in symptoms and signs, the NDT would be adjusted (titrated) to a higher or lower dose if needed. This titration process would continue based on the presenting symptoms and signs of the patient. This meant that the doctor would have to work with the patient and listen to what they were saying about how they were feeling in response to treatment. There were no laboratory tests to get in the way between the doctor and the patient in front of them. The improvement in the well-being of the thyroid patient was the primary goal prior to the 1970s. This approach worked pretty well a lot of the time.

What Happened from the 1970s Onwards?

In the 1970s, the TSH test became the standard way to assess whether thyroid treatment was working. Levothyroxine/Synthroid/T4 became the standard medication for treatment. Both of these required almost no effort on the part of the doctor or endocrinologist compared to what had happened in the past. It vastly reduced the work of the physician. The reliance on the

TSH test and the use of T4 medication also virtually guaranteed that no patient would ever be over-medicated.

This sea-change was the beginning of conveyor-belt thyroid treatment, optimised for the doctor, and far less likely to result in over-medication of the patient. However, it was much more likely to result in the under-medication of the patient!

Unfortunately, it is a method that frequently results in improperly treated hypothyroidism. Patients are often under-medicated and do not have enough T3 thyroid hormone. It is a broken paradigm.

Why is this a broken paradigm?

I have written about this in many other articles, but here is a resume:

1. Research has shown that it is safe for TSH to be totally suppressed when on thyroid treatment, i.e., near zero. This is fine and it does not mean the patient is hyperthyroid, if they show no symptoms or signs of hyperthyroidism. Many doctors believe that once TSH gets into the laboratory reference range that the patient must be properly treated. This leaves many thyroid patients under-medicated!

2. TSH does not track symptom improvement. So, seeing TSH get lower after an increase in T4 medication does not mean that the patient is doing better.

3. FT4 does not track symptom improvement either. A higher level of FT4 does not mean that the patient will be feeling better. Taking more T4 medication just to get FT4 into a good part of the reference range may not work well for poor converters of T4 to T3. Some thyroid patients do far better with low in the range or even below range FT4. A very few thyroid patients cannot get well with any FT4 at all. I know many patients in this last category, including myself.

4. Free T3 does track symptom improvement. However, FT3 is not the measure that most doctors focus on. Often FT3 is not tested and the FT3 level is not considered to be important – even though it is critical.

5. The reference ranges for FT4 and FT3 are population ranges. These are far too wide to conclude anything about whether a patient is well-treated or not. Real individual reference ranges (which cannot be known before treatment) are much narrower than the large population ranges. Individual ranges of FT4 and FT3 required for a person to be well have been shown to be around 38% the width of the wide laboratory population ranges that most doctors are using.

6. Reverse T3 (rT3) may or may not be an issue, and there is no ideal FT3/rT3 ratio for all patients. Just as the lab ranges are wide population ranges, people all have their own individual requirements for their labs. Very high rT3 is usually an issue but that is about all you can say about it in isolation. Symptoms and signs of the patient say more.

7. T4 does not work for all patients. Some patients cannot get well using T4 medication.

8. We also know that the thyroid gland itself is responsible for around 25% of our T3 (and much more in some people), mostly through conversion, so tissue damage through

Hashimoto's, or through the removal of the thyroid, loses a huge amount of ability to convert from T4 to T3. This can often not be compensated for with T4 alone. There is also a great variation in the amount of T3 produced by the thyroid gland itself, and in people who do not convert T4 to T3 very well, the thyroid gland is able to make more of its own T3 thus compensating for this. So, in cases of Hashimoto's or thyroidectomy, the loss of T3 can be even more dramatic for some individuals who are more reliant on their thyroid gland for T3 production.

9. Research has shown that the loss of conversion capability of the thyroid gland in thyroidectomy patients, causes the loss of the ability to achieve a balance of thyroid hormones and good conversion rate (homeostatic balance).

10. We also know from research that some people have genetic defects that reduce the capability to convert from T4 to T3 (DIO1 and DIO2 gene defects).

Moreover, we know from the experience of an immense body of thyroid patients, that many of them need different medications to get well: T4, NDT, T4/T3, or in some cases T3-Only.

Logic and patient experience also suggest that once a thyroid patient is on a combination of T4 & T3 treatments, the laboratory reference ranges can break down. The ranges are based on people with no thyroid issues or those on T4 treatment. They are not based on those on combined T4/T3 or T3-Only. It is not reasonable to hold a thyroid patient's T3 medication level down in order to satisfy the need to keep FT3 within the range if the patient has no indication at all of being over-medicated. On T3-Only in particular, the patient often has to have FT3 at or above the top of the range before they feel well (for good reasons I have explained in my books.)

So, the current paradigm of thyroid treatment is broken, and the research has shown this.

The Consequences of the Broken Paradigm.

This is the really sad aspect of all of this.

Thyroid patients are being left improperly treated in many cases. They are either on the wrong medication for them, or they are being left under-medicated.

Both doctors and thyroid patients are now incredibly focused on lab test results. This alone is liable to waste vast amounts of time, and not lead to good treatment and outcome. Both thyroid patients and doctors are chasing some ideal set of laboratory test results. We know from the research that it is virtually impossible to use just the lab test results to determine if someone is either on the right medication or the correct dosage of it.

The shift to this broken paradigm of lab-test-focused treatment and T4 medication has caused generations of doctors and patients to become fixated with lab test results. It has caused both doctors and patients to believe that these test results will reveal something amazing. It is sad because the lab-test-focused approach will not work – the research has proven this.

What Ought to Happen?

Lab test results should only be used in a supportive role during treatment.

You do need to have the lab test results, but watching how they change in relation to each other and to symptoms and signs is the most important thing.

The medical history of the patient and their presenting symptoms and signs should always be centre stage. If changes in signs and symptoms and in lab test results, with changing treatment, can be observed then it easy to make good changes to treatment. This has the caveat that lab test ranges are not being worshipped. The focus should be on improving how well the patient feels.

Here are two examples:

1. For a thyroid patient on natural desiccated thyroid (NDT), if the NDT was increased and the patient felt they had more energy, and FT3 also increased, and TSH lowered and FT4 raised a little, this would indicate that the NDT was being absorbed. It would also suggest that the treatment was resulting in higher FT3, which we know tracks symptoms. Because the patient said they had more energy, it would be clear that they were actually responding to treatment. This process of adjustment could continue until the patient felt well. Even if TSH went close to zero, it would not be a concern as long as the patient does not feel hyperthyroid, and FT3 does not go over the top of the reference range. If treatment was done like this, many more patients would get well. (Note: on T3-Mostly or T3-Only therapy, FT3 may sometimes need to be over the top of the range.)

2. For a thyroid patient on T4 medication, or even NDT medication, if this dosage was adjusted and FT3 was mid-range, FT4 was mid-range, and TSH only 2.0, many doctors would say that the patient was properly treated, even if the patient continued to have serious symptoms. It is common for doctors to say that the thyroid patient is adequately treated, and to suggest that something else must be causing the symptoms, e.g., chronic fatigue syndrome (CFS). This 'some other problem' excuse is used far too often by doctors. What ought to occur is that the labs should not be used to determine if the medication is sufficient. The medication should be increased, even though the lab tests are in the middle of the range. On thyroid treatment, TSH can be suppressed, and many patients do better with high in the range FT3. But the main thing, in this case, is that the patient does not feel adequately treated. In many cases, T4 medication will not fix all the symptoms. A T4/T3 combination of some kind might be needed. In a small percentage of cases far more T3 may be needed. Unfortunately, in many cases, the thyroid medication is never increased or changed.

The clinical response of the patient to changes in treatment (the medication type or the dosage of it) should be paramount. Symptoms and signs should be at the forefront of treatment assessment.

Treatment should be patient-centric, not lab-test-centric, once again. Just focusing on lab tests as the most significant thing and looking for some mythical good level is not what doctors or patients should be doing.

Laboratory tests should be used only to assess how the labs are changing in response to treatment and they should not be used to state whether the treatment is adequate or not.

The clinical presentation – the SYMPTOMS and the SIGNS are the most important things, with the labs being subservient to these.

The change in the way thyroid treatment is managed that occurred in the 1970s has been the biggest step backward that we have ever seen with the treatment of this disease.

Doctors and thyroid patients are both too focused on chasing 'ideal' thyroid laboratory test results. This has been the road to nowhere for some time and it continues to lead there.

The advent of thyroid lab tests for TSH, FT4 and FT3 ought to have made thyroid treatment far better and easier. However, in the process of using them, they have become the main focus and T4 medication has become the main treatment. This is where it has all gone wrong.

Both groups of people (doctors and patients) have been mesmerised by what could be viewed as the 'biggest confidence trick' in the history of treating thyroid problems.

4. ENFORCING NORMALISED THYROID LAB TEST RESULTS IS HARMFUL

Here is another great article about the flawed use of thyroid laboratory tests and lab reference ranges.

It talks about how endocrinologists and doctors want thyroid patients' lab results to conform to their standard lab ranges.

The article illustrates how this is harming the health of many thyroid patients.

I have written a lot about the poor use of thyroid lab testing – this speaks to this point totally.

Here is the article:
https://thyroidpatients.ca/2020/02/15/biochemical-bigotry-the-drive-to-normalize-thyroid-lab-results/

Being on any T3 medication, even a small amount combined with T4, begins to make the thyroid lab ranges too restrictive. The ranges were developed based on healthy people, or those on T4-Only therapy. They often do NOT apply to people on T3/T4 or on T3-Only. There are good reasons for this, and reasons that most doctors have not considered.

On T3-Only, people sometimes need to have an FT3 level which is at or just over the top of the FT3 reference range. The FT3 reference range is therefore not suitable for those on T3-Only. This is because these people have very little T4 and there is no on-going, hidden T4 to T3 conversion occurring in their cells. See Article 8 in this chapter for more details on this.

I believe for all medications, symptoms and signs ought to be the predominant method of assessing thyroid dosage efficacy. Thyroid lab test results must include FT3 because it is the most important measure but these results should only be used as an indication of whether the numbers are changing correctly with dosage changes.

Thyroid lab results should not be used to control patients' medication levels, as this is 'bio-chemical bigotry' as Dr Smith has written about so eloquently.

The current approach is definitely harming the health of thyroid patients.

5. REVERSE T3 (rT3) – WHAT IT IS AND WHAT IT MEANS TO THYROID PATIENTS

Reverse T3, also known as rT3, is a possible marker of poor conversion and potentially blunted T3 action. This makes it useful to test in some cases.

T4 is a relatively inactive hormone. T4 only becomes useful to the body after one of the D1 or D2 deiodinase enzymes converts it into the biologically active T3 hormone. Another deiodinase enzyme (D3), is able to convert some of the T4 into reverse T3 (often shortened to rT3).

T3 cannot be converted into rT3. Only T4 can be converted into rT3.

The deiodinase enzymes can be up-regulated or down-regulated depending on the need to increase conversion from T4 to T3 or reduce it, and increase or decrease rT3 (in order to manage T4 clearance).

The conversion process of T4 to rT3 occurs on an ongoing basis within the cells, in order to clear excess levels of T4 from the body.

RT3 is eventually broken down by other enzymes and converted into T2, which in turn is converted into T1. T2 and T1 are simpler molecules with fewer iodine atoms. The body then eliminates these molecules within roughly twenty-four hours. T3 is also converted into T2 and then into T1. So, even on T3-Only therapy, the body creates enough T2. Natural desiccated thyroid (NDT) users often cite the T2 content of NDT as being an advantage over using T4/T3 - but it is not. You get all the T2 that you need from T3 medication.

RT3 is an isomer of T3, which means that it has the same molecular formula as T3, but the atoms are arranged in a slightly different internal structure. For those who have a working thyroid, or are on medication containing T4, rT3 is a natural bi-product because the body needs a way to clear excess FT4. So, having rT3 is natural and is not necessarily a bad thing. Once FT3 is produced from FT4, it cannot then be converted to rT3. Once rT3 has been produced from FT4 it cannot then be converted into FT3.

Let me be very clear rT3 cannot bind to any thyroid receptor. RT3 itself does not block T3. There is no particular level of rT3 that is suddenly a special concern. RT3 does not have to be below mid-range. There is no FT3 to rT3 ratio that is either bad or good. There is much information out on the Internet that is clearly very incorrect with respect to rT3. However, this does not mean that excessively high rT3 cannot indicate a problem – because it can.

It is the D3 deiodinase enzyme that converts T4 to rT3. This is important to be aware of because high levels of D3 deiodinase enzymes can inhibit some of the T3 hormones from connecting with thyroid receptors in the cell nuclei. For this reason, elevated rT3 can be a potential marker of slower metabolism. Some doctors say rT3 has no importance at all, but research has shown that there is value in assessing rT3 under some circumstances. Elevated rT3 does indeed slightly reduce the number of D2 deiodinase enzymes that are present, which lowers FT4 to FT3 conversion. Moreover, because it is D3 deiodinases that convert T4 to rT3, very high rT3 can be a marker that these D3 enzymes may be interfering with T3 action in the cells (even though it is not rT3 that does this directly).

So, high reverse T3 can be a marker of T3 being blocked in both ways – through slightly lower conversion (less D2 deiodinases) and blocked T3 (high D3 deiodinases). Note: the words 'can be' in the last sentence. You have to look at the complete picture with the thyroid lab test results and especially at the clinical presentation of the patient (signs and symptoms).

It is true then, that in some circumstances you can view reverse T3 as a 'T3 blocker'. See this research paper that shows that reverse T3 (rT3) is a T3 blocker and not an irrelevant metabolite:
"Qualitative and quantitative differences in the pathways of extrathyroidal triiodothyronine generation between euthyroid and hypothyroid rats.". J E Silva, M B Gordon, F R Crantz, J L Leonard, and P R Larsen 10.1172/JCI111313. https://www.jci.org/articles/view/111313

RT3 exists in order to provide a dynamic mechanism to match the amount of available T3 to the body's needs. RT3 also provides a mechanism for slowing down the metabolism in the event of starvation, serious illness or high stress. In these circumstances, the conversion rate of T4 to T3 decreases and more rT3 is made. As rT3 increases, it also reduces the effect of FT3 through the D3 deiodinase enzymes. The reduced T3 level that occurs during illness, fasting, or stress slows the metabolism of many tissues. Because of the slowed metabolism, the body does not eliminate rT3 as rapidly as usual. The slowed elimination from the body allows the rT3 level in the blood to increase considerably.

Some studies show that most people convert over 50% of their FT4 to rT3 and therefore, they convert less than 50% of FT4 to the metabolically active hormone FT3. The levels of reverse T3 fluctuate up and down through the day. There is no ideal level for rT3 or any perfect ratio of FT3 to rT3.

Having said all the above, it is obvious to me, from my own experience and from working with thousands of thyroid patients, that a few thyroid patients cannot tolerate T4 medication and even low levels of rT3. This cannot be determined from laboratory test levels of rT3 or FT4. It has to be determined based on the symptoms and signs of the patient during treatment. These patients need to be on T3-mostly or T3-only therapy.

The late Dr John C. Lowe provided some excellent information on reverse T3, and he talked about whether it can actually be used to diagnose hypothyroidism:

"… I'm never confident of coming to the conclusion that someone has a problem with high reverse T3, not unless the person has had multiple measures of the reverse T3 over a 24-hour period. Like the TSH, free T4, free T3, reverse T3 levels vary dramatically every 30 minutes or so. Depending on when a person's blood is drawn or saliva is taken. Sometimes the levels will vary enough so that a clinician will give the patient a different diagnosis from the one that he or she would have given 30-minutes before or after the blood or saliva sample was taken. So, blood levels vary rapidly. Because of this, I do not believe the reverse T3 or the other lab tests, in general, are very useful. However, I do believe the reverse T3 is useful under one circumstance: when we have enough measures to get averages over time, and when the levels are regularly way out of range. So, in my view, the reverse T3 can be useful, but I think its usefulness is limited, which is true of the TSH and other thyroid hormone levels."

There are many conditions that can upset the balance of T3 and reverse T3. These include iron issues, taking too much T3 with T4, poor conversion of T4 due to lack of important nutrients like selenium, infections, tumours, damaged heart muscle, ageing, chronic alcohol abuse, diabetes, liver disease, kidney disease, severe illness, stress, surgery, a number of drugs, genetic defects affecting deiodinase enzymes (DIO1 and DIO2 gene defects), or other key components that may affect the pathways involved in thyroid hormone metabolism. Many more issues may be added to this list over time.

Once a decision has been taken by a doctor and patient that it is time for the patient to have a trial of T3 replacement therapy, the decision has been taken that T4 based medication should no longer be the predominant thyroid hormone being used. After this decision, there is little point in having any real interest in reverse T3, as correct titration of T3 thyroid hormone can only be done through using symptoms and signs.

Consequently, I believe the only real scenarios where rT3 may have some use, are in treatments that are predominantly T4 based, i.e., with T4, T4/T3 (where only small amounts of T3 are used), or NDT replacement therapies.

In predominantly T4 based treatment, rT3 is quite useful to test.

If a patient is using NDT or T4 medication (even if in a combination with T3), and their symptoms are not improving with medication increases, then checking rT3 as well as the other thyroid labs of TSH, FT3 and FT4 can be very insightful.

So, what should a patient who is on T4 based medication or a T4/T3 combination be on the lookout for with respect to rT3? Well, having T4 go into a lot of rT3 can mean the T4 is not converting into the necessary level of FT3. Only improving FT3 levels, track the improvement of symptoms.

Consequently, for someone on T4 or T4/T3 (including NDT), they need to be assessing:

1) Does the FT3 level increase? AND

2) Do they feel their symptoms and signs have improved?

If either FT3 does not improve OR symptoms and signs do not improve, then any rising rT3 may signal a conversion issue.

This assessment can be made whether the T4 or the T3 has been increased in any T4/T3 combination. Testing rT3 can help in making the assessment.

Any issues with the conversion of T4 to T3 could be due to the unsuitability of the type of thyroid treatment being used or due to something else like low iron or cortisol levels.

Note: in many cases, the type of thyroid treatment being used is limited in its success simply because a doctor fails to increase it to a high enough level, due to fear of low or suppressed TSH. This is frequently a huge mistake because the patient is neither over-medicated nor hyperthyroid. This is a very common error and it stops many thyroid patients from recovering.

It is also important to remember that in some cases rT3 may appear normal and yet the patient may still have problems with processing the T4 thyroid hormone and getting sufficient levels of the T3 hormone. RT3 can provide some additional insight. Also a few thyroid patients simply cannot cope with even low levels of FT4 and rT3.

RT3 is only a guide and has to be put into perspective with patient symptoms and signs being the most important focus, along with how FT3 changes with changing treatment.

6. CAN SOMEONE HAVE FT4 AND RT3 WHEN TAKING T3-ONLY MEDICATION?

From time to time, a thyroid patient asks me the question: how can they have a reasonably high level of rT3 or FT4 when they take T3-only medication?

Let me be very clear. T3 cannot under any circumstance convert into rT3. T3 and rT3 are what is known as isomers. They have the same atoms making up their molecules but the atoms are connected in different ways.

T4 can be converted in the body into either T3 or into rT3. But once T3 or rT3 is made, the body has no mechanism to take elements from a T3 or rT3 molecule and reorganise them together in a different way. So, rT3 cannot be converted to T3. Equally, T3 cannot be converted to rT3. This is impossible. It would be a bit like saying we could take all the cells that make up a tiger and rearrange them to create a lion. It just cannot be done.

So, if someone is on T3-Only, and they still have some measurable FT4 and rT3 there are only a few ways that this can be caused:

1) There is still some circulating T4 from any T4 medication that was being taken prior to the person going on T3-Only. Normally, after stopping all T4 medication and being on a TSH suppressive dose of T3 medication, it takes up to a further 12 weeks to clear all the FT4. During this time, it is even possible for rT3 to increase as more FT4 is converted into rT3 due to a suppressed TSH. A TSH suppressive dose of T3 might be 40 mcg for some people and well over 100 mcg for others.

2) The person is not on enough T3 to cause TSH to be zero over the full 24-hours. Sometimes TSH can rise at night – so testing TSH in the daytime may not detect that TSH is not suppressed. If TSH is not zero all the time, and the person still has some thyroid tissue left (even after a thyroidectomy), then some T4 will be produced and much of this T4 may go into rT3. In some cases, after a total thyroidectomy that shows there is no thyroid tissue left, new nodules can be produced – hence the need for regular check-ups.

3) In rare cases, someone might have a neuroendocrine tumour. These are benign hormone-producing tumours. Some neuroendocrine tumours produce hormones and some produce neurotransmitters like serotonin. Even though they are not cancerous, they can be incredibly difficult to diagnose and detect and require sophisticated scanning techniques. In rare cases, someone could have a neuroendocrine tumour that produces T4 (which can then be converted to rT3) even if the person has no thyroid gland. This is included here for completeness only, as it is very rare.

4) Lab error. This is unusual but it actually does happen. Sometimes the results of a thyroid lab test may make no sense. If this is the case, it may be worth questioning the

laboratory staff about the results. I have definitely heard of cases when either rT3 or other lab test results have been mistakes and the test has needed to be repeated.

The other obvious conclusion from all of this is that if a thyroid patient is on a T4/T3 combination and has continued high rT3, the best solution is to reduce the T4 content of the combination and possibly to increase the T3 content (based on symptoms & signs and lab test results). It is always the T4 that is the source of the rT3.

7. CAN FT3 BE USED TO MANAGE LIOTHYRONINE (T3) THYROID TREATMENT?

Many doctors and thyroid patients think that the Free T3 (FT3) thyroid lab test can be used to assess whether the dosing of Liothyronine (T3) is at the right level for the individual.

Testing FT3 can be useful if the thyroid patient is on Levothyroxine (T4-Only), or on T4 with a tiny bit of T3. In these cases, the FT3 level is relatively stable over twenty-four hours. If a thyroid patient is only using small T3 doses (< 10 mcg), then testing FT3 within 12 hours of taking a T3 dose may show an FT3 result that is in range.

However, the situation changes dramatically if the patient is on mostly T3 therapy (with some or no T4 medication). These are the patients for whom this article is relevant.

FT3 is the laboratory test of the bio-available level of T3 within the bloodstream at the time of the test. Remember, only FT3 can enter the cells and be biologically active.

On T3 therapy, this FT3 level is far from stable. It is about as stable as a rollercoaster!

After taking a dose of T3 medication, the T3 absorbs very quickly into the body. It absorbs far faster than T4 based medication. 2.5 hours after a dose, the FT3 reaches peak levels in the bloodstream – which means that most of the T3 dose has been absorbed.

Here is a link to the research study:

https://www.ncbi.nlm.nih.gov/pmc/articles/PMC5167556/

Important note: the volunteers in this study were euthyroid, i.e., normally they were not on any thyroid medication. They had a working thyroid gland and so their FT3 would never crash to extremely low levels 10-20 hours after the T3 dose. Many of us would see a more severe drop off of FT3 to a level that would not be good!

The research study included this chart that shows how rapidly FT3 rose after the Liothyronine (T3) dose and how FT3 fell after the dose:

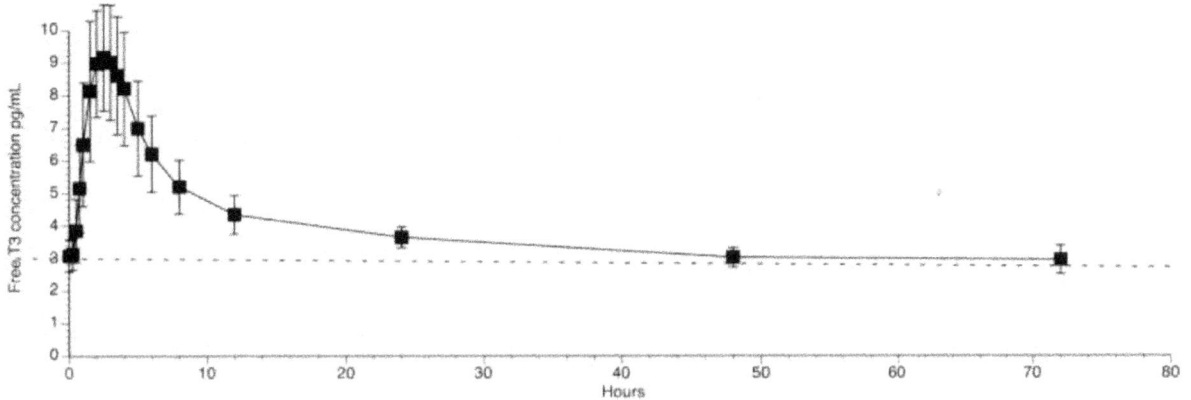

Figure 2b.

The study still illustrates the peaks and troughs of FT3 induced by Liothyronine dosing. But does that matter?

FT3 changes too dramatically following T3 dose administration to use it to manage medication dosage.

Many thyroid patients, including me, can sense a T3 dose has been taken within 20 minutes of taking it. So, we know that T3 begins to be digested and absorbed into the bloodstream within 15-30 minutes. It reaches peak FT3 levels in the blood at about 2.5 hours and will gradually decline in the bloodstream after this. All the T3 will be absorbed from the T3 tablet within 3-4 hours. By then, the level of FT3 in the bloodstream will be lower, because much of it will have entered the cells.

So, FT3 levels fluctuate. For those on T3 therapy, the length of time between the last T3 dose and the blood draw for an FT3 test is the biggest single factor in what level of FT3 shows up in the results. If the time varies, the FT3 result will vary. Testing FT3 within a few hours of a T3 dose will show a much higher level of FT3 than the trough level that will be reached from the longest gap a thyroid patient has between two T3 doses. For this reason, I prefer to see people testing FT3 at trough levels versus peak levels – it is a fairer test and more stable than testing anywhere close to peak levels.

However, the higher the amount of T3 in a dose that the person is on, the longer it will take to fall. For example, I know many people who would have over the range FT3 if they tested it 12 hours after a T3 dose. But at 18-24 hours they may well be in-range for FT3 (and have fewer issues with a doctor who was reviewing their results). Individuals do vary a lot though – even absorption rates vary, so FT3 will fall faster in some people than in others.

Furthermore, some people need T3 doses that take them over the FT3 range even when tested 12-18 hours after a dose of T3. This again makes using the FT3 range when on T3-Mostly or T3-Only very difficult.

Note: It can be helpful to test FT3 in order to check that FT3 does change with changing T3 dosage and to check if the T3 is absorbing. However, I do not think that testing FT3 is going to show that a thyroid patient on T3 therapy is adequately treated. The following explains why I think this.

Here is a strong statement and I really do believe this:

For those on mostly T3 therapy, blood levels of FT3 do not reflect how patients feel and how well they are treated/medicated!

The T3 thyroid receptors at the cell nuclei are where most of the action of thyroid hormone occurs. The T3 needs to arrive at the receptors for the action of thyroid hormone to make any real difference to how our cells work. I am not going to go into how this all works but it involves something called 'gene transcription' that is enabled by the T3 arriving at the T3 thyroid receptors. T4 cannot do this. It has to be the T3 thyroid hormone – the only biologically active thyroid hormone. The right level of gene transcription ensures our cells all perform the particular functions that they are designed for. Muscle cells have a different function to brain cells etc.

What is the most important thing that a T3 dose needs to achieve?

What matters most is that the T3 receptors in the cell nuclei have had enough T3 so that the cell nuclei can continue to function well for some time. To do this, the cells do not need to have stable levels of FT3 in the blood. This last point is very important. This is why, for many people, 3 doses of T3 per day work really well. In most cases, it is better to multi-dose the T3 because of the rapid nature of how fast it peaks in the blood and then declines again. Many thyroid patients need to multi-dose T3 so that the T3 gets to the thyroid receptors in several reasonably sized pulses over 24 hours.

Taking T3 in multi-doses, when the doses are the right size for the individual, is like rapid charging of a battery with each T3 dose. The 'battery' then has enough charge for quite a long time. Even after the 'rapid charging' is complete, there is still enough T3 left within the bloodstream and within the cells for some trickle charging to continue for some hours.

An example of this last point is that I take a T3 dose at about 3:00 am in the morning and no more until 11:00 am – a gap of 8 hours. This gap will be in the presence of peaking FT3 at about 5:30 am and a steady decline in FT3 all the way to 11:00 am. I have often completely forgotten to take any T3 until the early afternoon and still have not noticed any degradation in how I feel. This is because my T3 receptors in the cell nuclei have had 'a rapid charge' of T3 with the previous dose.

I hope this goes some way to explaining why, when we do exercise, we do not simply 'run out of T3'. Once we have enough T3 at the thyroid receptors in the cells, the effect of the T3 will continue to enable the cells to work well for a considerable amount of time.

Let me put the above a different way. On T3-Mostly or T3-Only therapy we know that TSH is often very low or suppressed and that low TSH on thyroid treatment does not mean someone is hyperthyroid. We also know that those people on mostly T3 are likely to have a below range or even near zero FT4 and consequently near zero rT3. So, we already have most of the thyroid labs that do not comply with the reference ranges. Why should FT3 be any different? Why would anyone assume that someone on T3 ought to comply with an FT3 reference range designed for healthy people or those on T4? It does not make any real sense.

I have worked with thousands of patients over the past 17 years who never get well unless they are on individual doses of T3 that are large enough to make an impact on their symptoms and signs. This often takes them over the FT3 reference range if the FT3 blood test is done too close to the last T3 dose. Frequently these people need to leave 24-hours after the last T3 dose if they are to have any hope of getting an FT3 result within the FT3 reference range. Basically, the FT3 test becomes far less useful the higher the T3 doses are.

For those patients that are certain, from signs and symptoms, that they are not over-medicated, it is important to find out whether their doctor insists on in-range FT3 and in-range TSH. If they do, then the patient needs to do a private test first (for their eyes only) leaving an 18 or 24-hour gap with no T3 prior to the lab test. If the results are well in range, then you know that this will work for you and you can let the doctor see the result or do the test again for the doctor. If the results are still a little out, then the private test needs to be repeated, with a slightly longer gap. The alternative is to risk having your prescription level reduced or even stopped.

So how can we tell if a thyroid patient has had enough T3?

To assess whether a thyroid patient has had the right T3 dosage, what we need to know is whether their cell nuclei have had enough T3 in order for the cells to run at the right metabolic rate. There is no test for this right now and I cannot foresee a time when such a test will exist.

For a thyroid patient on T3 therapy, trying to test whether they are on the right dosage of T3 based on a highly unstable level of FT3 is a flawed and misleading exercise. It is also flawed to attempt to assess T3 dosage based on the pituitary hormone TSH.

However, while a thyroid patient's T3 dosage is being adjusted, it can be very helpful to have occasional FT3 tests just to check that the T3 medication is being absorbed. More T3 medication ought to induce some level of increase in FT3 (as long as the same length of time from the last T3 dose to the time of the blood draw is maintained each time). However, FT3 is not going to inform anyone about whether the correct dosage has been achieved, and neither will TSH or FT4.

On T3 therapy when the patient is on T3-Only, or T3-Mostly with only a little T4 medication, the FT3 level could be in range, at the top of the range or even over the range. It is impossible to conclude whether the patient is under-dosed or over-dosed from any of these results. If the patient on T3-Only or T3-Mostly therapy has suppressed TSH or extremely low FT4, it is not possible to conclude that the patient is hyperthyroid, or requires the addition of T4 medication.

However, on the positive side, once a thyroid patient feels really well, knowing what their FT3 lab result is after a fixed time from the last T3 dose can provide some future value, if for instance, their symptoms worsen and they need to get some clue as to why this is. Testing the FT3 again, with the same period of time since the last T3 dose, could provide a much-needed clue.

The current laboratory ranges are not fit for purpose for patients on T3-Only or T3-Mostly thyroid medication.

The current laboratory ranges are designed for healthy people on no thyroid medication or for those on T4 monotherapy. These people have FT3 in the bloodstream but they also have on-going intra-cellular conversion of T4 to T3. They have more T3 than shows in the bloodstream than those patients on T3-Mostly or T3-Only.

The lab ranges are not designed for patients on T3-Only or T3-Mostly therapy, so why would anyone in their right mind attempt to apply the lab ranges in this case?

It makes no scientific or logical sense to attempt to apply the ranges developed for healthy or T4 medicated patients, to those patients who are on T3-Only or T3-Mostly.

If there was a need to have lab ranges for those on T3-Only or T3-Mostly thyroid medication, then this population of people on T3 therapy would have to be studied and ranges would need to be developed specifically for this usage of thyroid medication. Any range developed for patients on T3-Only or T3-Mostly therapy is definitely likely to be a lot higher at both the bottom and top end of the reference range. Force fitting the current labs for use with T3-Only or T3-Mostly patients cannot work and is likely to leave the majority under-medicated.

None of the current lab ranges are useful in assessing whether the T3 dosage is too high or too low or just right in T3-Only or T3-Mostly therapy – not TSH, not FT4 and not even FT3. These lab results are only useful in how they change as the T3 is being adjusted. The changes in TSH, FT4 and FT3 only show trends during T3 dosage adjustment. They cannot be used to assess the adequacy, inadequacy or excess of the T3 medication. The absolute values of the thyroid lab results cannot answer the question of whether the patient is on the right T3 dose.

Thyroid patients who have a doctor or endocrinologist who simply will not accept an FT3 result over the top of the reference range, even though they are on T3 therapy, need to be particularly careful about when the lab test is done after the last T3 dose.

So, how can someone assess whether their T3 therapy is dosed correctly for them? The answer is not simply by 'going how they feel'. This is far too vague and it is too easy to be misled by what you think is going on. We need a better, more objective approach.

So, what is the best way to assess whether the T3 therapy dosage is right or not?

I recommend the use of both Symptoms and Signs. Symptoms are subjective assessments of things like energy level, mental clarity, digestive system, skin and hair condition etc. However, Signs are more objective measurements. Signs include things like body temperature, heart rate, blood pressure, cholesterol level, calcium level etc., The Signs are numbers and they take the guesswork out of assessing T3 doses if the right ones are recorded at the right times.

Symptoms and Signs assess the response of a thyroid patient's body to the T3. This is actually the closest measurement we have to how the cell nuclei are responding to the T3.

My book, Recovering with T3, has a full protocol for doing this.

When I was first trying to get well, I got too confused trying to assess my T3 dosage based on how I felt (my symptoms alone). I gave up trying to do it that way after 6-12 months. This is when I began to create the method that is now written about within the Recovering with T3 book.

It is the pattern of the SIGNS before and after doses that is most helpful. Subtle changes in these can be informative. This approach stops people from going on hunches and also alerts them to dosing that is too high.

If someone were trying to manage T3 doses using FT3, I would say that this is a recipe for disaster, unless it is only a small amount of T3 combined with T4.

Symptoms and signs need to be used. The 'cellular batteries need to be recharged' and only symptoms and signs can tell us if this has actually happened. After a T3 dose, 'trickle charging' of the cellular batteries should occur. Perhaps, at some time in the future, technology will provide better support for the dosing of the biologically active thyroid hormone T3.

Here is a summary of the points made in this article:

- If a doctor or endocrinologist is planning to test your FT3 level, then any patient on T3 treatment needs to be careful about how long they leave after the last T3 dose before the blood test. I often recommend 18-24 hours to try to ensure that the FT3 result is in range. Ideally, the patient would test this privately first and see if this time delay provides the desired result. Having FT3 over range runs the risk of the patient's T3 dosage being reduced or even stopped.
- A T3 dose peaks rapidly in the blood and FT3 takes many hours to slowly lower.

- The size of the T3 dose determines how high the peak of FT3 is and how long it takes for FT3 to fall within the FT3 reference range.
- Small T3 doses e.g., 10 mcg or so, may allow FT3 to fall back within the FT3 reference range within 12-15 hours. But this varies by person and cannot be guaranteed 100%.
- Larger T3 doses that some patients require may take 18-24 hours or even longer for FT3 to fall back within the FT3 reference range.
- For those thyroid patients who wish to test their own thyroid labs. privately for their own viewing, testing after 12-18 hours of the last T3 dose is completely fine. The FT3 result would not be being used in this case to potentially reduce or stop the patient's T3 prescription.
- Knowing that FT3 changes when the T3 dosage is adjusted is helpful and it can show that the T3 medication is absorbing (and of good quality).
- However, the FT3 reference range is not designed for those on T3-Mostly or T3-Only therapy. Both the low end of the FT3 reference range and the top end of the FT3 reference range are too low. The peaks of FT3 due to T3 doses are high. In addition, these patients lack the on-going, hidden extra T3 that is constantly being converted within the cells from T4 that healthy people have (or those on T4-Only meds have).
- The bottom line is that it is not possible to use the FT3 test result to determine if a T3-Mostly or T3-Only thyroid patient is on the correct T3 dosing-regime for them. It can be used carefully to see how FT3 changes with different doses as long as the interval from the dose to the blood draw is the same and the laboratory testing it is also the same. Symptoms and signs need to be used to really assess how the T3 dosing is performing.

Note: I cover all of this in both The Thyroid Patient's Manual and in Recovering with T3.

8. WHY THE FT3 LAB RANGE MAY NOT BE HELPFUL FOR THOSE ON T3 OR T4/T3

Why is it foolish to rigidly apply the FT3 lab reference range to people on T3-Only, and probably for those on T4/T3 and NDT too?

Almost all doctors think the FT3 reference range should always be abided by, i.e., an FT3 result should always be in range. Most patients agree with this approach too, as it is what they are told.

However, the effect of doing this is that the patient's T3 medication is often not increased to a therapeutic dose, or it may even be reduced, if FT3 is above the top of the range.

There are some extremely good reasons why this is not acceptable. Note: the reasoning I use within this article has been discussed with several thyroid researchers and they agree with me.

Let us start with people on T3-Only, as the argument is more obvious in this case.

The first reason why the FT3 lab range is not sensible to apply in a rigid way, is that T3 doses cause extremely high peak levels of FT3 within a few hours of taking the T3 dose. In Article 7, in this chapter, there is a diagram that shows that shortly after a T3 dose the FT3 can rise to over three times the pre-dose level. Eventually, after many hours, the FT3 levels lower. However, depending on the size of a T3 dose, within 10-15 hours FT3 could still be over the top of the FT3 range, or at the top of the FT3 range or it may have fallen inside the top of the range. This depends on the size of the T3 dose, how well the patient absorbs the T3 and other factors that are patient specific. When should the FT3 be tested then in order to get a useful result? That is hard to say. In any event, the FT3 blood level is not representative of how effective a T3 dose is within the cells and we have no method of assessing this apart from observing signs and symptoms.

The second reason is due to how the FT3 reference range is created. The FT3 lab range is created from the lab test results of healthy people or those on T4 therapy.

However, healthy people, or those on T4 treatment, have T4 to T3 conversion constantly going on inside their cells. All of our cells do some level of conversion of T4 to T3. They make either D1 or D2 deiodinase enzymes in order to do this conversion. The liver and kidneys make D1 (the liver uses D1 to clear a lot of rT3) and the rest of the tissues make D2 (which is actually more efficient at converting T4 to T3). This T4 to T3 conversion occurs inside the cells and not in the bloodstream.

Much of this intracellular converted T3 is never returned to the bloodstream. So, these healthy people, or those on T4, have the measured FT3 in the blood, PLUS some amount of extra FT3 being constantly converted within the cells. The FT3 they have in the blood is moving into the cells on a constant basis, PLUS they have some hidden FT3 from conversion.

So, for healthy people, or those on T4, the FT3 lab range only represents the blood level of FT3 and does NOT include the extra, 'sneakily converted' FT3 that is also present in the person's cells.

Now, on T3-Only therapy thyroid patients often have very low FT4 levels (I have virtually zero). So, we get limited, or no, extra FT3 from conversion that is hidden away inside our cells. Some of the FT3 is moving into our cells all the time. However, we lack the extra converted T3 inside our cells that healthy people, or those on T4 medications have.

So, the FT3 range, that is developed based on healthy people or thyroid patients on T4 treatment, only makes allowance for the blood level of FT3. The intracellular converted FT3 is a bonus. People on T3-Only, or T3-Mostly, have no such bonus FT3. The problem is that doctors do not want our FT3 to go over the top of the FT3 reference range. We are being unfairly held to keeping FT3 in range! The same argument is true of the bottom of the FT3 reference range – it is too low for those on FT3-Only or FT3-Mostly. So, this situation sometimes needs to be compensated with both a higher bottom and top of the FT3 reference range for those on T3-Only or T3-Mostly.

If a patient on T3-Only gets told by a doctor that FT3 cannot go above the top of the FT3 reference range, the patient may never be given enough T3!

My own FT3 is sometimes 2-3 points above the top of the range (depending on when the blood draw is taken relative to the last dose of T3). I am NOT hyperthyroid, or thyrotoxic, in any way, which is what most doctors would interpret from an FT3 above the reference range.

If someone is on T3-Only, and the FT3 reference range is being used to manage the treatment, then the thyroid patient may end up being very under-dosed. The T3 dosage required might be higher than doctors or other thyroid patients might suspect.

Practical experience suggests 40 to 80 mcg per day of T3 is a fairly typical replacement dosage for most people when they use it as a T3-Only therapy. A few people need a little less and a few may need more. I have personally been taking 60 mcg of T3 for well over ten years and I can happily cope with higher levels without any issues.

Consequently, when patients who are on T3 therapy contact me and say they still do not feel well, but their lab test results say their FT3 is at the top of the range, I am not at all surprised that they do not feel great.

T3 therapy needs to use the patient's symptoms, and signs, like body temperature, heart rate and blood pressure in order to find the optimal T3 dosing. Symptoms are especially critical. If a patient has no hyper symptoms at all, has normal body temperature, has not got an elevated heart rate and has good blood pressure, they are extremely unlikely to be hyper – regardless of an FT3 result that may be a little over the top of the reference range.

On T3-Only, multiple sets of these measurements over the day, before and 2-3 hours after each T3 dose, provides good information, that virtually guarantees there is no hyperthyroidism present if the measurements are all normal. To be even more secure a doctor could occasionally run an ECG, and blood calcium, or other actual measures of true body function.

Laboratory tests are of far less value when a thyroid patient is on T3-Only therapy, apart from observing how FT3 changes as doses are altered.

This topic is thoroughly discussed within the Recovering with T3 book.

The above argument applies, but to a lesser extent, to T4/T3 therapies and NDT.

The top of the reference range may be too restrictive for some of these thyroid patients also. This argument becomes more relevant the more T3 is in the T4/T3 combination being used.

I have worked with many thyroid patients who have never recovered until they reached near zero rT3, near-zero FT4 and higher than range FT3.

In summary, the laboratory tests and their reference ranges are of little value on T3-Only therapy. In the early stages of treatment, it is useful to see FT3 rising and FT4 and rT3 getting lower. This confirms that the T3 is being absorbed properly and the body is responding correctly. Beyond that, assessing that TSH is getting lower and FT4 and rT3 are clearing can be very useful.

An FT3 result when on T3-Only therapy, will not tell a doctor or patient whether they are on the correct T3 dosage for them! Moreover, FT3 should not be used to restrict the level of T3 medication for a thyroid patient on T3-Only. These last two points may also apply to those on T4/T3 or NDT.

The above knowledge is in all my books, but I have not seen anyone else write about it… yet.

It is not surprising that the FT3 reference range is unhelpful for those on T3-Only or T4/T3 therapy. The lab reference ranges were never developed with these therapies in mind, or based on collections of data from patients who are successfully treated whilst on these therapies.

9. THYROID LAB RANGES – CAN THEY BE USED FOR ALL THYROID MEDICATIONS?

I have written about this topic in various articles and in my books, especially The Thyroid Patient's Manual. I am going to speak very frankly and from 35 years of experience, research and working with thyroid patients.

Let us start with the 'belief system'.

Doctors and endocrinologists are trained to believe that all people must conform to thyroid lab results that fit with the laboratory reference ranges. The ranges are based on an assessment of mostly healthy people and some thyroid patients. The thyroid patients are invariably those on T4 medication.

The reference ranges are 'normal ranges' and this is a statistical term that can also be written as 'Gaussian ranges.' This means that most people fit somewhere within it. The spread of a population of tested patients will range from only a tiny number at the bottom of the range, with far more around the middle of the range and some at the very top of the range. This is why a 'normal range' is often described as a 'bell shaped curve'. The important thing is the range represents a distribution of people. Therefore, having results somewhere within the reference range for something important like FT3 does NOT mean you are correctly treated. You have to be in the right place within the reference range for you.

Thyroid patients have to be in the right spot in the reference range for them – for both FT3 and FT4.

The belief system that is currently being used by most doctors is that a thyroid test result within the range means the thyroid patient is 'normal' because the range is a 'normal range'. This is wrong and a misunderstanding of what the reference ranges actually are.

In addition to the above, most doctors and endocrinologists do not think that the thyroid patient's Free T3 (FT3) level is crucial. Most of the time, doctors do not even test FT3 – they test TSH, or TSH and FT4. FT4 and TSH can look fine, but the active hormone FT3 can still be far too low. If they test FT3 at all, then having it fall inside the 'normal range' is 'good enough'.

Having an FT3 result which is at a good point for the individual is critical. Why is this? T3 is the active thyroid hormone – see Article 2 in Chapter 7. TSH and FT4 do not mean much in terms of the thyroid patients health but FT3 does. Only T3 is the active hormone in our cells. Only T3 helps to improve symptoms – see Article 5 in Chapter 9.

So, we start with a belief system amongst doctors and endocrinologists that having thyroid test results within the reference ranges means 'normal'. Even low in the range or mid-range FT3 is considered fine. Changing thyroid medication dosages in any way that might make TSH low (suppressed) or not keeping FT4 and FT3 in range, is seen as totally unacceptable. In fact, doctors and endocrinologists often call patients in to see them to adjust their thyroid medication if their lab test results fall outside the ranges.

The belief system extends to completely embracing the lab testing method where the results are looked at and then the thyroid medication is adjusted almost entirely based on manipulating thyroid results somewhere within the reference ranges. It is almost like a game. The focus is rarely on how the patient feels, on their signs and symptoms or on their FT3 result (unless to lower thyroid meds because FT3 has got too high).

Sadly, doctors and endocrinologists during meeting after meeting with the thyroid patient convince him/her of these beliefs. Over time, the thyroid patients come to accept the same belief system. Frequently, at the start of the process, thyroid patients feel that the appointments with their doctor or endocrinologist to review the latest set of lab test results are actually going to help them. Thyroid patients begin to think that they actually need these lab tests and regular reviews to ensure that they are properly treated. It is often only when thyroid patients have been sick for many years that they begin to question all of this. It is a very, very sad state of affairs, and it continues as I write this article. This belief system has infected most of the medical profession and it has also been passed on to many thyroid patients. Hopefully, at some point soon, more thyroid patients will come to realise this.

So, the belief system is flawed. That is the first thing I needed to say.

So, what can we say about TSH, FT4 and FT3 values and their reference ranges during thyroid treatment?

Let me start with TSH. I make it very clear in The Thyroid Patient's Manual that, once someone is on thyroid treatment, the use of laboratory test results is not the same as during diagnosis. We know from research that during thyroid treatment, it is acceptable for TSH to be low or close to zero/suppressed. Most doctors still mistakenly believe that this means the patient is hyperthyroid or thyrotoxic – this is simply not true. If the patient shows no clinical presentation (symptoms or signs) of being hyperthyroid, and as long as FT3 is not over the very top of the reference range, a suppressed TSH is acceptable and not a concern – see Articles 3 and 6 in Chapter 6.

I also make it clear in The Thyroid Patient's Manual that only the FT3 lab test value correlates to patient symptoms, i.e., if the thyroid treatment can be adjusted so that symptoms improve, it is the FT3 that has invariably risen. So, during treatment FT3 ought to rise and as it rises, without high Reverse T3 (rT3), the patient should feel better.

FT4 is not correlated to symptoms at all – so tracking FT4 with the view that if it goes up the person must feel better, is a flawed concept. It should not be assumed that increases in FT4 mean the treatment is working. FT3 is the only thyroid lab correlated to symptoms and as such, is the important value to track.

The thyroid labs are useful to track but the patient's response in terms of symptoms and signs should be the most important thing a doctor tracks. The clinical presentation of the patient is more important than thyroid labs. Thyroid lab test results are useful to look at during treatment but they should not be the main guide during it.

Those on T4 treatment that are responding well to T4, can, of course, use the current lab tests and lab ranges, with the caveats explained above in the 'belief system' section.

However, once T3 is added, things change. T3 is added to T4 treatment in some cases, because T4 medication does not always resolve symptoms.

As the T3 aspect of the combination is increased, the T4 content often has to be reduced in order to avoid excess rT3 and to actually increase FT3.

As this happens, TSH can become low or suppressed and FT4 can fall close to the lower end of the reference range (or even below it). As more T3 is added to thyroid medication, FT3 is so influenced by the time the last T3 medication was taken that it becomes a far less useful measure (other than to know that the T3 medication raised FT3). In order to be able to compare FT3 test results, thyroid patients ought to always leave the same length of time between the last T3 dose and the blood draw.

However, be aware that any lab tests done within 12 hours of the last T3 dose can risk a high FT3 result. This is why I often recommend an 18-24-hour gap between the last T3 dose and the blood draw to avoid a doctor decreasing the needed T3 medication due to a short-term raised FT3. It is also best to do a private blood test first to be certain that your guessed interval with no thyroid meds prior to the blood draw is actually enough to keep your doctor happy with the TSH and FT3. Until the medical community have a better understanding of how T3 (even in T4/T3 or NDT therapy) can change the situation with the lab test results, this is the type of thing that patients need to do to get well and stay well. Ideally, the FT3 reference range would be different for those on T3 treatment – see Articles 7 and 8 in this chapter.

It is possible as the patient is given more T3, and potentially less T4, that both FT3 and FT4 do not conform to the reference ranges any more, i.e., they may both fall outside of them. TSH might also be very low. The lab tests themselves and any attempt to adjust thyroid medication to ensure that the results fit into the reference ranges can, at this point, result in extremely poor choices being made. As more T3 and less T4 is used, there comes a point where the value of even doing the laboratory testing of thyroid levels becomes questionable.

I will not discuss T3-Mostly or T3-Only therapy here as this can be even more extreme.

So, can thyroid lab test results and ranges be applied with all treatments?

My answer to this is, "No!" The laboratory reference ranges have to be used as a guideline. Lab test results that fall within these ranges do not mean a thyroid patient is correctly treated. Lab test results that fall completely outside the lab test ranges do not mean the thyroid patient is incorrectly treated. Signs and symptoms need to guide the treatment.

Thyroid patients need to put less trust in these highly trusted lab test results and references ranges. The medical profession – endocrinologists and doctors – need a massive upgrade in their knowledge, understanding and treatment practices. Many of them feel handcuffed by guidelines and would do things differently if they could. This really has to change if thyroid patients are going to get better treatment.

All the thyroid hormones have to be available for clinicians to use in the treatment of their patients. And it is important not to worship the lab results in the same way once T3 is added to treatment. Seeing changes occur in labs is a good thing – it means the way that the levels are changing is working. But trying to force fit people on T4/T3 or T3-Only into the same lab result straight-jacket using the same reference ranges is not going to work.

Doctors who always insist on keeping all thyroid lab test results within the reference ranges will actually ensure that some patients remain sick.

Some thyroid patients can only get well through not conforming to the rigid ranges that are designed for healthy people or those on T4 medication. This is the bottom line.

Much is not right in current thyroid treatment practice. I hope this provides more insight to those of you who are trying to make sense of lab tests and ranges.

10. USING PERCENTILES IN ASSESSING THYROID TREATMENT EFFECTIVENESS

This is a very simple article about thyroid blood test results that I was prompted to write as a couple of thyroid patients seemed to find this information helpful. It is basic maths and I have always found it quite useful.

What is the Percentile of the Range for any result?

The percentile of a range is how large the result is when expressed as a percentage of the entire width of the reference range. As an example, for a reference range of 1 to 4, a result of '4' is 100th percentile (100%), a result of '1' would be 0 percentile (0%) and a result of '2.5' would be 50th percentile (50%).

How Can Percentiles be Useful for Thyroid Patients?

When patients get thyroid blood test results like Free T4 (FT4) and Free T3 (FT3), it can be very obvious that they are low in one of the results, or high in some cases. However, over time the results might seem to change but it can be very hard to spot whether the changes are significant or not. Using percentiles can clarify where the test result is in the reference range. It is also significantly easier to see if the thyroid hormone has actually improved or deteriorated over time.

Note: Free T3 is the bio-available measure of T3, the active thyroid hormone. FT3 is the T3 in the bloodstream which is not bound to protein (thyroid binding globulin). Total T3 can be measured also, but this includes the bound T3 and as such, it is not very useful.

Sometimes, a thyroid patient needs to change the laboratory that is being used to do the test. This almost always means that the reference range will be slightly different. It can then be very hard to see if the test result is better, worse or the same as with the previous laboratory. Using percentiles makes the comparison a lot easier, although different laboratories have different assays (the actual testing method in the lab.) and this can also change the result.

Very often a doctor or endocrinologist will look at the laboratory test results and tell the thyroid patient that all is well, using the famous phrase, "Your results are in range", or even more annoyingly, "Your results are normal", even though you feel like death! Using percentiles can quickly show very low results, especially for the active hormone FT3.

So, using percentiles can be very helpful.

How is a Percentile Calculated?

Let us use some actual thyroid test results to make this more realistic. Here are some results from an actual thyroid patient, who converts quite well and is on a combination of T4 and T3:
TSH 0.001 mIU/L
FT4 18.20 (9.01-19.05) pmol/L
FT3 5.40 (2.62-5.70) pmol/ L

I do not use percentiles for TSH. I do not worry about low TSH. I only pay attention to TSH when it is high or it is changing during treatment.

I always use percentiles for FT3, as it is the active hormone.
I use it for FT4 and for Reverse T3 (rT3) if it is available.

Here is how the percentile for FT3 is calculated:
The bottom of the FT3 reference range is 2.62, and the top of the FT3 reference range is 5.70 in this case. The length of the reference range is known as the Reference Interval and this is $5.70 - 2.62 = 3.08$ for FT3.

We also need the amount above the bottom of the range that the actual FT3 result is $5.40 - 2.62 = 2.78$.

So, all we do now is divide the amount of FT3 above the bottom of the range by the FT3 reference interval x 100%.

FT3 percentile of the range = $(2.78 / 3.08)$ x 100% = 90.25%.

Clearly, this very simple formula also lends itself to being put into a spreadsheet for those thyroid patients that are tracking their thyroid labs over time with medication changes.

Here is the same process for calculating the FT4 percentile:
For the above results, the FT4 reference interval is $19.05-9.01 = 10.04$.
The amount above the bottom of the range of the FT4 result was: $18.20 - 9.01 = 9.19$.
So, the FT4 percentile is $(9.19 / 10.04)$ x 100% = 91.5 %.

Clearly, if there were an rT3 result, then the rT3 percentile could be calculated in the same way. For completeness, you can be below the range for a thyroid test result, i.e., a negative percentile, and it is also possible to be above the range and have a percentile which is > 100%.

For those of you who are more visual, here is a simple graphic that explains it:

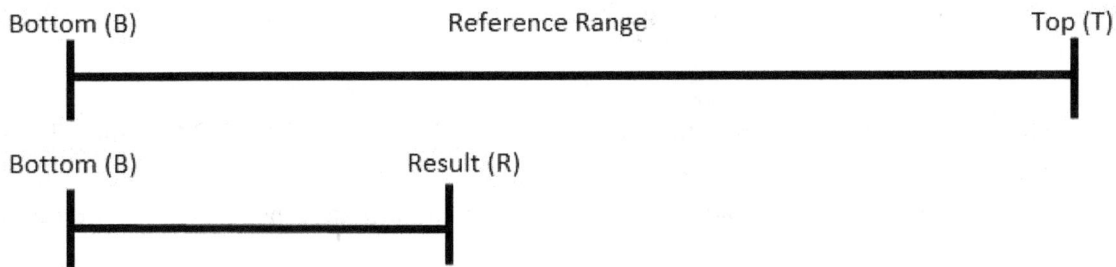

Bottom (B)   Reference Range   Top (T)

Bottom (B)   Result (R)

$$\text{Percentile Formula} = \frac{R - B}{T - B} \times 100\%$$

How can Percentiles be used?

I have already mentioned that it is far easier to see if the thyroid lab results have changed by using percentiles.

However, it is critical to be aware that only changes in FT3 affect symptoms in a meaningful way. If FT3 stays the same but FT4 goes up, it is unlikely that you will experience improvement. FT4 is not a proper thyroid hormone and it does not connect to the thyroid receptors within our cells. Only FT3 is the active hormone and tracks symptoms. See Article 5 on this in Chapter 9.

The other thing to be aware of is that having results that fall within the reference range is not sufficient to feel well. Every thyroid patient needs to have results that fall in the right part of the reference range for them, individually, in order to feel well. See Article 6 in Chapter 9.

So, tracking FT3, FT4 and rT3 results and their percentiles can be very helpful.

I prefer NOT to generalise, as thyroid patients are individuals and therefore have different needs. But in general, thyroid patients do better with an FT3 result that is in the upper half of the FT3 reference range or even the upper quartile. So, in general, they do better with FT3 > 50% of the range and often >75% of the range or even nearer the top of the range. Frequently, this also has to be matched by an rT3 percentile that is NOT high.

11. BASELINE THYROID TESTING FOR YOUNG PEOPLE

I think all young people who have one or more parents who have thyroid disease should have baseline thyroid hormone testing when they are 18 years of age (and possibly even younger).

The baseline tests I am thinking of are TSH, FT4, FT3, TPOAb and TGAb autoantibodies and rT3 (if you can get it tested).

Thyroid disease and thyroid hormone issues often have a genetic aspect and run in families.

Often the genetic connections that are present mean the condition develops in an adult in their late twenties or thirties.

Knowing the values of thyroid hormones for young, healthy adults would really save a huge amount of time, effort, stress and cost later on if the individual developed a thyroid issue.

Lab test population ranges are too wide to assume that any result within them is normal. I know this is what doctors think. However, research has shown that simply having thyroid lab results somewhere within the laboratory reference range does not guarantee that the person is healthy and has no hypothyroid symptoms. We know that 'individual person ranges' are narrower than the large population ranges.

I am proposing the routine testing of young adults with a full thyroid panel (including FT3) if either parent or grandparent has any history of thyroid problems. With the state of our current medical systems, this is unlikely to happen of course. However, my suggestion is that parents who know there are thyroid issues in the family should organise private, full thyroid panels for their children once they are 18 years of age.

I asked some thyroid patients what they thought about this. This is what I heard back:

"Yes, I am planning on having all of my children having a baseline done. My baselines have proved invaluable now. I can look back and see how my thyroid functioned on its own over 20 years ago, before Hashimoto's set in."

"I wish I'd had mine all the years that I fought with the doctors about my poor response on T4. It may have saved me years of poor treatment."

"Oh, and I found out that around 15 years ago they did some thyroid tests but the hospital letter just says normal with no numbers. Not one of the doctors I have seen have even referred to it and I only found it by accident when reviewing my notes."

"I'm assuming that if you had a baseline when in good health, the differences would at least be obvious and it would make the argument for more or different treatment easier."

"Yes, I think it's great!"

"Unfortunately, this makes way too much logical sense for the medical community to adopt into practice. So, therefore, it will never happen…lol."

"Definitely! all 3 of my children are showing signs of being hypo. I've made sure they've had tests since being around 13 xxx"

"Oh dear! I have had my two daughters tested. Neither has hypothyroidism but my eldest has put on weight inexplicably and is always tired, always has something wrong, has a very short fuse. I wonder sometimes…"

"I hadn't thought of this but it sounds like fine advice. Thanks!"

"I think that sounds like a great idea."

"My daughter was diagnosed with Hashimoto's aged 17 – I just knew she had it but they wouldn't believe me – they did a thyroid function test and tested antibodies when she was younger, which showed her TPO as 30 and I knew they would rise. They were 400 on the last count! My youngest, aged 13, also had a test at my insistence. Her TPO is 28 – let us just wait and see – I can tell by personality alone!"

"My daughter is moving to Chicago and I plan on getting her started with a doctor there. It is obvious that it can happen in younger children as well. I feel good that I have resources to go to for information. When I first was diagnosed, I felt so alone. It can be very difficult."

"It seems like a lot of people develop thyroid disease at an earlier age than 18, so wouldn't it make sense to start the testing process sooner? Would it be reasonable to start getting tests at an earlier age to establish a baseline?"

"Definitely at 18 would've worked for me. However, my kids around age 8 -10 were bad, 14-16 were bad and still continue at 20, 21. Still working on getting myself sorted and with knowledge comes the awful truth about what has ailed my kids most of their life with different illnesses/symptoms and poor treatment for conditions that "don't exist" or are "normal"."

Clearly, my question struck a chord with them. I think doing this type of baseline testing would be very helpful.

Chapter 6

Suppressed TSH & Dogmatic Views

1. THYROID PAPER ON THE NEED FOR INDIVIDUALISED TREATMENT

There is a need for far more individualised treatment of hypothyroidism. There is no 'one size fits all' in either treatment or necessary lab values, and patient symptoms need to be kept clearly in focus.

The paper highlights that:

- The TSH measure alone is really not sensitive enough to tell a doctor when a patient is properly treated.
- Each patient has to be in the right range for them for TSH, FT4, FT3 and rT3.
- Being somewhere in the lab range for FT4 and FT3 does not mean the patient is correctly treated.
- T4 leaves many patients unwell and with remaining symptoms.
- T3 often needs to be included in the treatment, as many conditions and thyroid tissue loss leaves patients low in the conversion of T4 to T3.
- Many issues get in the way of conversion including loss of thyroid tissue, deiodinase defects, etc.
- Patient symptoms need to be at the forefront of treatment – not placed after lab results which only include TSH and FT4.
- There need to be other biochemical markers of being adequately treated – TSH, FT4, and FT3 are not enough.

Here is the link to the paper by Hoermann, Midgley, Larisch and Dietrich: "Individualised requirements for optimum treatment of hypothyroidism: complex needs, limited options". Hoermann, Midgley, Larisch and Dietrich. Drugs in Context DOI 10.7573/dic.212597
https://www.drugsincontext.com/individualised-requirements-for-optimum-treatment-of-hypothyroidism:-complex-needs,-limited-options/
(You can download the full paper from the link within the abstract)

Note: I have grouped these articles on low and suppressed TSH together, as I realise that many patients have doctors and endocrinologists who refuse to have below reference range TSH. Even if the patient remains with severe hypothyroid symptoms that go away with more thyroid medication, many doctors will not allow TSH to go below the bottom of the reference range. They assert that low TSH will result in bone loss or heart issues and is unacceptable.

There is research that disagrees with these views on TSH – some of this is presented in this chapter. Moreover, some doctors ignore the fact that remaining severely hypothyroid is linked to cardiovascular issues, diabetes, depression and a host of other undesirable health issues.

Having said all this, no matter what research links or arguments are presented to some doctors and endocrinologists, there is often no shaking their opinion, so strong is the dogma that has developed during their training. All I can do in this book, is to present the alternative case.

Many thyroid patients now refuse to have their health ruined by a doctor or endocrinologist who is content to leave the patient with severe hypothyroid symptoms. I know I would not hand my hormone health over to a doctor ever again – I lost far too much by doing that for too long the first time.

For those patients that know they have a doctor, or endocrinologist, who is fiercely dogmatic about not allowing low TSH, there is one approach that can work. If the patient is certain that they are not hyperthyroid at all in terms of signs and symptoms, and they feel far healthier on the current dosage of thyroid medication, then private lab testing can help. By stopping thyroid medication, especially T3, for 18-24 hours prior to the private laboratory test of TSH and FT3, the patient can get the results and determine whether this time gap with no T3 medication is going to be sufficient to get TSH and FT3 in range. If it is still a problem, then it can be repeated with a longer gap. We should not have to do this. However, it is better than having the thyroid medication withdrawn or reduced.

2. TSH USE SHOULD BE SCALED BACK TO A SUPPORTING ROLE

The way TSH is currently used by endocrinologists and doctors treating thyroid patients is wrong.

The way people are treated, as if they are all the same, is wrong. Simply being 'in range' on levothyroxine monotherapy is not going to guarantee a good outcome. We are not all robotic machines that have come off a production line. Treating us as if we are, is not working well for some patients.

I include two research papers in this article.

The first piece of research is undoubtedly one of the most important studies done in the last ten years.

It finally begins to be clearer that TSH is one of the least useful tools in assessing thyroid hormone levels and whether someone is actually getting enough T3 in the cells:

"Homeostatic Control of the Thyroid-Pituitary Axis: Perspectives for Diagnosis and Treatment." Hoermann, Midgley, Larisch, Dietrich. Front Endocrinol 2015 Nov 20;6:177. doi: 10.3389/fendo.2015.00177.
Abstract: https://www.ncbi.nlm.nih.gov/pubmed/26635726
Full Article: https://www.frontiersin.org/articles/10.3389/fendo.2015.00177/full

This second research paper concludes that getting TSH into the reference range is no guarantee of good health. It shows how simplistically and poorly TSH is being used today. TSH is not something that should be relied upon in the way it is being done at the present time:

"TSH Measurement and Its Implications for Personalised Clinical Decision-Making" Rudolf Hoermann and John E. M. Midgley. Volume 2012 Article ID 438037 https://doi.org/10.1155/2012/438037
https://www.hindawi.com/journals/jtr/2012/438037/

3. SUPPRESSED TSH ON THYROID TREATMENT DOES NOT MEAN HYPERTHYROID

There is a new research paper out which again shows that the current use of TSH when thyroid patients are on thyroid hormones is flawed.

The paper shows that patients who have had a total thyroidectomy are very likely to require a suppressed TSH in order to be able to give them enough T4 hormone replacement to correct their symptoms. In these athyreotic (no thyroid) cases, it is clear from the study that a suppressed TSH does not mean the patients are hyperthyroid. In fact, it is often necessary to have a suppressed TSH in order to provide enough T4 medication to get a sufficiently high FT3 level that the patient feels well.

It is also clear from the research that athyreotics (people without a thyroid, also referred to as 'thyroidless'), are just one end of the spectrum to those with reduced thyroid hormone production. It IS a spectrum and it should be clear that simply having a very low or suppressed TSH cannot mean automatically that a thyroid patient receiving thyroid treatment is hyperthyroid.

One of the big takeaways from this is that endocrinologists and doctors should stop assuming that, every time a thyroid patient has very low or near zero (suppressed) TSH on thyroid treatment , this means the person is hyperthyroid, or that they will develop heart issues or bone-loss. It simply is not true.

If someone is NOT on thyroid treatment but has a suppressed TSH then this situation is utterly different to when a patient is under treatment.

It is usually not a problem at all for a thyroid patient who is receiving thyroid hormone treatment to have a suppressed TSH, as long as they do not have actual hyperthyroid symptoms (or elevated FT3).

The practice of automatically reducing thyroid medication due to suppressed TSH is quite wrong. That is just a numbers game and makes no allowance for either the research or the clinical presentation of the patient.

This practice of never allowing a suppressed TSH when on thyroid medication is making the flawed assumption that you can treat thyroid patients receiving thyroid medication as if they are on no medication at all and hyperthyroid. It is quite wrong.

For those on thyroid treatment, the clinical presentation must be paramount and the use of simplistic thyroid labs must come secondary.

Here are the details on the paper:

"Heterogenous Biochemical Expression of Hormone Activity in Subclinical/Overt Hyperthyroidism and Exogenous Thyrotoxicosis". Rudolf Hoermann, John E.M. Midgley, Rolf Larisch, Johannes W. Dietrich PII: S2214-6237(19)30152-8

DOI: https://doi.org/10.1016/j.jcte.2020.100219

Reference: JCTE 100219

https://www.sciencedirect.com/science/article/pii/S2214623719301528

Many thanks to Dr John Midgley for letting me know about the paper.

Note: for those on treatment containing T3 (T3/T4 or NDT or T3-Only), TSH can easily be suppressed to near zero even though FT3 and FT4 can be in range. This is one of the flaws of the TSH test.

Even Dr Robert Utiger who created the TSH test in the first place acknowledged the highly suppressive effect of T3 containing medication.

So, attempting to use TSH for those on T3 therapy in the same way as it is used for those on T4 medication is flawed.

4. ONE REASON WHY TSH CAN BE SUPPRESSED WHEN TAKING SOME T3

This article explains one reason why TSH can often be very low or suppressed when taking reasonably high doses of T3 thyroid hormone.

I have explained many times that TSH being low on thyroid treatment is not necessarily a problem if the person does not have extremely high levels of FT3 and has no hyperthyroid symptoms or signs. Being on thyroid treatment is an entirely different situation from not being on any thyroid treatment. There is already plenty of research available that shows that suppressed TSH on thyroid treatment does not have to be an issue. See my other articles in this chapter.

However, this article explains why using T3 can raise levels of the thyroid hormone metabolite Triac for a short while. Triac is known to powerfully suppress TSH. So, it should be no surprise to see that people on NDT or on reasonable levels of T3, have low or suppressed TSH.

Here is the article:

https://thyroidpatients.ca/2020/01/02/when-dosing-t3-you-get-higher-levels-of-triac/

Here is another research article that talks about T3 suppressing TSH more powerfully than T4. The essence of this article is that when T4 enters the circulation it gets converted to T3 through the process of deiodination. T4 and T3 can then exert negative feedback on TSH levels (high levels of T3/T4 decrease TSH release from the anterior pituitary, while low levels of T3/T4 increase TSH release). T3 is the predominant inhibitor of TSH secretion.

Here is the article:

https://www.ncbi.nlm.nih.gov/books/NBK499850/

Note: Here is more support for not caring about suppressed TSH, when the thyroid patient is not showing any signs or symptoms of hyperthyroidism and FT3 is not high. It is a quote by Dr G Foresman, MD in the USA:

"Studies from decades and decades ago indicated that a suppressed TSH might be an issue. What they used to do more than twenty-five years ago was to give high doses of Synthroid (T4) to patients with the intention of suppressing their TSHs in order to shrink thyroid gland nodules. A very bad, outdated protocol that doctors no longer practice. At the time, they used such high doses of T4 that they were making some people chronically hyperthyroid and of course, they were seeing bone loss, arrhythmias, etc. The medical community stopped implementing that practice because of those outcomes. But unfortunately, as a result of that antiquated practice, there are still doctors who think that a suppressed TSH is dangerous to the patient.

All of the studies in the last few decades indicate that TSH suppression has no association with some of those feared results, like osteoporosis. Interestingly enough, my patients with the lowest TSH values have the best bone density scores. I have had patients move to another state, and their new doctor refuses to prescribe desiccated or compounded. And as soon as the doctor sees a suppressed TSH, the doctor freaks out and lowers the patient's thyroid medication.

It's an antiquated belief system based upon the decades-old history of using suppressive thyroid hormone to shrink thyroid nodules. As a result, doctors are still afraid of suppressing TSH, even though the literature has shown for decades now that you can suppress TSH with no metabolic consequences whatsoever. A suppressed TSH does not lead to heart failure, it does not lead to arrhythmia, and it does not cause osteoporosis."

5. LOW TSH DOES NOT CAUSE BONE LOSS IN THYROID TREATMENT

Many guidelines strongly caution against the risk associated with low TSH.

Some doctors and thyroid patients have jumped to the conclusion that a low TSH 'causes' osteoporosis.

Some even believe a low TSH must be avoided at all costs during thyroid therapy, even if lowering their thyroid hormone dose causes chronic hypothyroid symptoms in a patient (which in turn may cause osteopenia and then osteoporosis).

But, as of 2019, the truth is that real science still indicates that suppressed TSH is not responsible for bone loss.

In 2007, Bassett et al stated, "Thyroid hormone excess rather than thyrotropin (TSH) deficiency induces osteoporosis in hyperthyroidism". Note: this means too much thyroid hormone for the patient is a risk for osteoporosis, but this means they would usually have hyperthyroid symptoms. Low TSH itself is not an issue.

Here is the 2007 study:

"Thyroid hormone excess rather than thyrotropin deficiency induces osteoporosis in hyperthyroidism". Bassett, J. H. D., O'Shea, P. J., Sriskantharajah, S., Rabier, B., Boyde, A., Howell, P. G. T., … Williams, G. R. (2007). Endocrinology (Baltimore, Md.), 21(5), 1095–1107. https://academic.oup.com/mend/article/21/5/1095/2738372

In 2018 Van Vilet et al stated, "We found no evidence for a causal effect of circulating TSH on BMD (Bone Mineral Density)".

Here is the 2018 study:

"Thyroid Stimulating Hormone and Bone Mineral Density: Evidence from a Two-Sample Mendelian Randomization Study and a Candidate Gene Association Study". Van Vliet NA, Noordam R, van Klinken JB, et al. J Bone Miner Res Off J Am Soc Bone Miner Res. March 2018.

https://www.ncbi.nlm.nih.gov/pubmed/29544020 and full article:

https://onlinelibrary.wiley.com/doi/full/10.1002/jbmr.3426

A full discussion of this topic has been written by thyroid patient advocate Dr Tania S. Smith: https://thyroidpatients.ca/2019/07/12/as-of-2019-still-no-proof-that-low-tsh-causes-harm-to-bones/

Apart from hyperthyroidism, one of the reasons that some doctors have jumped to the conclusion that there is a link between low TSH and bone turn-over is because bone cells express a functional TSH receptor on their surface. So, the TSH can connect to this receptor.

However, any potential TSH effect is interwoven with other signals such as by thyroid hormones and estrogens. There is redundancy in the system. This means that what happens is highly dependent on the specific condition and combinations, not a sole influence. It is also very difficult to isolate the TSH effect, because it is not the same in everybody.

Furthermore, it is extremely difficult to create a proper controlled experiment when thyroid hormones and estrogens are all perfect, yet TSH is low. There has to be an individualised approach, as outlined in the following review: Hoermann R, Midgley JEM, Larisch R, Dietrich JW. Individualised requirements for optimum treatment of hypothyroidism: Complex needs, limited options. Drugs Context. 2019;8:212597. doi:10.7573/dic.212597.
See: https://pmc.ncbi.nlm.nih.gov/articles/PMC6726361/

The biggest causes of bone loss, potentially leading to osteoporosis in women are:

1) Low oestrogen.

and

2) Low thyroid hormones, especially low FT3.

So, testing oestrogen, progesterone, TSH, FT4, FT3 and ideally rT3 is important so that any potential cause of bone loss can be identified and corrected. Testing vitamin D levels is also important, as low vitamin D results in poor calcium absorption. My book, The Thyroid Patient's Manual, shows you how to interpret the vitamin D result and what supplements to use to correct low vitamin D.

Addressing low oestrogen is essential, whilst balancing with progesterone. Remaining clinically hypothyroid is in itself a big risk of bone loss, which may develop into detectable osteopenia and ultimately osteoporosis. Going simply on TSH and FT4 is a big mistake.

Having low FT3 and clinical signs/symptoms of being hypothyroid are what should tell the person and their doctor that this needs to be treated. Hypothyroidism requires treating with the right level and combination of thyroid hormones for the individual (not just being put on levothyroxine and monitoring TSH level). Remaining with hypothyroid symptoms is a big risk for osteoporosis.

The level of TSH is not linked to osteoporosis when a thyroid patient is receiving thyroid medication that is properly managed for them, i.e., with the right level of FT3 thyroid hormone.

Treating any low oestrogen issue and any clinical hypothyroidism issue can halt and sometimes reverse bone loss in women.

I actually know of thyroid patients who have built bone when their T3 doses have become optimal for them, even when they had low TSH.

6. IS IT SAFE FOR TSH TO BE LOW OR SUPPRESSED ON THYROID TREATMENT?

I often get asked the question of whether it is safe to have low (or suppressed TSH) when on T4/T3 treatment (or any thyroid treatment).

Recent research is quite clear. A suppressed TSH when on thyroid treatment is usually NOT a concern, as long as:

- The person has no hyperthyroid symptoms and
- FT3 is not above the range (but this last point also has caveats).

The above statement is true on T4 and I will provide the research references below to back this up.

What about T4/T3 or T3-Only therapy?

Firstly, it is important to know that for those on treatment containing T3 (T3/T4 or NDT or T3-Only) TSH can easily be suppressed to near zero even though FT3 and FT4 can be in range. This is one of the flaws of the TSH test. Even Dr Robert Utiger who created the TSH test in the first place acknowledged the highly suppressive effect of T3 containing medication on TSH. So, attempting to use TSH for those on T3 therapy in the same way as it is used for those on T4 medication is extremely unlikely to be helpful.

Secondly, sometimes people need a high level of T3 in their medication in order to get well. In fact, on any T4/T3 based treatment, I believe FT3 can creep up to and even over the range. There is a very clever, but complicated explanation for this. It goes like this:

People who are healthy, or on T4 medication, have on-going T4-to-T3 conversion happening within their cells. Much of this intra-cellular-T3 that is converted from T4 remains in the cells and is used there. Little gets returned to the bloodstream. This is an IMPORTANT point. The FT3 population reference range is created by measuring blood levels of FT3.

So, for people who are healthy, or on T4-therapy, they have the FT3 that can be measured. However, they also have the EXTRA FT3 that is being constantly converted from T4 within their cells.

So, the FT3 reference range does not account for the extra intra-cellular FT3.

As soon as someone uses T4/T3 treatment or NDT, they have extra T3, but usually less T4 than they previously had. So, the FT3 measured in blood is almost certainly going to be higher for someone on T4/T3 therapy than someone on T4 treatment. There will also be less intra-cellular T3 being converted from T4. The net result is that T4/T3 therapy patients are much more likely to have/need a higher blood FT3 – possibly close to the top of the FT3 reference range.

The thyroid lab ranges have not been developed based on a population of thyroid patients who are on some T3 – so this should not be a surprise.

The situation gets a whole lot worse for people on T3-Only. They have NO intracellular T4-to-T3 conversion at all. Their FT3 level is often pushing the top of the FT3 reference range. This is necessary in order to compensate for the lack of intracellular T4-to-T3 conversion.

Our UK reference range for FT3 is typically 3.3-6.6. My FT3, when tested, is often at or just above the top of the FT3 reference range. I have near-zero FT4 and near-zero TSH. I am NOT hyperthyroid. This makes lots of sense when you understand the real endocrinology.

This is a great paper that describes how, even on Levothyroxine only (T4-Only) therapy, TSH can be low for some patients:

> "Problems with the assessment of thyroid function and levothyroxine replacement levels in pituitary disease" The Pituitary Foundation.
> https://www.pituitary.org.uk/problems-with-the-assessment-of-thyroid-function-and-levothyroxine-replacement-levels-in-pituitary-disease/

In addition to all the above, some thyroid patients have central hypothyroidism. This means that, either due to a maladjustment of the pituitary or of the hypothalamus, they tend to always have low TSH – even if their FT4 and FT3 are low. In these cases, it would be positively dangerous to attempt to use TSH to manage medication levels. The patient's signs and symptoms must be the primary focus, as well as FT3 and FT4 levels.

I said at the start that I often get asked questions about whether a low TSH is acceptable. This is a typical question from a patient, followed by my answer:

Patient:

"I have sub-clinical hypothyroidism. I take Levothyroxine & Liothyronine. All my doctors get freaked out at my very low TSH numbers and want to lower my Levothyroxine dose. I'm a bit sceptical".

My response:

"If FT3 is not high, and you have hypothyroid symptoms remaining, you are not hyperthyroid. If FT3 is low and you still have hypo symptoms then you cannot be hyperthyroid – regardless of TSH.

What about people with central hypothyroidism that have a pituitary gland that never has anything but low TSH? Do those people have hyperthyroidism even though their FT3 is low? No, of course they do not.

Doctors always work on the assumption that the pituitary is perfectly accurate. The scientific reality is completely different.

The pituitary gland is a very small spherical gland that has only the view of the FT4 and FT3 that flows into it in the bloodstream. It is also one of the best converters of FT4 to FT3 in the body, as it makes both the D1 and D2 deiodinase enzymes. The pituitary has the highest concentration of FT3 out of all the glands and tissues in the body. So, the pituitary's only view on your thyroid status is what it sees inside its own little sphere, and it has no idea whether the rest of your body is hypo or hyper. The pituitary gland cannot see inside your brain, your liver, your digestive system, your cold feet and hands etc.

In addition to the above, every other gland, organ, body tissue we have can have malfunctions. We might need to wear glasses, or hearing aids. We have digestive system disorders, liver issues, thyroid gland issues, diabetes, joint problems… you get the picture. Why do doctors think the pituitary gland, with its already extremely limited perspective, can always be absolutely spot on correct? Nonsense! It is not always correct.

Plus, when people take thyroid medication, and especially T3, this changes the normal balance of free hormone levels in order to compensate for any lost conversion ability of T4 to T3. This also confuses the normal algorithm that the pituitary uses to assess the hormones and produce a TSH level. The more T3 we take, the more likely TSH will be suppressed. It just is not designed to work like this. The level of TSH produced, even by a non-malfunctioning pituitary gland is designed for those with healthy thyroid glands, and normal-for-them thyroid hormone levels. TSH needs to be ignored to a certain extent when someone is on thyroid meds. This is especially true if the person is still hypothyroid and has low or sub-optimal FT3, or they are on a fair amount of Liothyronine (T3). Even on T4-based meds, with poor conversion, often the T4 dosage has to be raised very high, in order to create enough FT3 to stop the patient being hypothyroid. TSH is often suppressed in these cases too.

You are right to be sceptical – TSH can be very low and you may still be either on the right medication level, or even under-medicated.

Here is one final point on this subject, before I list some relevant research papers:

Patients occasionally ask me for peer-reviewed research papers that show why a low TSH is safe. It might seem a reasonable question on the surface but when you think more deeply about it several aspects are problematic:

1) Peer review is no longer a guarantee of the quality of the research and the experimental quality.

2) Most research on suppressed TSH requires high levels of thyroid hormones to do the suppression. The contention by many researchers, and myself, is that it is excess thyroid hormone that causes issues like atrial fibrillation (AFib) and bone loss, not low TSH. So, any experiments done like this must be immediately discounted.

3) There is already research that shows that low TSH itself is usually not an issue.

4) The only proper experiment with humans to see if low TSH causes issues in a population would be to engineer low TSH in a set of subjects that have normal-for-them thyroid hormone levels. So, this would involve having two sets of subjects:

a) a set of control subjects with in-range TSH and normal-for-them thyroid hormones, and

b) a set of subjects with TSH levels engineered to be suppressed to zero, whilst their thyroid hormone levels are artificially maintained at the normal-for them-levels. Now, whilst some medications are known to lower TSH, e.g., steroids, they are unlikely to suppress TSH, plus they have effects on the heart and bones independently. So, the only way I can think of to do this would be to surgically change the pituitary gland to have no TSH generating capability, without affecting other hormones. The experiment would have to only have low TSH, with all other hormones and body chemistry unaltered. This is both unethical and near impossible to do.

Apart from hyperthyroidism, one of the reasons that some doctors have jumped to the conclusion that there is a link between low TSH and bone turn-over is that bone cells express a functional TSH receptor on their surface. So, the TSH can connect to this receptor. However, any potential TSH effect is interwoven with other signals such as by thyroid hormones and estrogens. There is redundancy in the system. This means what happens is highly dependent on the specific condition and combinations, not a sole influence. It is also very difficult to isolate the TSH effect, because it is not the same for everybody. Furthermore, as explained above, it is near impossible to create a proper experiment when thyroid hormones and estrogens are all perfect yet TSH is low. There has to be an individualised approach, as outlined in the following review (also listed in the research references – 7). This was peer reviewed btw.: Hoermann R, Midgley JEM, Larisch R, Dietrich JW. Individualised requirements for optimum treatment of hypothyroidism: Complex needs, limited options. Drugs Context. 2019;8:212597. doi:10.7573/dic.212597

Many of the other so-called 'research papers' on TSH and issues, seem to have just focused on TSH and not accounted for the reason the TSH is suppressed, which is hyperthyroidism. For the patient with low TSH, the doctors are often not accounting for whether the thyroid patient is well treated for hypothyroidism in terms of the right balance of T4 and T3 medication for them. They also often ignore the status of the patient's estrogen levels.

I come back to the point that when a patient is still hypothyroid, or is only on enough thyroid medication to resolve symptoms, and FT3 is not high, then TSH is not something to be concerned over, if the patient is well and other hormone levels are good. e.g., estrogen."

Here are some further research papers on this subject:

1. "Symptomatic Relief is Related to Serum Free Triiodothyronine Concentrations during Follow-up in Levothyroxine-Treated Patients with Differentiated Thyroid Cancer" Larisch, Midgley, Dietrich, and Hoermann. https://www.researchgate.net/publication/322914153_Symptomatic_Relief_is_Related_to_Serum_Free_Triiodothyronine_Concentrations_during_Follow-up_in_Levothyroxine-Treated_Patients_with_Differentiated_Thyroid_Cancer

This paper clearly proves that FT3 concentrations are the most important in clinical decision making, as they are most closely linked to residual hypothyroid symptoms in T4-Only treated patients. It also shows that in-range TSH is not sufficient for symptom relief.

2. "Homeostatic equilibria between free thyroid hormones and pituitary thyrotropin are modulated by various influences including age, body mass index and treatment" Hoermann R1, Midgley JE, Giacobino A, Eckl WA, Wahl HG, Dietrich JW, Larisch R. See: Clin Endocrinol (Oxf) (2014) 81:907–915. doi:10.1111/cen.12527 URL: https://www.researchgate.net/publication/263321383_Homeostatic_Equilibria_Between_Free_Thyroid_Hormones_and_Pituitary_Thyrotropin_Are_Modulated_By_Various_Influences_Including_Age_Body_Mass_Index_and_Treatment

This is a great paper, although complex. It shows that it is the relationships of the thyroid hormones, and how they adjust during treatment, that counts. It also makes it crystal clear that TSH should only have a supporting role in the assessment process during treatment.

3. "Recent Advances in Thyroid Hormone Regulation: Toward a New Paradigm for Optimal Diagnosis and Treatment" Hoermann, Midgley, Larisch, Dietrich. https://www.frontiersin.org/articles/10.3389/fendo.2017.00364/full

This paper talks about the need for a new paradigm of thyroid treatment that accepts that the relationship between TSH and thyroid hormones are individual, dynamic and can adapt, i.e. the current practice of simply looking at numbers that do or do not fit in the population ranges is not sufficient.

4. Thyroid hormone replacement – a counterblast to guidelines – Dr A.D. Toft. See: http://www.rcpe.ac.uk/sites/default/files/jrcpe_47_4_toft.pdf

5. Consensus statement for good practice and audit measures in the management of hypothyroidism and hyperthyroidism – M P J Vanderpump, J A 0 Ahlquist, J A Franklyn, R N Clayton, on behalf of a working group of the Research Unit of the Royal College of Physicians of London, the Endocrinology and Diabetes Committee of the Royal College of Physicians of London, and the Society for Endocrinology.
See: https://www.ncbi.nlm.nih.gov/pmc/articles/PMC2351923/pdf/bmj00557-0041.pdf

6. A Dialogue with Utiger: T3 based thyroid therapy over-suppresses TSH – Thyroid Patients Canada.
See: https://thyroidpatients.ca/2019/09/10/a-dialogue-with-utiger-t3-over-suppresses-tsh/

7. Hoermann R, Midgley JEM, Larisch R, Dietrich JW. Individualised requirements for optimum treatment of hypothyroidism: Complex needs, limited options. Drugs Context. 2019;8:212597. doi:10.7573/dic.212597.
See: https://pmc.ncbi.nlm.nih.gov/articles/PMC6726361/

I said at the start that many patients have doctors and endocrinologists who refuse to allow below reference range TSH. For these doctors, it is acceptable for patients to remain with severe hypothyroid symptoms. This is still true even if these symptoms are eradicated with more thyroid medication. These doctors and endocrinologists will not allow TSH to go below the bottom of the reference range. They assert that low TSH will result in bone loss or heart issues and is unacceptable.

There is research that disagrees with their views on TSH, and they ignore the fact that being severely hypothyroid is linked to cardiovascular issues, diabetes, depression etc.

It is worth being aware that in some cases, no argument will work with these doctors. Many thyroid patients now refuse to accept poor treatment, and find other physicians, or other ways to avoid being left with severe hypothyroid symptoms. I know I would not let any doctor damage my health ever again.

As mentioned earlier in this chapter, doing a private laboratory test, to determine how long thyroid medication needs to be stopped in order to get TSH and FT3 in range can be helpful. Finding a suitable, time gap from the last thyroid dosage to the blood draw could save the thyroid patient from having their medication reduced or stopped. Clearly, this is only sensible if the patient feels well, has no hyperthyroid symptoms at all and has good signs and symptoms.

Chapter 7

Thyroid Hormones, Dosing, Conversion Etc.

1. EVERYTHING CHANGES WHEN YOU HAVE A THYROID GLAND ISSUE

Below is an excellent article that explains in detail how important the thyroid gland is to maintaining healthy T3 levels.

It shows how the loss of thyroid gland tissue is a game-changer. Losing the thyroid gland causes the thyroid patient to lose a lot of conversion ability from T4 to T3, and it loses the thyroid's ability to switch more production to T3 if this is required. Loss of the thyroid gland can be complete with thyroidectomy, RAI, or long-term Hashimoto's or Atrophic Thyroiditis. Partial loss can also be present but this still loses significant thyroidal contribution to T3 production.

It shows why conventional thyroid labs that have been developed from testing healthy people, are no longer applicable when you have a thyroid gland damage or loss.

It discusses the importance of the thyroid gland itself to maintaining good T3 levels, and in maintaining a healthy conversion rate of T4 to T3.

It introduces a term that I have avoided using, just in case it confuses people. This term is the T3-Shunt or TSH-T3 Shunt. Basically, this is all about the importance of the thyroid gland itself, in both producing and converting large amounts of T3 in a way that contributes to overall T3 levels, without detracting from peripheral T3 generation in the rest of our cells. The term is used to describe the way that sufficient functional thyroid gland tissue is able to produce more T3 in order to keep the individual alive and healthier than they would otherwise be.

Note: there is not a special piece of tissue within the thyroid gland that is called the T3-Shunt. This term is just intended to describe the way that the thyroid works and is able to exhibit independence in making additional T3 if the individual requires it, as long as the thyroid gland is health. Clever thyroid gland!

It is a good read and explains some of the research papers in slightly simpler terms. Here is the link: https://thyroidpatients.ca/2019/10/21/the-tsh-t3-disjoint-in-thyroid-therapy/

It is definitely worth a read through a few times.

2. T3 IS THE BIOLOGICALLY ACTIVE THYROID HORMONE

T4 is a prohormone, or storage hormone. T4 is only truly useful if it can be converted to enough T3. T3 is the only biologically active thyroid hormone.

People can be totally healthy, for their entire life, using T3-Only, or T3-Mostly, medication on its own. People cannot be well on T4 medication if the T3 that is converted from it is too low.

No cells in the body work as intended without sufficient T3. Hence the range of symptoms caused by low T3 levels are vast. T3 affects our entire body, so symptoms caused by low T3 can include fatigue, brain-fog, digestive system issues, the skin, cardiovascular issues like high heart rate and high blood pressure, weight gain etc.

So, is it essential to take some T4 medication in some form?

From time to time someone puts forth an opinion that everyone needs to take some T4 (Levothyroxine, Synthroid or NDT), i.e., that it is critical to have some T4 medication. However, T4 is not really a thyroid hormone. It has an extremely weak effect and is mainly there to convert to T3. T4 mainly binds to receptors on the cell wall. T4 enters the cells but when it does, the T4 is only inside the cells in order to be converted into T3. Many thyroid patients are entirely well without any T4 at all. I have had zero T4 in my body for well over thirty years! It is not essential to take T4. However, for someone who converts T4 to T3 efficiently, then T4 medication is very easy to dose and to manage.

In this article, I provide more information on why T3 is the only truly biologically active thyroid hormone.

Genomic and non-genomic action of thyroid hormones.

Thyroid hormone receptors are present in the cell nuclei. T3 binds easily to these receptors. Researchers would say that T3 has a 'high affinity' to them. T3 affects gene transcription within the cell nuclei. This means that it is T3 that causes some genes to be active in fulfilling their purpose. It is by this process that the cells perform their function and produce whichever proteins they are designed to make. This is the main way in which thyroid hormone exerts its influence on our cells. The more T3, the faster this process occurs up to a certain limit. It is the main way in which metabolic rate is maintained.

Make no mistake here; the genomic action of T3 IS the main action of thyroid hormone, and the thyroid receptors are designed for T3.

T4 only has a very weak ability to bind to the nuclear thyroid receptors and when it does, it has only a very weak effect. Researchers would say that T4 has a 'very low affinity' for the nuclear thyroid receptors. Importantly, even if T4 does bind to the thyroid hormone receptors, its effects there are very weak indeed compared to T3. T3 is at the very least 10 times more potent than T4, even if T4 does manage to connect to the cell nuclei. The genomic effect of T4 is negligible compared to T3.

Now, in addition to this, there are thyroid receptors (integrin αvβ3 receptors), on the cell membranes. T4 can bind to these and exert non-genomic effects. These can be faster than the genomic effects, but they are not as powerful and do not result in the same regulation of cell function. Reverse T3 can also bind to the cell membrane receptors but cannot bind to the nuclear thyroid receptors. Note: there is also concern that the T4 and rT3 binding to the integrin αvβ3 receptors is linked to cancer proliferation. I cite research papers in articles in Chapter 9. So, high levels of T4 and/or rT3 are also health risks.

It seems, from research, that T3 can also bind to the cell membrane receptors and create these non-genomic effects but it may need to be at a higher concentration than normal to do this, i.e., as happens in people on T3-Only or T3-Mostly.

It is clear that the best combination for stability in the system, and to have it work as it is designed to do, is to have both T4 and T3. I have never argued that this is not the case. What I have argued is that you do not have to have T4 in order to be completely well, as T3 can replace the function of T4 if the situation requires it. It is important to be aware that some people cannot handle some, or even any, T4. So, trying to achieve a 'normal' T4 and T3 balance will simply leave some proportion of thyroid patients extremely unwell. So, striving to achieve a balance of thyroid hormones that include reasonable FT4 levels will be highly detrimental to some thyroid patients.

In addition to all the above, there is redundancy built into the system, i.e., the body compensates when needed. This is very important. It also explains why it is NOT a good idea to get into 'religious arguments' about whether someone on T3-Only therapy should have to take T4 also. For example, if conversion from T4 to T3 is poor, the direct uptake of T3 into the cells, via active transporters, can be increased. This means more T3 will be taken into all cells and used there. Thus, for people on T3-Only, more T3 than normal will enter all cells and will regulate cell function, compensating for any missing T4 to T3 conversion, that would have come previously, before thyroid problems, from T4. In the higher concentrations of T3 that exist when someone is on T3-Only therapy, the T3 will also bind to the cell membrane receptors, thus compensating for any lack of T4.

The body adapts and compensates when someone is on T3-Only.

If T4 is not present, the critical genomic effects of T3 will continue, and some of the T3 will also act non-genomically at the cell membrane. Active transporters will also carry more T3 into the cells.

There is no loss of function due to having no T4 present. This is why people on T3-Only feel completely well when it is dosed correctly. It has to be dosed correctly though, as described in the Recovering with T3 book.

This is one of the big flaws in the arguments of people that say everyone has to have some T4. They look at studies that show how a normal balance of T4 and T3 works. Then they extrapolate this to a situation when someone might not have any T4, but they do not allow for any compensatory changes in the system. Their logic is flawed. It is often because they themselves got well using T4/T3 or NDT. There is always a big danger of assuming that whatever treatment worked for one person, will work for others. The expression that seems to fit well for those people who believe that what worked for them should work for others is, "When all you have is a hammer, everything you see is a nail."

What about T2 and T1?

This is another argument that is made at times by those who use or promote the use of natural desiccated thyroid (NDT). They state that NDT also contains T2 and T1. However, there are only trace amounts of T2 and T1 in NDT – hardly anything. The main flaw in the argument of the pro-NDT lobby is that when T3 connects to the thyroid receptors in the cell nuclei and begins to be used, it produces all the T2, and then T1, that we need. This is where most of the T2 and T1 is made – by the use of T3. So, anyone on T3 therapy, or those on T4 therapy that convert well to T3, will have all the T2 and T1 that is required. There is no good argument for the use of NDT because of T2 and T1 content.

Conclusions on the use of T3-Only, and on T3 vs T4 thyroid hormones.

So, what does all the above mean to those people on T3-Only?

Yes, we are missing the non-genomic action of T4. Does this matter? Almost certainly not. T3 in higher concentrations will compensate for what the T4 was doing.

We also know from pragmatic experience that people on T3-Only, even after thyroidectomy, feel completely well. That alone should prove it.

However, for those people who are still sceptical of this, you have to remember that there is redundancy in the system. Alternate active transporters are expressed to transport more T3 into the cells if that is more readily available than T4. T3 itself has a non-genomic effect at the cell membrane, and in higher concentrations will compensate for lack of T4.

This means that when studies are done that find particular functions of T4, it does not mean that those on T3-Only lack these. That is a wrong conclusion. On T3-Only the higher concentrations of T3 and the adaptation of the system will actually meet the need that the specific function of T4 was providing. Our system has compensatory mechanisms within it.

I have spoken with thyroid researchers at some length on this topic, and have not just read research studies and made my own conclusions. It is clear to thyroid researchers that T3-Only replacement generally works as well as T4 or T4/T3.

T4/T3 replacement is ideal, and is often simpler to manage, but if it does not relieve symptoms, it is of little value. There is no point in taking the 'ideal' combination of medication if it leaves you feeling ill! However, until the medical profession stops being opposed to T3 medication, there will not be enough proper research done that explores T3-Only treatment.

My perspective on the various thyroid hormone medications has never changed.

I am in favour of using T4 replacement if it works well. If it does not, then T4/T3 or NDT should be tried. T3-Only is a good choice if the person remains sick on the other treatments and no other explanation can be found and fixed.

T3-Only is hard to dose, and it should be the therapy of last resort. But when the other treatments do not work, T3-Only therapy can be the route to amazingly good health. I took that route and have never regretted it.

T3-Only does work well, is safe, and is very effective when the other treatments have been shown to leave the patient unwell. T3 is the main biologically active thyroid hormone. T4 remains, in essence, a pro-hormone, with almost no effect at all compared to T3.

I hope the above further clarifies my views on this subject. I have remained consistent with the above throughout the years and throughout my books.

When asked why I or others do not take any T4 medication, I have three ways of answering:

1. "Why would I? I feel great on T3-Only, and feel ill when I add any T4" – this is the short answer.
2. "T3 is the active thyroid hormone. T4 is just a prohormone, with weak, or negligible effects until it is converted to T3". This is the typical answer I give, and the way I usually express it in my books. It is simple and accurate but does not include all the details and discussion.
3. This article – the more full and complete answer.

However, most of the people that raise the T4 issue with me, tend to be quite argumentative and sometimes even aggressive in their opinions. They do not appear to be open to any answer that is not the one that they had to begin with. So, I rarely go to a deeper level.

3. MORE ON THE POWER OF THE T3 THYROID HORMONE

T3 is the only true, biologically active thyroid hormone.

This always needs to be remembered during thyroid hormone assessment and thyroid treatment.

Doctors and endocrinologists who believe that they can optimise a thyroid patient's medication by looking only at TSH, or TSH and FT4 are missing the entire point. It is T3 that works to keep us well. FT3 is the most important thyroid hormone level to assess.

I had a conversation with a patient recently who had begun to have symptoms of hypothyroidism again after an inadvertent, slight reduction, in her T3 medication. This had occurred due to switching T3 brands. It made me realise that I probably need to say a little more about how T3 works and why even very small changes can make such a large difference.

In 2010, I wrote in one of the early drafts of Recovering with T3, in Chapter 14, that T3 could be viewed as a wave:

"Imagine a sandy beach, which is sheltered from the sea by large rocks. Only a wave that is large enough and powerful enough is capable of striking the rocks and sending a spray of seawater over them, to drench the sand beyond.

Each T3 divided dose is like a wave, the intracellular targets of T3 are akin to the beach and the rocks represent all the possible biochemical barriers that the T3 has to overcome. I do not believe that this is just some idle analogy. This is definitely how T3 replacement appears to feel and work within my own body. A small dose of it (2.5 or 5 mcg) might not do very much, because only some of it will become properly active within the cells.

A little more might enable more T3 effect to occur."

I also wrote in the protocol chapters that it was important to only change one dose at a time by 2.5 to 5 mcg at most, OR change a timing. I already knew that a small change could cause profound effects.

I knew that T3 affected the cell nuclei and caused the basic function of cells (through gene transcription) to work and speed up. I also knew that T3 caused the mitochondria to work more efficiently and to multiply within cells. I found research that proved that the number of mitochondria per cell decrease in the presence of low FT3, and increase with increased FT3. The mitochondria improve their performance and provide more cellular energy (ATP) when T3 and cortisol are at good levels. I also knew that T3 tended to increase cortisol levels and the effectiveness of cortisol.

Very shortly after the Recovering with T3 book was published, I began to see the research that showed that T3 improved the level of cortisol through the hypothalamic-pituitary system being more stimulated, thus enabling the adrenals to make more cortisol.

We now know that cortisol works synergistically with T3. Without enough T3, cortisol does not work well. Without enough cortisol, T3 does not work well. Both cortisol and T3 work at the cell nuclei and the mitochondria.

As you can see – there are a lot of connections. So, when one key hormone is low, there are a lot of systems that are affected.

So, in summary, T3 – works to improve the performance of:

- Cell nuclei.
- Mitochondria.
- Hypothalamic-pituitary system – thus helping to improve cortisol production from the adrenal glands and
- Cortisol-effect itself within the cells (just as cortisol helps to improve the effect of T3).

T3 thyroid hormone is potent and needs to be handled carefully. My protocol for using T3 recognised this potency when I first developed it nearly 30 years ago, and when I wrote about it in my first drafts of Recovering with T3.

It is not just the effect of T3 on cell nuclei. But it is the combined effect of an increase in T3 on the nuclei, the mitochondria, the hypothalamic-pituitary system and how cortisol and T3 enhance each other's effect.

Note: because T3 affects the nuclei in all of our cells, the range of symptoms caused by low T3 are vast. All the systems of our body can be affected.

This is why so many thyroid patients are sick. They are deficient in T3 throughout their body. This is also why T3 needs to be handled with some degree of reverence and care. A good protocol needs to be used. I think that the safe and effective protocol that I created and wrote about in detail in the Recovering with T3 book is still the best way to use T3.

When thyroid patients do not respond to T4 therapy or to T4/T3, or NDT therapy, more T3 or even T3-Only therapy can be truly helpful.

Used skilfully, and when required, T3-Only can have profoundly good effects and help someone who is still ill and struggling with hypothyroidism symptoms to recover.

4. PHARMACEUTICAL EQUIVALENCY OF T4, T3 AND NDT

I have now worked with thousands of thyroid patients over many years. In my books, Recovering with T3 and The Thyroid Patient's Manual, I make it very clear that I believe that it takes between 40 and 80 mcg of Liothyronine (T3) to correct hypothyroidism in most thyroid patients who are using T3-Only. A few patients may need a little less and some need more. My conclusion is based on endocrinology texts and also on a lot of my experience working with thyroid patients who need to use T3 in order to recover from hypothyroidism. I still stand by this view.

Here is an article that refers to various studies that suggest a typical replacement dose of T3 that is very close to the 40 – 80 mcg range that I have mentioned. One study concludes that a full replacement dose of T3 is 50 – 100 mcg, and another concludes that 50 – 120 is required to achieve a euthyroid state. These numbers are totally consistent with the information that I provide in my books.

The title of the article, and much of the content, is about the equivalency of T3 to T4 medication.

It is clear from the research studies that there is not a fixed mathematical equivalence.

We are not robots, and as human beings we vary considerably in our ability to convert from T4 to T3. However, the past studies referred to suggest that in many cases it requires 25 – 35 mcg of T3 to replace 100 mcg of T4 medication. There will of course be some people that might need more or less T3. In all cases, only the use of the patient's clinical presentation (symptoms and signs) would actually reveal if the individual is on the correct dosage and is effectively euthyroid.

I thought the article was very well written and interesting. I hope that you will too.

Here is the link: https://thyroidpatients.ca/2019/09/19/no-25-mcg-of-t3-liothyronine-isnt-equivalent-to-100-mcg-t4/

5. IT IS NOT POSSIBLE TO USE RATIOS OF T4/T3 OR RT3 TO PREDICT T3 DOSAGE

I have never been a fan of putting a lot of reliance on particular reverse T3 (rT3) levels to assess thyroid treatment. However, rT3 does have value. This is especially true if the thyroid patient continues to have symptoms and signs that suggest they still have low thyroid hormone issues. For example, when rT3 is very high then a T4 to T3 conversion issue might be interfering with treatment. RT3 can be viewed as a 'T3 blocker' when present in high levels. Note: it is the D3 enzymes that converts FT4 to rT3 that is responsible for any T3 blocking effect – see Article 5 in Chapter 5 for more specifics on rT3.

On various Internet sites, and in many books, you will find comments about the need for specific levels of rT3, or FT3/rT3 ratios.

This article puts rT3 in its real context and debunks a lot of the mythology that has been spread around on the Internet. Here is the article:

https://thyroidpatients.ca/2019/11/17/principles-practical-tips-for-reverse-t3-ft3-ft4/

In my book, The Thyroid Patient's Manual, I wrote this about rT3 during treatment:

"Reverse T3 – if progress is not going well, a conversion problem might be considered as a possibility. So, if FT3 is not increasing enough, or symptoms are not improving, testing FT3 and rT3 at the same time (same blood draw, so they are consistent in time), might be a good idea. A mid-range (or lower) FT3, and high rT3, would suggest there was a conversion problem, especially if someone is not improving after dosage increases. However, I do not believe there are any specific target levels for rT3, or an ideal ratio of FT3:rT3. You have to use common sense when interpreting the FT3 and rT3 levels together, perhaps seeing how they change during treatment, together with symptoms and signs."

Here is another article that highlights how the confusion surrounding rT3 may have arisen:

https://thyroidpatients.ca/2019/11/16/rt3-versus-a-dose-of-anti-thyroid-medication/

6. T3-ONLY TREATMENT: USING SYMPTOMS & SIGNS INSTEAD OF BLOOD TESTS

Thyroid patient's on T3-Only treatment, or T3-Mostly with some T4, should not rely entirely on thyroid blood tests to try to check if their dosage of T3 is correct

I believe there is too much importance placed on using thyroid blood test results to manage the dosage of T4/T3 combinations. As patients increase T3 and decrease T4, the usefulness of thyroid blood tests to determine if the treatment is correct, declines further. The thyroid laboratory ranges for FT4 and FT3 also become inapplicable to T3 therapy. These lab ranges are developed for healthy people or people on T4-only medication. They do not work well for those on T3-Only or T3-Mostly medication. When doctors try to manage a patient's T3 treatment to conform to thyroid lab ranges, this often leads to the patient remaining with symptoms. See Chapter 5 for more articles on the limitations of thyroid blood test results.

However, it is important to reiterate that thyroid blood tests still have an important role in the diagnosis of hypothyroidism.

My typical thyroid blood test results back in 2012 looked like this when tested around 12 hours or less after my last T3 dose (on my 60 micrograms of T3 per day – which is quite a modest amount compared to some patients):

- TSH was often near zero (but by leaving a gap of 18 hours or more between the last T3 dose and the blood draw, TSH can sometimes become higher and a prescription reduction avoided).
- FT4 was 0.3 pmol/L (lab reference range 12.0–22 pmol/L).
- FT3 was 8.9 nmol/L (lab reference range 3.1–6.8 nmol/L) (but by leaving a gap of 18 hours or more, my FT3 could get close to being in the reference range – often 18-24 hours or more might be needed for some patients).

My thyroid is now dead and atrophied, having had Hashimoto's for around 30 years, and Atrophic Thyroiditis. I take no T4 medication, hence my FT4 is near zero. I use T3-Only, hence the high FT3.

Most patients on T3-Only have:

- High FT3 (close to or sometimes over the top of the reference range).
- Low FT4 (often below the bottom of the reference range due to low TSH).
- A suppressed or very low TSH.

See this link to some 2016 research which shows the effects on TSH of a T3 dose: https://www.ncbi.nlm.nih.gov/pmc/articles/PMC5167556/

Often patients on T3-Only are in a long-running battle with their doctor or endocrinologist to add some T4 or to reduce their T3 dose because of their low TSH, or high FT3. However, the reduction of their T3 dosage, or the addition of T4, usually makes their symptoms worse.

Once a year, I have a thyroid blood test, as my doctor has to do that to conform to administration rules of the local health authority. We do not necessarily act on these results. Some doctors might assume I was thyrotoxic given my FT3 level, but I am not remotely close to this.

Thyroid blood tests are only a rough guide as to whether our cells are getting and using the thyroid hormone they need. They are an accurate estimate of blood levels but can be desperately inaccurate in terms of cellular levels of thyroid hormones.

In particular, thyroid blood test results sometimes do not reflect how well or unwell the thyroid patient actually feels. Attempting to use thyroid labs alone is likely to result in the thyroid patient remaining hypothyroid, especially if FT3 is too low for the individual person.

Only the active cellular level of thyroid hormone counts, and we cannot measure this with any laboratory test yet. High blood levels of thyroid hormone cannot cause bone loss or heart problems or any other problems, as thyroid hormone in the blood does nothing until it reaches the cell nuclei and the thyroid receptors within the nuclei.

However, there are ways to assess the effect of the biologically active T3 thyroid hormone within our cells

Many years ago, doctors would have used a complicated apparatus to measure Basal Metabolic Rate (BMR). In fact, this BMR measurement used to be the only diagnostic method for detecting hypothyroidism, apart from the patient's symptoms and other signs like heart rate and body temperature. The BMR measures the energy consumed by the body when completely at rest. If a patient had hypothyroidism, then their basal metabolic rate would have been very low.

However, now we have to adopt a simpler, but still effective, approach to provide data on how well thyroid hormone is regulating cell function.

Symptoms and signs are indicators of cellular levels of thyroid hormone.

We have not got a laboratory test that indicates how well thyroid hormone is actually regulating our cells. So, what can we do?

All we can do is measure the effect of these thyroid hormones on our bodies. This is what I have done for well over twenty years. I use symptoms and signs.

A doctor describes a sign as something that is objective and can be measured. A symptom is a subjective assessment of something.

So, a patient may say, "I feel cold". Feeling cold is the symptom and body temperature is the sign.

Anyone who suspects that they are still hypothyroid can track symptoms and signs every day and build up a diary record of these, which can be used to determine if they are hypothyroid at the cellular level. But only an open-minded doctor is likely to accept this approach.

However, for someone on T3-Only, this is currently the ONLY reliable method, to manage the T3 divided doses, until a researcher comes up with a proper test of thyroid hormone that shows how well thyroid hormone is actively regulating cell function.

Anyone on T3-Only who has a doctor who is attempting to manage their T3 dosage entirely with thyroid blood tests (TSH, FT4, FT3), needs to be aware that this is likely to fail. It is likely to result in very bad decisions being made that could easily keep the thyroid patient hypothyroid. If this is the case, the patient should consider changing their doctor. This may also be true of people who take predominantly T3 with some T4.

Note: when beginning to use T3 therapy checking thyroid labs from time to time does make sense. It is helpful to know that FT3, FT4, TSH and possibly reverse T3 are all adjusting as you would expect them to.

Here is the list of symptoms and signs that I use on a regular basis:

Symptoms:

- Mood.
- Anxiety (including restlessness, hyperactivity or irritability, being anxious, edgy, tense, and unable to relax, usually means too much thyroid hormone).
- Mental ability and clarity.
- Energy level.
- Muscle weakness.
- Digestive system performance.
- Condition of skin, hair, and nails.
- Heat or cold sensitivity.
- Muscle aches or pains.

Signs:

- Resting heart rate.
- Blood pressure.
- Body temperature.
- Weight gain/loss.

I have been very brief with the list of symptoms and signs, and not explained fully how I use them, but the list should give a pretty good indication that dosage management with T3 is not as simple as T4. However, it is still possible to do it well.

It is also important to use symptoms and signs to determine when each T3 dose is due during the day - taking a T3 divided dose too early is just as bad as taking too much. The Recovering with T3 book has a T3 dosage management process, designed to determine only the amount of T3 needed to regain good health and no more than this. Symptoms and signs often show patterns over the day. It is possible to recognise these if tracking is done before and a few hours after thyroid medication doses. The patterns of change in symptoms and signs are incredibly helpful in determining an optimal T3 dosage. The Recovering with T3 book goes into detail on this.

Until thyroid researchers develop new laboratory tests of how well thyroid hormone is regulating the function of our cells, the use of symptoms and signs is the only reliable way of managing the dosage of T3-only replacement.

The Recovering with T3 book emphasises safety and caution. The T3 dosage management process which is described in detail within the book, allows the patient's T3 dosage to be determined safely and effectively. I continue to hope that over time some of the more open-minded doctors and endocrinologists will read it and find some value in it also.

See Article 7, which is next in this chapter, for more details on using signs and symptoms.

Even if your own doctor is unwilling to take the approach of using symptoms and signs on board, you can still do your own tracking. In this way, you can form a clear view of whether you are under-dosed or over-dosed, and which thyroid medication dose(s) needs adjustment. This information will provide useful data that can help in thyroid medication discussions with your doctor.

7. TRACKING SYMPTOMS & SIGNS (VITALS)

When using T3-Only, or T3-Mostly, it is not possible to use thyroid blood tests to manage the T3 dosage. Finding the daily amount of T3 needed, the right number of doses, and their sizes and timings will not be possible from thyroid blood testing.

The Recovering with T3 book describes a protocol, for determining doses of T3, and for slowly and safely increasing the T3 doses in order to find the optimal overall dosage for the individual patient. The protocol uses both Signs and Symptoms, which I discuss in all of my books. Tracking signs and symptoms is useful regardless of the type of thyroid medication. However, the more T3 that is being used, the more critical the reliance on signs and symptoms needs to be.

Signs are measurements that are not subjective, i.e., not based on an opinion. An example of a sign is body temperature, measured by a thermometer. Signs are sometimes also known as 'vitals' (or vital signs). Signs provide an objective, in-arguable measure of how the body is responding to thyroid treatment.

Symptoms are subjective. An example of a symptom is whether someone feels their energy level is good or not (there is no device to measure this).

When using T3-Only/T3-Mostly it is critical to track both signs and symptoms in a rigorous way and record them. This is so that BOTH the TIMING of the doses and the SIZES of each dose can be adjusted and tailored to be ideal for the individual.

If this is done EVERY DAY, it is the best way to assess T3 dosage changes and any subtle alteration of signs or symptoms. Blood tests will tell you very little indeed and are often not worth doing when on T3-Only medication. The process can also be helpful for those on T4, T4/T3 or NDT medication. See The Thyroid Patient's Manual for more information on managing T4, and T4/T3-based medications.

Here is a summary of how to go about tracking signs and symptoms.

When to collect sets of signs/symptoms for those on T3 (or T4/T3 or NDT):

1. Do not attempt to measure signs (vitals) around the time of a CT3M dose (if one is being used), as this will disrupt sleep.
2. On waking/getting up, or within 30 minutes of getting up (which is probably more ideal). Do not assess signs in bed. Actually, get up, get dressed then do it.
3. Just before (5-15 minutes before) the first daytime T3 dose – so you can see what the situation is before the dose was taken. Alternatively, if another T3 dose is not being taken in the morning, take some measurements at least once during the mid-late morning or 2-3 hours after the first morning measurements of signs.
4. 2 hours (3 at the most) after the first daytime T3 dose – which is when it ought to be helping to raise metabolism. The comparison between the results of this measurement and the previous one can be very helpful in assessing dosing.
5. Just before (5-15 minutes before) the second daytime T3 dose.
6. 2 hours (3 at the most) after the second daytime T3 dose. Alternatively, if there is no afternoon dose of T3 being taken, take some measurements in the mid-afternoon.
7. If you have a third daytime dose of T3 then repeat 5) and 6) for that third daytime dose of T3.
8. Once in the evening e.g., 7 or 8 pm.

For those NOT on Thyroid Treatment yet, take them:

1. Within 30 minutes of getting up.
2. Late morning.
3. Mid-late afternoon.
4. Early to mid-evening.

Note: for those people who are still in the process of detailed adjustment of dose sizes and timings, more frequent measurement can be helpful. From more frequent measures before a T3 dose and after a T3 dose you can observe the pattern of changing signs (temperature, HR, BP). This can show if a dose is too soon, too late, too high or too low. The pattern of change is often more helpful than absolute values. This is especially helpful if it is not clear what is going on. More frequent assessment of signs will show how BP, HR and body temperature fluctuates running up to a T3 dose, then after it, until the next dose is due. It is often possible to understand far more from this than from just one measurement before and after a T3 dose.

THYROID HORMONES, DOSING, CONVERSION ETC.

HERE IS AN EXAMPLE OF A PATIENT'S SYMPTOMS AND SIGNS IN THE RIGHT FORMAT:

*** START EXAMPLE ***
DATE: 8th March 2021
Date any T4/NDT Meds were Last Taken: 7 weeks.
GET-UP TIME (we need to see if CT3M was being used): 7:00 am.
T3 (and other thyroid medications)
Dosage:
25mcg T3@07:00 am;
12.5mcg T3@11:00 am;
12.5mcg T3@16:00 pm.

SIGNS / VITALS:

TIME	TEMP	HR	BP
07:30:	36.7	95	107/64
09:30	36.9	90	110/70
10:45:	36.8	97	101/65
11:30:	36.8	92	105/63
12:30:	36.9	90	110/69
13:30:	37.0	97	109/65
15:30:	37.0	94	109/66
16:30,	37.0	88	110/70
18:00:	37.0	92	106/63

If there had been any new laboratory test results done, the results should be included after the vitals, along with reference ranges and units – as laboratory test results are also signs.

SYMPTOMS SUMMARY: Tired in the morning with a headache. I did not sleep well the previous night. Felt warm from 12 noon & a bit on edge in the afternoon. Had energy in the afternoon, my body feels 'lighter' & head feels clearer.
*** END EXAMPLE ***

The above is clear, organised and only has the essentials in it. This thyroid patient created a diary with time-stamped (dated) entries with this type of information, which made it easy for her to track progress after any thyroid medication change (in this case it was T3-Only medication).

Too much information, with many detailed descriptive comments, is almost as bad as too little, making it very difficult to interpret. Summarising the symptoms and signs collected into a few lines also makes it easy to create a diary that the thyroid patient and their doctor (if they can be engaged in the process), can easily assess. Pages of information with many detailed descriptive comments are much more difficult to use. When the information is summarised tidily, and in a short amount of space, then any obvious patterns or results may be found far more easily.

The format above is ideal and has been proven to be quite easy to interpret.

The get-up time is very important to have as it shows if someone is using CT3M.

Note: Waking temperatures can be lower when a woman's period is due.

Making a good recording of symptoms and signs before and after T3 doses, and at key times of the day can help to assess whether there is the right number of T3 doses and whether the doses are too high or too low.

What is most important is the pattern of how the symptoms and signs change before and after T3 doses. This pattern often provides the most information on what might not be optimal in the dosing of T3.

What if things get very confusing and you are not sure if a dose is too high, too low, too early or too late?

In this case, the thyroid patient can record symptoms and signs more frequently in the hours before a dose is due, and in the hours following it. Sometimes doing this every hour is sufficient, but in very confusing situations then recording the information every 30 minutes can begin to make the pattern of change in symptoms and signs more obvious. By recording the signs especially every hour or 30 minutes in the hours before a T3 dose and in the hours following a T3 dose, the patterns will become obvious.

Sometimes signs worsen as the T3 dose is due and then improve after it. This can indicate that the previous dose was too low or the time between the doses was too large. This diligence is extremely important if someone wants to fine-tune their T3 doses and feel really well.

I understand that people are busy but when the T3 dosing is confusing, using a quieter day to record signs and symptoms every hour during that day, can really be helpful.

All this information is discussed in more detail in the Recovering with T3 book. I recommend reading Recovering with T3 before anyone even begins to use T3 thyroid hormone, even if it is being used in combination with T4 or in natural desiccated thyroid (NDT). Recovering with T3 can be bought on any Internet bookseller site including Amazon in your own country or in a country near you.

8. THE HYPOTHYROIDISM NUMBERS TRAP – THYROID PRODUCTION OF T4, T3, & CONVERSION RATE ARE HIGHLY VARIABLE

I have heard so many pieces of nonsense over the years about how much T4 and T3 is produced by the thyroid gland and what the ratio of this T4 to T3 is. This is often mistakenly assumed to be 80% of T4 and 20% of T3 from the thyroid gland

I have also heard too many times that conversion from T4 to T3 in the peripheral tissues (non-thyroid) is in a fixed ratio.

Both the fixed thyroid production ratio of T4 to T3 and the fixed T4 to T3 conversion ratio are utter rubbish. These ratios vary hugely between individuals. They are also variable for every individual and can vary with the thyroid medication dosage.

Poor assumptions about T4 & T3 production and conversion ratios, leads to bad treatment practices. This frequently causes thyroid patients to have insufficient T3, i.e., they remain symptomatic at best, and sometimes very ill.

These incorrect beliefs assume that we are all robots that fall off a production line. These beliefs assume we all have identical thyroid gland production levels of T4 and T3 that never alter with circumstance or disease. These flawed beliefs assume that we all have the same conversion ratio from T4 to T3 in the peripheral tissues and that this conversion ratio never alters. The beliefs are utterly flawed, but many doctors are using them routinely in their medical practices. Note: It is not just endocrinologists and doctors who are doing this. It is also thyroid patients, as they try to assist other patients using this errant information.

Let me provide a couple of common examples of what often happens:
- When a thyroid patient is undergoing treatment, their doctor often assumes that they will always get ideal conversion from T4 to T3 and that simply replacing missing thyroid hormones with T4 will work. This is clearly not always true.
- If a thyroid patient wants to add one type of thyroid medication to their treatment, e.g., adding 10 mcg of T3 to T4 medication, they may be told to reduce the T4 level by 40 mcg. This is because some doctors or patients believe that 40 mcg of T4 will convert to 10 mcg of T3. This information might come from a doctor or another patient on a patient forum.

    I could list many other examples.

There is a large variation of thyroid secretion of T3 between individuals. There is also a large variation of FT4 to FT3 conversion capability between individuals. The conversion rate from FT4 to FT3 is also regulated for each individual, i.e., it will change depending on thyroid medication dosage and other factors.

Every healthy individual has the ability to make more or less thyroid hormone and convert more or less T4 to T3 in a dynamic way. In a healthy person, with a working thyroid gland, the thyroid hormone system is variable and regulated for them as an individual.

The variation between individuals of other biochemical issues that affect thyroid hormone medication absorption, conversion, and utilisation in the cells (where it counts most) is also LARGE.

This is all frequently made worse when an endocrinologist or doctor insists that TSH can be used to monitor and determine when the 'treatment' is adequate.

Every individual needs a unique approach to treatment that is tailored to them and driven first and foremost by symptoms and signs.

Here are some implications for thyroid treatment:

People without a healthy thyroid gland are missing half the equipment (the thyroid gland itself) needed to balance the right secretion and balance of thyroid hormones and the right balance of conversion.

Thyroid-disabled people do not have the equipment to manage metabolic flexibility.

If our body needs to reduce the T3 supply, that is pretty easy. It is easier to destroy than create. All our body needs to do is to make more Deiodinase Type 3 (DIO3 / D3), which happens as FT4 and FT3 rise. This D3 enzyme will increase the rate of conversion of T4 to Reverse T3 and of T3 into T2.

On the other hand, people without a fully working thyroid gland cannot enhance both secretion and conversion at the same time, when our bodies need to increase our metabolic rate in response to environmental or health challenges.

For example, in the mid-winter cold season, some thyroid patients without thyroids need a little more T3 hormone as their FT3 can fall lower. Whilst healthy people get a boost to their FT3 because they can turn up the thyroid hormone thermostat to stay warm. Therefore, some thyroid patients may need a backup supply of T3 thyroid hormone. This does not apply to all thyroid patients, as their daily dosage can absorb the shock of minor to moderate bumps in the road.

The article below explains how endocrinologists and doctors have mistakenly used some older research and have come to invalid conclusions. Individuals have such a massive variability of thyroid hormone production and conversion that simplistic levels and ratios result in extremely poor treatment. Unfortunately, many thyroid groups and individuals offering advice on these have also fallen into the same trap.

Here is the actual post with the details. It is quite long and detailed but worth the read when you have time to sit down and go through it carefully:

https://thyroidpatients.ca/2020/05/04/t3-compensates-conversion/

9. A HEALTHY THYROID COMPENSATES FOR POOR T4 TO T3 CONVERSION

I have listed a link below to an article by Dr Tania S. Smith. It contains an analysis of the classic 1990 thyroid science article by Alessandro Pilo and team, and it supplements it with insights from more recent thyroid science.

The article debunks the commonly held view about the 20/80 origin of T3 hormone in the body; the view that, on average, our T3 supply arises from a 20:80 secretion to conversion ratio. The reality is more wide-ranging and diverse. It also reveals the flexibility of the healthy hypothalamic-pituitary-thyroid axis.

My own main interest is always about what a scientific paper means in terms of proper and effective thyroid treatment. It will be obvious to the reader, that for some people on thyroid treatment, Levothyroxine (T4) therapy is never going to work. This is especially true for those who have lost some, or all, of their thyroid through various conditions. Those thyroid patients who have had a thyroidectomy or have lost significant thyroid tissue due Hashimoto's, or Atrophic Thyroiditis, are at a huge disadvantage to other patients. They are far more likely to fail to resolve their symptoms with T4 medication alone.

It is important to be aware that the diversity of individuals is such that some are far more reliant on their thyroid gland to compensate for poor peripheral tissue conversion than others. When these people develop a thyroid condition, they will only ever return to being healthy by being given a significant amount of T3 in their treatment.

Many thyroid patients are well aware of the variation between people, but sadly, the majority of the medical profession operates as if all our thyroid glands and thyroid hormone processing were identical. We are treated as if we are identical robots that have come off a production line. This is not true, as the article carefully and methodically explains.

One of the big implications of the article to me, is that T3 (Liothyronine) treatment must always be available as an option for use, if the patient does not respond symptomatically to T4 treatment.

The article is quite long and has three separate parts to it. It is definitely worth spending the time to read it. However, there is also a summary of the article for those who are short of time or want a good idea of what it is about before reading the full version.

Here is the link to the summary of the article:
https://thyroidpatients.ca/2020/05/27/summary-t3-secretion-conversion/

Here is the full article:
https://thyroidpatients.ca/2020/05/04/t3-compensates-conversion/

10. WHY T3-ONLY SHOULD BE THE LAST TREATMENT THAT PATIENTS CONSIDER

I developed Hashimoto's thyroiditis (an autoimmune thyroid disease) around thirty years ago. I was given the standard T4 (Levothyroxine/Synthroid) thyroid treatment. However, despite still feeling unwell, I was told by endocrinologists and doctors, "You are cured!'.

So, I asked them, "Why do I still have all the symptoms of hypothyroidism?"

The answers to the question varied depending on the doctor I spoke to:
- I was told I had some unknown disease that appeared to have symptoms similar to hypothyroidism.
- I was' told that I had a psychological problem – likely depression. I was refused any more blood tests or referrals by one GP unless I took a course of Prozac (antidepressants).
- I was consistently told I could no longer have any problems with thyroid hormones because my thyroid hormone levels were 'normal' as determined by laboratory testing.
- I was asked to join a growing number of patients in an ME/CFS support group by one endocrinologist. Many of them had also been his thyroid patients. It seemed that he was happy to stick a ME/CFS label on me, and push me into a room to commiserate on my bad luck, and lack of a future, with others that he had similarly failed to help!

Far too many thyroid patients who do not feel well on just T4 thyroid hormone medication have encountered these ridiculous attempts to justify poor diagnostic work and even poorer treatment. Some have even more unpleasant diagnoses, having been told that they are lazy, eating too much or simply getting old.

I did not believe any of the doctors or endocrinologists who tried to explain away my symptoms. So, I did my own research and I read endocrinology books.

I concluded that a trial of T3 (Liothyronine) was necessary because my hypothyroidism was not fixed by using Levothyroxine (T4).

I needed to learn more about what was 'broken' inside me. I knew something was broken because such a wide range of T4 dosages had been tried and all had failed. I also knew that this had all occurred after the advent of my autoimmune thyroid problem - Hashimoto's thyroiditis. I was totally healthy prior to developing Hashimoto's.

Eventually, I found a doctor who allowed me to try natural desiccated thyroid (NDT) and then T4/T3. We also used hydrocortisone and prednisolone. None of these treatments made any difference. Eventually I got the T3 trial that I had wanted for so long.

With T3, the lights went on. Within a week, I could get up the stairs at home more easily. My digestive problems all vanished within days. I began to think more clearly and function once again. Within a few weeks I felt like I was a different person − not the shambling wreck of a human being who was old before his time. T3 on its own was the answer and the clue. I still had a lot of fatigue issues but these arose from my continuing low cortisol, which I had yet to resolve.

My problems had definitely been occurring at a cellular level and beyond the ability of any blood test to see them or make them obvious.

I now know that there are many causes for this. Although at the time I was not really able to pin down any one specific reason.

It took me nearly three years to completely finalise my dosage and understand how to use T3 correctly. I had to apply all my background in science and applied research in order to do so. I also had to discover how to use T3 in order to raise my cortisol levels and recover fully.

I have now been using T3 (Liothyronine) for over thirty years and am fit and well. I have no weight issues or any other symptoms of hypothyroidism or low cortisol.

So, why have I chosen the title for this article?

T3 is far more difficult to use and find the right dosage, compared to other thyroid hormone treatments. Doctors are also far less keen to prescribe it.

When I first began to discuss T3-Only use on forums, many years ago, I frequently met ignorance, defensiveness, and incredulity. I even received abusive and rude comments from other thyroid patients. Some thyroid forums are still like this today. There was so little discussion about T3, and so few people who had good experiences of using it that I found the Internet forums to be quite difficult places to inhabit. The situation is somewhat different today but it still happens. However, these days, far more thyroid patients are using T3 in order to recover from hypothyroidism.

Over the years, I have now spoken to thousands of thyroid patients who have managed to recover their health using T3-Only.

Many patients are now hungry for information about this under-prescribed thyroid medication.

However, I increasingly get questions from people who want to know if they might be able to get well by taking T3-Only instead of T4. Some people even consider switching directly from their current T4 medication to T3. This trend has provided me with the idea for this article.

T3 is not an easy drug to use. Any patient, or doctor, who begins to introduce T3, whether on its own or in combination with T4 or NDT, must know quite a lot about it before commencing its use.

Some of these thyroid medications are more difficult to use than others. The order of increasing difficulty to use is:

1. T4 (levothyroxine) – easiest to use.
2. T4 / T3 in combination.
3. Natural desiccated thyroid (NDT).
4. NDT / T3.
5. T3-Only (T3 on its own or pure T3) – hardest to use.

I am prepared to debate where 2 and 3 are relative to each other and possibly even 4. I only put T4/T3 ahead of NDT, because T4/T3 combinations allow for some change in the ratio of T4 and T3.

What is clear to me is that 1 (T4) is definitely easier to use than 2-4 (combos of T4 and T3). Number 5 (T3-Only) is harder to use than the others.

Why should I say this last statement? Once the nature of the T3 hormone is understood, and the reasons why people resort to it are also taken into account, it should become clear why T3 is a medication that should not be seen as a simple panacea.

In the human body, the biological half-life of T4 is approximately seven days, which means a patient can take their entire daily dosage of synthetic T4 in one go, without any issues, because it is used up relatively slowly.

In contrast, the biological half-life of T3 is believed to be twenty-four hours. A single dose of T3 is rapidly absorbed and reaches peak circulating concentration in just two to three hours (2.5 hours is typical), after ingestion. This will vary a little by person.

Blood serum concentrations of T3 may remain somewhat elevated for six to eight hours. After this, blood serum concentrations decline again, unless another dose of T3 is ingested.

So, for most thyroid patients, T3 has to be taken several times a day. Taking it all in one go, once a day, is far too potent in one dose for most thyroid patients.

THYROID HORMONES, DOSING, CONVERSION ETC.

The other interesting fact about T3 is that it arrives in the body extremely quickly and it has the effect of rapidly suppressing the TSH. Therefore, patients who are receiving only T3 replacement therapy should expect unusual laboratory tests of thyroid hormone levels. This makes it impossible to use thyroid lab tests to manage the T3 dosage. Many doctors are still very uncomfortable with this as they mistakenly think that the lab ranges developed for people on T4 medication can be used for ALL the thyroid medications.

Low FT4 levels should be expected. FT3 results could be low, normal or elevated above the top of the reference range, depending on how much T3 is being prescribed and the exact time of the thyroid blood test, in relation to the time that the last dose of T3 was taken. TSH could be highly suppressed or at the very least TSH is likely to fluctuate far more with the use of T3 medication than with T4.

The above information, on the rapidity with which T3 achieves peak serum concentrations and then declines again and the potential for unusual TSH, FT4, and FT3 results, is very important. This means that laboratory tests cannot assess the adequacy of replacement with T3.

Endocrinologists, doctors and thyroid patients may wish to use thyroid blood test results to check the T3 dosage – but this simply will not work!

Other methods need to be used to manage the T3 treatment and set the correct level of T3 medication. Symptoms and signs must be used but this is not as easy as the conventional way of looking at thyroid labs. It is crucial to realise that the T3 is being taken to overcome whatever the problems with T4 or T4/T3 are and that the goal is for the patient to feel well again, with normal symptoms and signs (including key measures like blood pressure and heart rate).

In order to achieve this, the right amount of T3 needs to be effective within someone's cells. When this occurs, the levels of hormones within the bloodstream are likely to be completely unrepresentative of the cellular activity of the T3. So, TSH, FT4, FT3, or reverse T3 in the bloodstream (which is the only place they can be measured currently) are very likely to be unrepresentative of actual cellular activities of these hormones.

Attempting to manage the dosage of T3 for someone who can only get well by using T3-Only can only currently be done effectively and safely by using indirect measures of thyroid hormones, as described in my books.

Attempting to do this by using thyroid hormone blood test results could even be dangerous, as all of these thyroid hormone test results may have no bearing on cellular activity. This point is highly relevant for those patients using T3 only and this is a major reason why using T3 is harder than the other hormones.

Someone new to T3 replacement therapy may believe that the medication can be taken in a single daily dose, just like synthetic T4. This may work for a very small number of people but for others, the daily dosage of T3 will need to be split up and taken in smaller doses, known as divided doses. This divided dose approach enables T3 to be taken at various intervals throughout the day, in order to provide a steady supply of T3 to the body.

The use of divided doses also ensures that no single dose of T3 creates an exceptionally high peak level of T3 in the tissues of the body. The majority of patients successfully using T3 use between three and four divided doses of T3 per day.

Using divided doses of T3 clearly adds a lot of complexity to the life of thyroid patients. A further complication of the use of T3-Only is due to the suppressive effect that it can have on TSH. The level of TSH influences the conversion of T4 to T3. A high TSH results in the maximum level of conversion of T4 to T3. A fully suppressed TSH will result in the conversion rate of T4 to T3 being reduced to the minimum level.

For the patient on combined therapy with T4 and T3, this is very significant indeed. Some doctors attempt to perform simple mathematical calculations when they add T3 to their patient's T4. They reduce their patient's T4 dosage when T3 is added. Often there is no understanding that the added T3 is likely to have a suppressive effect on TSH and this is likely to downgrade any T4 to T3 conversion rate. So, finding the right balance of T4 and T3 can be an extremely challenging task.

In summary, the use of T3 has a number of difficulties:

- The half-life of T3 is short and the drug is very potent. T3 usually needs to be taken in three to four divided doses per day. A few patients find that they can cope with just two divided doses.
- T3 acts quickly and powerfully and will distort thyroid blood test results of TSH, FT4, FT3, and rT3. For someone using T3-Only, these thyroid blood test results are not reliable measures to be employed for managing the treatment.
- Doctors may wish to try to manage the patient's T3 dosage using thyroid blood tests and the standard lab ranges – this will not work.
- T3 used in combination with T4 can also prove difficult. Blood test results can be distorted, divided doses of T3 need to be used and the conversion rate of T4 can deteriorate.

All of the above difficulties mean that using T3-Only is not something that anyone should want to do unless everything else has been tried and failed. Using T3 in combination with T4 is simpler but still has some issues, just not to the same extent as T3-Only.

As well as bearing the above in mind, investigations into deficient nutrients or low cortisol levels should be thoroughly performed and ruled out before ever considering the use of T3. T3 is harder to use, so other treatments should be explored first.

I have been known to refer to T3 as the thyroid hormone treatment of last resort – I believe it should be viewed like that. But, if all the necessary investigations have been performed, and all the thyroid hormone therapies have all been tried and shown to fail, then T3-Only can be a wonderful way of recovering your health. I know – I have done it, and so have thousands of other patients. However, a safe and effective protocol needs to be used – this is why I wrote Recovering with T3.

11. WHY T3 (LIOTHYRONINE) IS USUALLY TAKEN IN MULTI-DOSES PER DAY

This article discusses why multi-dosing with T3-Only, or T3-Mostly, medication is more effective and safer for most thyroid patients. It is not about dosing with mostly T4 medication and a little added T3. I am talking about full replacement daily dosages of T3, in the 40-100 mcg per day region. Smaller amounts of T3 than this are more easily managed in two doses or even one single dose per day.

Very occasionally, I hear of individuals advocating that thyroid patients should take all of their T3-Only medication in one single daily dose. I know that this approach does not work for most people.

Over the past fifteen years or so, I have worked with thousands of thyroid patients and have helped them to use T3 effectively. Whilst a handful of them can successfully take a single daily dose, the majority need to multi-dose the T3 in some way.

Here is how I came to this conclusion and how and why multi-dosing can work better for most people.

When I first started on T3-only, I tried taking my 50-mcg daily dose all at once in the morning. That left me extremely hypothyroid after about 8 hours. Over several weeks, I tried increasing the dose to make it last longer but I always became hypothyroid within 8-10 hours. It never lasted longer than this. By that stage, I had become expert at assessing not only my symptoms but also my vital signs of heart rate, blood pressure and body temperature. So, I could see quite clearly that my metabolism slowed down after 8-10 hours – it was not my imagination.

In this trial, I continued to increase the total daily dose of T3 from my normal 50 mcg until I eventually reached about 160 mcg of T3 per day.

Two things became apparent:
1) I still became hypothyroid after around 10 hours.
2) I felt hyperthyroid during the early and middle hours. My BP became high, my heart rate was elevated, my temperature was slightly high and I felt anxious and ill.

The bottom line was that I could find no single daily dose of T3 that either lasted for 24 hours or avoided some element of feeling hyperthyroid at some points and hypothyroid for a lot of the time.

Dr John Lowe and I discussed this many times. He and I knew each other well. I read his book The Metabolic Treatment of Fibromyalgia about 6 times. Dr Lowe proof-read and wrote the foreword to my Recovering with T3 book. He supported the book and was going to market it for me in the USA had he not died in an accident. We agreed on most things and we both saw that there were going to be different groups of people who would find one form of T3 dosing more effective than another.

John originally believed that, for a lot of people, taking T3 once a day was enough to provide a large genomic 'kick' to the cell nuclei. His view was that this would provide enough blood levels of T3, and intra-cellular levels, that there would be a T3 supply, albeit a lot lower than the initial 'kick', for long enough to just about get through 24 hours. Through our discussions, we both came to the conclusion that there might be different classes of people who have different needs.

The people that John treated were incredibly ill fibromyalgia patients. John himself had serious genetic resistance to T3 and this ran in his family. However, most people who need T3 do not have such deeply problematic issues, myself included.

John and I basically reached an agreement that it was fine to have different modalities of T3 use available to suit everyone. I still believed that the majority of people would be more safely and more effectively served with 3 to 4 doses of T3 per day.

I still believe, that the best way to provide enough T3 for a thyroid patient, over 24 hours, is to use multi-doses.

This does not require stable blood levels of T3 in order to be highly effective. In fact, the free T3 level in the bloodstream can fluctuate significantly. What counts is whether the genomic activity in the cell nuclei is sustained at a healthy rate over 24 hours.

My work with thyroid patients makes me very confident in saying that 3 to 4 doses of T3 over the day suits the majority of patients very well and avoids both hypothyroid periods and any risk of hyperthyroid episodes. However, I have always believed that there are some people for whom 2 doses of T3 per day or even 1 dose per day would be sufficient. We are all different and no one solution works for everyone.

The protocol I developed for using T3 safely and effectively is described in detail in the Recovering with T3 book. The book shows thyroid patients and their doctors how to go about finding the most effective T3 dosage that is very safe for the individual. I also discuss the principles behind multi-dosing.

Here is an extract from Chapter 11 of Recovering with T3:

"HOW T3 IS USUALLY TAKEN EACH DAY – DIVIDED DOSES

Someone new to T3 replacement therapy may believe that the medication can be taken in a single daily dose, just like synthetic T4. This may work for a few people. However, for most people, the daily dosage of T3 will need to be split up and taken in smaller doses, known as divided doses.

This divided dose approach enables T3 to be taken at various intervals throughout the day, in order to provide a steady supply of T3 to the body. The use of divided doses also ensures that no single dose of T3 creates an exceptionally high peak level of T3 in the tissues of the body. Through the careful use of divided doses, it is possible to avoid the risk of tissue over-stimulation by T3 (T3 thyrotoxicosis). Some people refer to the taking of divided doses as multi-dosing.

In the UK, T3 is only available in 20-microgram tablets. Unfortunately, this makes matters rather difficult for the patient.

In order to achieve a divided dose strategy, the UK-based patient may have to carefully break the tablet in half (to create two 10-microgram doses), or into quarters (for a 5-microgram dose). If a 2.5 microgram T3 dose change is required, the tablet has to be broken up even further, which can be difficult.

In some countries, specialist companies, known as compounding pharmacies, can produce sustained release T3 for patients. This releases the T3 in a slow way. The idea behind it is to avoid potential issues caused by large peaks and troughs in the circulating level of T3 throughout the day. Sustained release T3 is sometimes referred to as 'slow release T3'. However, there are mixed reports concerning sustained release T3. For those patients who require a full replacement of dosage of T3, sustained release T3 does not appear to work as well as pure T3. There may be many reasons for this. It is hard to tailor a sustained release T3 dose to provide enough T3 for many hours, without either providing too much, or too little T3, for some periods of time. This could explain why many of the patients who have tried to use sustained release T3 have chosen to go back to using pure T3.

When he initially prescribed T3, my doctor recommended that I split the daily dosage into two divided doses. I quickly discovered that two divided doses were not going to provide a steady enough level of T3 for me during the day. This is just one example of how limited the existing information on T3 was, as there were no recommendations to try smaller, more frequent doses, if the larger, less frequent doses caused side effects.

I have now communicated with many patients who use T3 replacement therapy. There are a small number of patients who do manage on two divided doses of T3 per day and a very small number, for whom one large dose of T3 appears to work perfectly well. However, the vast majority of patients using T3 replacement therapy appear to be using between three and four divided doses of T3 per day. I have also heard of some patients who use even higher numbers of divided doses but I would consider higher numbers of divided doses to be bordering on impractical.

I cannot emphasise how important it is for many people to employ T3 in divided doses. For a small proportion of people one or two divided doses of T3 apparently works very well.

However, the careful use of three to four divided doses of T3 appears to suit many people extremely well."

I strongly believe that the majority of thyroid patients do better, have more effective results, and are far more protected from any over-stimulation and any hyperthyroid symptoms or signs, with multi-dosing of T3. There are always going to be exceptions to that and I wrote this in the above text in my original draft of Recovering with T3 – the text is still the same as it was back in 2011.

12. MORE ON MULTI-DOSING OF T3

A few years ago, I wrote an article explaining why T3 (Liothyronine) is best taken in multiple doses during the day. This article is a follow up to that one, based on a series of questions and answers that happened recently between a thyroid patient and myself. You may find it interesting.

Patient:

Just something I'm curious to know. I have read that the half-life of T3 is between 6-8 hours. How does it maintain an optimal body temperature over 24 hours if that half-life is correct? Thank you.

Paul:

The blood half-life is about 24 hours. However, most people feel that a T3 dose only seems to last 4-8 hours. The blood half-life is largely irrelevant apart from lab testing considerations.

When someone takes a reasonable sized T3 dose, for example 10 to 25 mcg of T3, the FT3 peaks in the blood during the first couple of hours of swallowing it. The T3 begins to enter the cells and connects with the thyroid receptors in the cell nuclei. This begins to increase the rate of gene transcription within the chromosomes of the cell nucleus. As more T3 arrives from the dose, the rate of gene transcription increases. This makes the cell function properly and produce the proteins that it is supposed to. Even when the blood FT3 levels eventually begin to fall after 6 to 10 hours the effect on the cell nuclei continues.

One dose of T3 per day, taken at the size it would need to be to facilitate enough T3 to keep the cells working for 24 hours, is usually far too large for most people to deal with and some people have a much faster clearance of T3 which also makes it difficult to cope with one dose.

However, 2 to 4 doses over the day are usually enough to ensure that more T3 begins to rise in the blood again before the cell nuclei have lowered the rate of gene transcription – thus allowing the cells to chug along at a nice rate, even though the blood levels might fluctuate.

So, this is all about what happens in the cells and nothing at all about the blood levels. None of the interesting action can be measured directly unless we dissected you! All we can do is measure the effect of the T3 - hence signs and symptoms are our best assessment of how the cell nuclei are getting along. See my books for more about using signs and symptoms and managing T3 dosing (and the dosing of the various thyroid medications).

This is also why multi-dosing of T3 works so well and can work far better than slow release T3 when someone is using a good amount of T3 or T3-Mostly or T3-Only.

But basically, we can do really well over 24 hours once the cell nuclei have got their momentum up with the T3 doses and have the right rate of gene transcription in process. Yes, it can go a little slower during the night while we sleep but that is fine as we are not as active. Some need more T3 in the night to allow the pituitary to function well enough to make cortisol (hence the Circadian T3 Method – see my books for more on CT3M).

I hope that explains it.

Patient:

It's very nice to have this explanation. What I do not understand is, what is the blood FT3 doing?

Paul:

The blood FT3 is doing absolutely nothing. T3 does nothing until it is transported to the cells. Most of its work happens at the cell nuclei and also at the mitochondria. When someone has no T4, the T3 can also operate at the cell wall thyroid receptors. But in the blood - nothing at all. The T3 just circulates so that it can reach the cells of the tissues and organs throughout the body.

This is the problem with doing blood testing. Blood testing is a kind of surrogate measure of what might be happening at the cell nuclei. But we do not know how effective the transport into the cell nuclei through the cell wall is. We do not know how easily the T3 can reach the nuclear thyroid receptors.

But doctors think they can measure FT3 and FT4 and say we are ok - just based on a poor surrogate measure. Even though our signs and symptoms might suggest we are very hypothyroid still. Some doctors even think that TSH is a surrogate measure for FT4 and FT3 and rT3 – which is even more silly. Some do not even measure the active hormone FT3. The entire current paradigm of endocrinology practice is really flawed.

This is why my books focus on the use of signs and symptoms, with blood tests giving only an indication that dosage changes are moving things in the right direction. Even aiming for specific blood test targets of FT3 in the range or rT3 in the range is nuts. We do not know what this is translating to in terms of cellular effectiveness of T3 for an individual.

Some thyroid patients seem to put so much trust in their blood test results and think searching for some magic numbers for FT4 and FT3 is what they need to do. But these results vary from time to time and they really are only shadows of what the real picture is within the cells and the cell nuclei.

Patient:

Thank you for this extended explanation. When someone is on quite a lot of T3 they often have to avoid taking the medication for many hours prior to any FT3 test, just to avoid the FT3 result being over range and scaring the doctor, thus having their T3 dosage reduced. A question I have always had, is, why would we need our FT3 to be this high at all?

Paul:

The blood levels do not matter, especially when measured too close to a T3 dose. The FT3 does not do anything in the blood. If your signs and symptoms are fine then you're pretty much in good shape. FT3 fluctuates far too much after a T3 dose is taken and it can get very high for several hours before it eventually falls again. The lab ranges are designed for healthy people and those on T4 medication, so they are not really suitable for those on mostly T3 treatment when FT3 levels fluctuate violently in the blood after T3 doses.

Patient:

So, it's okay if we walk around every day with an FT3 level ABOVE range (if we feel good)? The only reason we disguise that is for the purpose of keeping the doctor happy?

Paul:

Yes this is true for some people, especially if they are taking a lot of T3 medication. If their signs and symptoms show no evidence of being hyperthyroid at all, then testing FT3 within hours of taking a T3 dose and finding it high is not a concern. If I tested my FT3 within 12 hours of a T3 dose, it would be around 9 to 10 and my local reference range is 3.4 - 6.7. So, I tend to leave 18 to 24 hours and test trough levels, by which time my FT3 is in range. Some thyroid patients may need to leave longer to get both FT3 and TSH in range. It is best to test this privately first – to avoid nasty surprises and having your much needed medication level reduced.

But you need to be certain your signs and symptoms are good and not suggesting that you are on too much thyroid medication. These include blood pressure, heart rate and body temperature. Checking blood calcium is also good as too much T3 can raise it. An ECG (EKG) is a good idea too during the period of titrating your T3 dose and maybe occasionally thereafter.

These comments would be heretical on many thyroid groups by the way. Even many of the patient groups have been conned into thinking they have to adhere to thyroid lab tests and ranges that are designed for healthy people or those on T4 based thyroid medication. The people in these patient groups often talk about being in the upper quartile for FT3 or lower half for rT3, but they are still playing the lab test game that the endocrinologists and doctors have told us we need to abide by – even if this keeps many thyroid patients in a permanent symptomatic state of hypothyroidism.

Patient:
Last question. We have discussed FT3 a lot, what about TSH level, especially for those taking T3. Is it ok for TSH to be very low – as a lot of doctors want you to reduce thyroid medication when it is?

Paul:
If FT3 is not high, and you have hypothyroid symptoms remaining, you are not hyperthyroid. If FT3 is low and you still have hypo symptoms then you cannot be hyperthyroid – regardless of TSH.

What about people with central hypothyroidism that have a pituitary gland that never has anything but low TSH? Do those people have hyperthyroidism even though their FT3 is low? No of course they do not. Doctors always work on the assumption that the pituitary is perfectly accurate. The scientific reality is completely different.

The pituitary gland is a very small spherical gland that has only the view of the FT4 and FT3 that flows into it in the bloodstream. It is also one of the best converters of FT4 to FT3 in the body as it makes both the D1 and D2 deiodinase enzymes. The pituitary has the highest concentration of FT3 out of all the glands and tissues in the body. So, the pituitary's only view on your thyroid status is what it sees inside its own little sphere and it has no idea if the rest of your body is hypo or hyper. The pituitary gland cannot see inside your brain, your liver, your digestive system, your cold feet and hands etc.

In addition to the above, every other gland, organ, body tissue we have can have malfunctions. We might need to wear glasses, or hearing aids. We have digestive system disorders, liver issues, thyroid gland issues, diabetes, joint problems… you get the picture. Why do doctors think the pituitary gland, with its already extremely limited perspective, can always be absolutely spot on correct? Nonsense, it is not always correct.

Plus, when people take thyroid medication, and especially T3, this changes the normal balance of free hormone levels in order to compensate for any lost conversion ability of T4 to T3. This also confuses the normal algorithm the pituitary uses to assess the hormones and produce a TSH level. The more T3 we take, the more likely TSH will be suppressed. It just is not designed to work like this. The level of TSH produced, even by a non-malfunctioning pituitary gland is designed for those with healthy thyroid glands and normal-for-them thyroid hormone levels. TSH needs to be ignored to a certain extent when someone is on thyroid meds. This is especially true if the person is still hypothyroid and has low / sub-optimal FT3, or they are on a fair amount of Liothyronine (T3). Even on T4-based meds, with poor conversion, the T4 dosage often has to be raised very high in order to create enough FT3 to stop the patient being hypothyroid. TSH is often suppressed in these cases too.

Many patients can never get well and be on enough thyroid medication if TSH is used to limit their medication level.

Even given the above arguments, patients still occasionally ask me for peer-reviewed research papers that show why a low TSH is safe. It might seem a reasonable question on the surface, but when you think more deeply about it, several aspects are problematic:

- Peer review is no longer a guarantee of the quality of the research and the experimental quality.
- Most research on suppressed TSH requires high levels of thyroid hormones to do the suppression. The contention by many researchers, and myself, is that it is excess thyroid hormone that causes issues like atrial fibrillation (AFib) and bone loss, not low TSH. So, any experiments done like this must be immediately discounted.
- There is already research that shows that low TSH itself is not an issue.
- The only proper experiment with humans to see if low TSH causes issues in a population would be to engineer low TSH in a set of subjects that have normal-for-them thyroid hormone levels.

  So, this would involve having two sets of subjects:

  a) a set of control subjects with in-range TSH and normal-for-them thyroid hormones, and

  b) a set of subjects with TSH levels engineered to be suppressed to zero, whilst their thyroid hormone levels are artificially maintained at the normal-for-them levels. Now, whilst some medications are known to lower TSH, e.g., steroids, they are unlikely to suppress TSH, plus they have effects on the heart and bones independently. So, the only way I can think of to do this would be to surgically change the pituitary gland to have no TSH generating capability, without affecting other hormones. This is both unethical and near impossible to do.

Apart from hyperthyroidism, one of the reasons that some doctors have jumped to the conclusion that there is a link between low TSH and bone turn-over is because bone cells express a functional TSH receptor on their surface. So, the TSH can connect to this receptor. However, any potential TSH effect is interwoven with other signals such as by thyroid hormones and estrogens. There is redundancy in the system. This means that what happens is highly depends on the specific condition and combinations, not a sole influence. It is also very difficult to isolate the TSH effect, because it is not the same for everybody. Furthermore, it is extremely difficult to create a proper experiment when thyroid hormones and estrogens are all perfect yet TSH is low. There has to be an individualised approach, as outlined in the following review – which was peer reviewed btw.:
Hoermann R, Midgley JEM, Larisch R, Dietrich JW. Individualised requirements for optimum treatment of hypothyroidism: Complex needs, limited options. Drugs Context. 2019;8:212597. doi:10.7573/dic.212597

Many of the other so-called 'research papers' on TSH and issues, seem to have just focused on TSH and not accounted for the reason the TSH is suppressed – hyperthyroidism. For the patient with low TSH, the doctors are often not accounting for whether the thyroid patient is well treated for hypothyroidism in terms of the right balance of T4 and T3 medication for them. They also often ignore the status of the patient's estrogen levels.

When a patient is still hypothyroid, or is only on enough thyroid medication to resolve symptoms, and FT3 is not high, then TSH is not something to be concerned over.

See Recovering with T3 for comprehensive information on using T3. See The Thyroid Patient's Manual for a broader review of thyroid hormones, diagnosis and treatment using all the different thyroid medication.

13. THYROID PATIENTS NEED ENOUGH T3 TO RESOLVE THEIR SYMPTOMS

Going by standard laboratory test range guidelines, and just seeing your results fall somewhere within the ranges, is often NOT going to tell you whether you are correctly treated. This is especially true if all your doctor is testing is TSH, or even TSH and Free T4 (FT4).

I frequently hear thyroid patients tell me that their doctor believes that they are properly treated with thyroid medication because they have TSH, FT4 and Free T3 (FT3) results that are within the laboratory reference ranges. I utterly disagree with this view. The patients that contact me usually go on to tell me that they have terrible ongoing symptoms of hypothyroidism.

This situation gets even worse if the doctor concerned is only judging treatment based on TSH and FT4 levels.

I also disagree with the view that there are ideal levels of Free T4 and Free T3 (and even Reverse T3) that can be applied to all thyroid patients.

T3 is the biologically active thyroid hormone. A single molecule of T3 is more than ten times more potent in making our cells work than T4. Recent studies suggest that T3 may well be over fifteen times more potent than T4. T4 is really a pro-hormone that is mainly there to be converted into T3.

T3 binds to the thyroid receptors in the cell nuclei. A thyroid receptor is a bit like a lock and the thyroid hormone is a bit like a key. There are multiple thyroid hormone receptors in the nucleus of each cell and in the many mitochondria, which make the energy needed for the cell.

Thyroid hormone is mostly bound to protein but some is 'free' which means it is unbound. When thyroid hormones are unbound/free, they are able to pass through the membranes into the cells. Only FT3 binds in great numbers to the nuclear thyroid receptors, but FT4 can be converted into FT3 within the cells. However, some people do not convert enough FT4 into FT3. We only feel well when enough FT3 is available to both the cell nuclei and mitochondria.

FT3 operates genomically at the cell nucleus, which means that it has the effect of making some genes go to work and begin their process of making proteins. This is through a process called 'gene transcription', which is the most profound way that thyroid hormone can affect the cell nuclei. T3 makes our cells work in the way they are intended to do.

The above is why it is imperative that FT3 is actually tested and focused on during treatment. FT3 needs to improve during treatment so that the patient's symptoms also improve.

FT4 does not operate genomically at all. FT4 can bind to receptors on the cell wall and acts non-genomically there.

FT4 also enters the cells and can be converted there to either FT3 or Reverse T3 (rT3).

RT3 can be seen as a T3 'blocker' or 'hinderer', i.e., the process that converts FT4 into rT3 can reduce the number of D2 deiodinase enzymes and thus lowers T4 to T3 conversion levels. RT3 is converted from FT4 by D3 deiodinase enzymes. High levels of D3 deiodinases are known to hinder the T3 hormone from binding to receptors in the cell nuclei, hence high rT3 levels can be seen as a hindrance to T3, or as a partial blocker. This is especially true if the individual is still experiencing less than optimal FT3 levels and/or hypothyroidism symptoms.

So, high rT3 can be a marker that T3 action within the cells is being hindered by high levels of D3 deiodinase enzymes.

RT3 is necessary, as it provides a means of clearing excess FT4 and lowering metabolism when needed. RT3 slows metabolic rate by lowering T4 to T3 conversion. When rT3 is being produced at high levels, in someone with a lot of T4, this means the T4 is being converted to rT3 and not to FT3, and so this is a marker that metabolism may be being slowed down. High rT3 does not automatically mean the person will be hypothyroid though. The entire situation with an individual would need to be assessed with rT3 only being a part of the data used.

FT3 speeds up metabolic rate.

RT3 is not a poison and it does not directly block T3 or completely stop T3 binding to the thyroid receptors. This is very misunderstood by a lot of thyroid patients and some doctors. In fact, for most people, rT3 is necessary if they have a lot of FT4 that needs to be cleared by the body - it is a means of removing excess FT4. However, rT3 in itself is absolutely not necessary for the body to function well. Neither is FT4 in many cases. However, rT3 is needed if there is too much FT4 that needs clearance. To clarify this further, people can be very healthy if they have only T3 and absolutely no FT4 or rT3 in their systems. I am one of these people and I know many others like me. The point is that some people process T4 well enough into enough FT3 that having some rT3 is not an issue.

However, some thyroid patients have very sensitive metabolisms and have a hard time coping if rT3 is very high. Some thyroid patients even struggle to cope with T4.

So, rT3 cannot bind to the nuclear receptors but can bind to the receptors in the cell wall. High rT3 levels will also cause fewer D2 and D1 deiodinase enzymes to be produced - so less conversion from T4 to T3.

However, as rT3 rises, as a result of poorer conversion to T3, the D2 and D1 conversion enzyme levels fall, and the D3 enzyme rises. D3 deiodinase actually does hinder T3 from accessing the cell nuclei.

Consequently, rT3 can be viewed as one marker that metabolism may be slowing. The real blocker of T3 is the D3 deiodinases and they may well be high if rT3 is very high. Although low FT3 levels would be the most obvious marker of slow metabolism.

However, there are no hard and fast rules over how high is considered too high for rT3. There are no rules about what the ideal levels are for FT3 or FT4 either. Nor is there a good or bad FT3/rT3 ratio. Good judgement has to be used. The patient's response to treatment has to be considered, i.e., their clinical presentation and the way thyroid lab results change as treatment is altered, needs to be assessed.

Every individual thyroid patient needs his or her levels to be where they need to be for them. Just having thyroid laboratory test results within the reference range is no guarantee that the person is well.

A healthy person will have good levels of FT3, FT4, and rT3, for them as an individual.

To Summarise:

- We cannot measure the levels of thyroid hormones within the cells. A thyroid blood test is just a measure of what is in the bloodstream.
- We cannot see the exact intracellular conversion rate and what level of FT4, FT3 and rT3 exists within the cells.
- We cannot see how well the hormones are transported into the cells, nor how well they bind to the receptors.
- The above information is invisible to thyroid laboratory testing, or any other form of testing currently available.

We know from patient experience that:

- Some people just cannot get well with T4 therapy (Synthroid, Levothyroxine).
- Some people cannot even get well with NDT or T4/T3 – but more do well with this than with T4 alone.
- A few people need T3-Only and almost no rT3 and FT4 in order to recover. This is not just about getting a high enough FT3. It is about having far less (or no) FT4 and rT3.
- Low FT3 or high rT3 can be red flags that the FT4 is not converting well enough. But the signs and symptoms of the patient need to be considered. How the patient's signs and symptoms change and how the lab results change as the treatment is adjusted needs to be assessed properly in order to judge if the treatment is moving in the correct direction.

In my own case, if I add any T4 to my working T3 dosage, my symptoms begin to come back (even if I increase the T3 dosage). I need an FT3 at, or just above, the top of the reference range to feel well. But I also need FT4 near zero and near zero rT3 and near zero TSH. I am not in the slightest bit hyperthyroid or thyrotoxic. Generalisations about a good FT4 and FT3 level can be misleading at times - for some people.

Consequently, for a few people, FT4 also seems to be a hindrance. For some, it is better to shift the balance towards more FT3 and far less rT3 and less FT4.

It ought to be incredibly clear from the above that FT3 absolutely has to be tested when checking thyroid laboratory tests. In an ideal situation, rT3 would also be tested. The full thyroid panel with TSH, FT4, FT3 and rT3 really does provide useful insights, together with the clinical presentation of the patient, as treatment is adjusted.

Hungry for sherbet lemons analogy:

The analogy I have used on forums is based on a shop selling sweets/candy for children. It is not a perfect analogy – but it gets the point across.

Imagine there are three groups of kids.

The group that YOU are in is really keen to buy some sherbet lemons in the sweet shop. The sherbet lemons represent successful binding with cell receptors.

A neighbouring, but friendly group, also wants to buy some sherbet lemons.

However, the bullies from the next town have turned up, and they want to buy some too.

The three groups are all there in the sweet shop.

You have to have enough presence in the sweet shop with all of your mates in your group, to have a chance of getting the attention of the 4 people serving behind the counter.

The bullies (if they turn up in numbers) will just elbow you and jostle you and your mates out of the way – these are like rT3. You hope that you do not have too many of them there.

The neighbouring friendly group are OK, but they have the ability to get in the way, and some might get converted into members of the bully gang.

If you really need to get those sherbet lemons for all of your mates, you really do not want too many of the neighbouring friendly kids turning up, as they can interfere and possibly even join the rival gang – they are like FT4.

Your group (the FT3 kids) really need to be dominating in numbers, if you are really hungry for sherbet lemons and want to buy a lot.

The takeaway is that we each need enough T3, for us as individuals, in order to feel well.

Healthy people, with perfectly normal thyroid hormone function, can tolerate the normal levels of the other hormones. It is Ok to have some bullies (rT3), and a good number of neighbouring friendly kids (FT4), even if they convert to a few more bullies. This is because the normal kids (FT3) are not so desperate for sherbet lemons (getting and being active at the receptors in the cells).

The trick is working out what 'type of kid' each thyroid patient is, and if they are a 'desperate for sherbet lemons kid' or not.

All thyroid patients are different and these differences can be quite significant. We are all unique and need unique solutions that suit us all as individuals.

Doctors and endocrinologists need a full toolkit of all the different thyroid therapies in order to choose the right solution for the individual.

Doctors also need to stop thinking of thyroid patients as all being the same and needing just to have their lab test results somewhere in the reference range. This does not respect the individual nature of every thyroid patient. It is very sad that in many cases, thyroid patients are being deprived of having sufficient T3, which leaves them symptomatic.

14. THE EFFECT OF TSH ON THE CONVERSION OF T4 TO T3

Why do so many thyroid patients feel slightly better for a few days, or a week, after an increase in thyroid medication (T4 or T3), and then they feel just as bad as they did before?

The answer to this question may well be linked to the effect of TSH on the conversion of Free T4 (FT4) to Free T3 (FT3).

The tissues in our body produce deiodinase enzymes that are critical in the conversion of FT4 to FT3.

D2 and D1 deiodinase enzymes convert FT4 to FT3.

D3 deiodinase enzymes convert FT4 to Reverse T3 (rT3).

Although rT3 itself only has a minor effect in reducing the level of D2 enzymes, it is a marker for problems. This is because when rT3 is high, there is likely to be a higher level of D3 enzymes. D3 enzymes prevent T3 from binding with receptors in the cell nuclei, i.e., they block the effect of T3.

Consequently, rT3 can be seen as a 'T3 blocker', but it is really the D3 enzymes that are doing this.

The more D2 and D1 deiodinase enzymes there are, the better the conversion rate from FT4 to FT3, i.e., higher FT3. The fewer D2 and D1 deiodinase enzymes there are, the lower the conversion, i.e., lower FT3.

The thyroid gland is also the biggest converter of T4 to T3 in the body. The thyroid gland produces less of its own T4 and T3 when TSH goes lower. The thyroid produces more T4 and T3 when TSH is higher.

Importantly, the thyroid also makes fewer D2 and D1 deiodinase enzymes when TSH is lower, and more enzymes when TSH is higher.

So, the conversion rate of T4 to T3 within the thyroid gland is lower with lower TSH. The conversion rate of T4 to T3 within the thyroid gland is higher with higher TSH. TSH is also used to regulate conversion rate within other tissues of the body.

Researchers call the process of adjusting the level of deiodinase enzymes up-regulation (making more) or down-regulation (making fewer).

Note: According to thyroid researchers, is it likely that there are many other tissues with TSH receptors. The cells of the heart, fat, bone and brown adipose tissue all have TSH receptors, and it is likely that more locations will be discovered over time. All of these tissue types will be subject to up-regulation and down-regulation of T4 to T3 conversion through the level of TSH.

What are the Implications?
What happens if a patient adds more T4 medication?

After an increase in T4 medication, the effect will usually be that the level of TSH over the next few days will tend to be lower. This effect may take several days to occur after an increase.

Until this change in TSH occurs, the patient will have more FT4 as a result of the increase in T4 medication. This increase in FT4 should produce more FT3. It ought to result in an improvement in the well-being of the thyroid patient.

However, as TSH lowers, this will tend to cause a lowering of the FT4 to FT3 conversion rate. So, after a few days, the FT3 level lowers again. This often leaves the poor thyroid patient right back where they started and feeling poorly again. It can bring FT3 down to where it was to start with, or even slightly lower. Do you recognise that pattern?

This entire theory does not apply to those patients who respond well to T4 medication, as these patients convert FT4 very well and can cope well with FT4 in their bodies.

However, for those that do not do well with T4 medication, this should go a long way to explain this phenomenon.

What happens if a patient adds some T3 medication?

The same thing occurs when T3 medication is added alongside T4 medication.

When a thyroid patient begins to add T3 to T4 medication, the first thing that happens is that free T3 levels increase. Lo and behold! FT3 levels rise and the thyroid patient feels better!

This is not a surprise. This improvement can last for 3 days, 5 days or even a little longer. It rarely lasts beyond this.

Thyroid patients often expect the improvement they feel when they add T3 to their T4 medication to LAST. It is a top-up of T3 after all - why should it not last? The thyroid patients experiencing this feel encouraged. Finally, this is an improvement in how they feel. They think that, finally, they are on the road to recovery.

However, it often does not last, due to the control system that is in place.

The lowering of TSH that comes with the increase in FT3 level, lowers the conversion rate of FT4 to FT3.

Consequently, for those patients who rely on some T4 medication (or some natural thyroid medication or some T4 from their own thyroid gland), adding T3 medication can create an initial great result. This is frequently followed after a short time by lower conversion of FT4 to FT3.

The net result is often a good improvement of symptoms, followed by FT3 dropping to a level that is just as low as it was to begin with. The initial improvement in symptoms is then undone and the patient is back to where they started. Is this a familiar pattern?

This is a frequent occurrence. It seems to occur in the majority of cases of thyroid patients who add some T3 medication to their existing T4 medication.

This mechanism is important to be aware of and can make all the difference in getting thyroid hormone dosage correct for the person. It can actually be an encouraging pattern, because it points the way forward to the real solution.

Excluding other common problems may be helpful. Running the full iron panel is a good idea. Having the cortisol saliva test and 8:00 am morning cortisol blood test is also sensible. Testing other nutrients that might be low like B12, vitamin D etc. may also be required.

However, if adding some T3, results in a clear improvement that then disappears, one has to suspect the above mechanism is operating.

What can be done to improve things?

Do not get disheartened. You already have your clue that you need a higher FT3!

Slowly increasing the T3 content of thyroid medication, using 2-4 divided doses, can frequently resolve the problems. The T3 content may sometimes be T3 or NDT (depending on which is most appropriate).

It may also be VERY necessary to reduce the amount of T4-based medication that you are taking and increase the T3 medication. This can switch the balance to more T3, without having the same suppressive effect on TSH. Lowering the T4 medication, means less FT4 will be available to be converted into rT3.

In addition, when TSH is fully suppressed, the mechanism ceases to operate (TSH cannot get lower) and further additions of T3 begin to actually add FT3.

Note: research has now shown that a suppressed TSH when on thyroid treatment is acceptable. It does not automatically mean the person is hyperthyroid or thyrotoxic. A suppressed TSH in a thyroid patient under treatment is an entirely different situation to a patient who is not on thyroid medication.

The Thyroid Patient's Manual covers both the mechanism described here and the research explaining that a suppressed TSH is not a concern when a thyroid patient is taking thyroid medication.

Sometimes the rT3 level of the patient is too high, and bigger reductions of T4 are needed.

It is a balancing act, but being aware of how the mechanism works is a real help when trying to add T3 to T4 meds.

Knowledge is power! In this case, it helps to set expectations and helps patients and doctors understand the response and what the next steps might be.

Here are some research studies that support the above:

"Effect of thyrotropin on conversion of T4 to T3 in perfused rat liver" Ikeda, K., Takeuchi, T., Ito, Y., Murakami, I., Mokuda, O., Tominaga, M., Mashiba, H. Life Sciences, Volume 38, Issue 20:1801-1806, 1986
http://www.ncbi.nlm.nih.gov/pubmed/3010024

"Effect of TSH on conversion of T4 to T3 in perfused rat kidney" Ikeda, T., Honda M., Murakami, I., Kuno, S., Mokuda, O., Tokumori, Y., Tominaga, M., Mashiba, H. Metabolism, Volume 34, Issue 11:1057-1060, 1985.
http://www.ncbi.nlm.nih.gov/pubmed/4058310

"Effects of Thyrotropin on Peripheral Thyroid Hormone Metabolism and Serum Lipids" Beukhof, Massolt, Visser et al. Thyroid. 2018 Feb;28(2):168-174. doi: 10.1089/thy.2017.0330. Epub 2018 Feb 1
https://pubmed.ncbi.nlm.nih.gov/29316865/

I mention the mechanism of TSH affecting T4 to T3 conversion and the above research in Recovering with T3. I have also successfully used this knowledge for many years when helping thyroid patients.

Note: These research references are based on isolated, perfused rats' livers and kidneys. Perfused means that the livers and kidneys are being maintained outside of the body and are acting only in response to the stimulus provided. This means that any change in FT4 to FT3 conversion that was measured within these tissues, when TSH was injected into them, proved that conversion rate change was entirely due to the change in TSH. Liver and kidney tissues are not supposed to have TSH receptors within them, so more research in this area is required (but it also supports my view that TSH does have a great effect on the regulation of conversion to FT3 and rT3).

The implications of this research fits very well with my own experience of observing the response of patients to treatment. It also confirms why, on so many occasions, my suggested thyroid hormone adjustments for thyroid patients have worked so very well.

15. MORE THYROID MEDICATION MIGHT NOT RAISE FT3 LEVELS

This article may well be one of the most important ones that I have ever written. It is especially relevant to those thyroid patients who plan on introducing some T3 into their treatment.

I discuss the content of the article in Recovering with T3, and even more so in The Thyroid Patient's Manual. However, this article devotes a lot more space to this important topic.

Why do I say it is one of the most important things that I have written? When thyroid patient's medication is being adjusted, it may be that some extra T4 medication or a little T3 medication might be added. It frequently takes a knowledgeable thyroid patient a long time to persuade their doctor, or endocrinologist, to consider adding some T3 thyroid hormone.

However, whether it is T4 or T3 that is added, the patient may get some benefit for a short time and then the symptoms return and they often feel just as bad as before the change. In some cases, there may not even be any benefit, or symptoms might quickly worsen.

The next meeting with the doctor frequently prompts the response, "Well, I did say that your thyroid hormones are already optimal", or "I told you that the T3 would not make any difference".

In defence of the doctors, or endocrinologists, some may simply not know any better. They do not understand what is going on, because no one has explained it to them.

This article explains WHY the change in thyroid medication can FAIL, and HOW to FIX it. As such, it is VERY IMPORTANT, as this occurs VERY FREQUENTLY.

Sometimes 2 + 2 does not equal 4 when dealing with thyroid hormones.

This article is relevant to those patients who are trying to feel healthier by increasing their thyroid medication, but find that this does not seem to work and can sometimes even make their results worse than they were before.

It also applies to those who are beginning to receive thyroid hormone treatment.

Patients that have ongoing hypothyroid symptoms often need a higher FT3 level. This usually needs to be achieved by raising thyroid medication. However, there are some things to be aware of that may help avoid confusion and enable the patient to make the correct choices.

The typical pattern.

I have frequently observed two types of confusing responses that may follow an increase in any type of thyroid medication:

1. Some patients may feel a lot better immediately. This can be more obvious when someone adds T3/Liothyronine. The individual is often convinced that this increase is going to be wonderful for them and that they will now continue to feel so much healthier. However,

after 3-5 days, this initial benefit can disappear and they feel just as bad as they did beforehand.

2. For some patients, an increase in T3 thyroid medication may make the patient feel more hypothyroid very quickly. This can also be due to the same mechanism as in 1.

Sometimes, when patients in either of these categories repeat their laboratory tests, they find that FT3 has not increased and it can even be lower than it was to begin with. Why is this?

This pattern is easy to understand when you realise that the conversion rate of FT4 to FT3 is not fixed - it is variable and regulated and different by individual. I hope that this article will help you to understand why this can happen and how to avoid it.

Conversion from T4 to T3.

Only unbound (free) thyroid hormones are able to enter our cells. Therefore, only Free T4 (FT4) and Free T3 (FT3) can enter cells. Once inside the cell walls, some of the FT4 will be converted to additional FT3.

FT4 to FT3 conversion occurs within every cell of the body. Most of the T3 in the blood comes from conversion within the cell walls of the thyroid gland, liver, kidneys, peripheral tissues, and the gastrointestinal tract.

All cells depend on taking some FT3 from the bloodstream and/or taking in FT4 and converting it to FT3. The cells vary substantially in their ability to convert FT4 to FT3, depending on what tissue they are part of.

This process of conversion requires the removal of an iodine atom from an FT4 molecule, so it is referred to as deiodination. There are enzymes produced in certain tissues (cells of the body), called deiodinase enzymes. It is through the action of two of these enzymes (D1 and D2 deiodinase) that FT4 is converted to FT3.

The brain, pituitary, heart, thyroid gland and skeleton muscle (peripheral tissues) use D2 to convert FT4 to FT3. The liver, kidneys and thyroid gland use D1.

D2 is significantly more efficient in converting FT4 to FT3, than D1. However, D1 deiodinase is very important in the clearance of Reverse T3 (rT3) by the liver. The liver clears rT3 through the deiodination of rT3 into T2, then T1 and T0 (which is excreted within a day). In some people, genetic defects associated with these enzymes can hamper conversion from FT4 to FT3, and rT3 clearance.

The thyroid gland contributes about 25% of our circulating T3. This occurs partly through T3 production and mostly through FT4 to FT3 conversion within the thyroid. Consequently, the thyroid production of T3, and its conversion of FT4 to FT3, provide a large proportion of the available FT3 in the body. Even if the thyroid gland produced no hormones of its own, it would still convert some of the FT4, that is present in the blood that flows through it, into FT3. The thyroid gland is like a little machine that sits in the blood flow, converting FT4 to FT3.

FT4 to FT3 conversion requires adequate amounts of the right deiodinase enzymes. These enzymes are heavily dependent on the mineral selenium in their construction. Consequently, it is important to have enough selenium in the diet or through supplements. The FT4 to FT3 conversion process is also dependent on levels of B12, zinc, ferritin, and iodine.

D3 deiodinase enzymes convert FT4 into Reverse T3 (rT3). Although rT3 itself only has a minor effect in reducing the level of D2 enzymes, it is a possible marker for problems. This is because when rT3 is high, there is likely to be a higher level of D3 enzymes. D3 enzymes hinder FT3 from binding with receptors in the cell nuclei, i.e., they block the effect of FT3. In some ways, rT3 can be seen as a 'T3 blocker', but it is really the D3 enzymes that are doing this. If the thyroid patient is not improving in terms of their symptoms after thyroid medication raises, and rT3 appears to be rising without much improvement in FT3, then this suggests that the T4 medication may not be converting well to T3.

Both the levels of TSH and of FT3 have an effect on the regulation of the deiodinase enzymes and therefore on conversion rate.

Let me deal with TSH first. The thyroid gland has TSH receptors within it. The thyroid uses TSH to regulate its production of T4 and T3. The thyroid produces less of its own T4 and T3 when TSH goes lower. The thyroid produces more T4 and T3 when TSH is higher.

Importantly, the thyroid also makes fewer D2 and D1 deiodinase enzymes when TSH is lower, and more enzymes when TSH is higher. So, the conversion rate of FT4 to FT3 within the thyroid gland is lower when TSH is reduced. The conversion rate is higher with higher TSH. Researchers call the process of adjusting the level of deiodinase enzymes up-regulation (making more) or down-regulation (making fewer).

The takeaway here is that the more D2 and D1 deiodinase enzymes there are, the better the conversion rate from FT4 to FT3, i.e., more FT3 is produced from conversion of FT4. The fewer D2 and D1 deiodinase enzymes there are, the lower the conversion, i.e., less FT3 is produced from conversion of FT4. This is the process that up-regulates and down-regulates conversion. So, the conversion rate is not fixed at all - it is variable and regulated.

The thyroid is not the only tissue which has TSH receptors. There is evidence that brown adipose tissue, the heart, bones and fat tissue also contain TSH receptors. Some research studies strongly suggest that TSH also regulates FT4 to FT3 conversion in the liver and kidneys. So, many of the body's organs and tissues also up-regulate and down-regulate their FT4 to FT3 conversion rate with higher or lower TSH level. Less FT3 will be produced from FT4 conversion when TSH is lower, and more FT3 will be produced from FT4 conversion when TSH is higher.

According to thyroid researchers, is it likely that there are more tissues in the body with TSH receptors, and it is likely that these will be uncovered over time.

TSH is not the only factor involved in how the cells decide to regulate conversion. As FT3 levels increase D2 enzymes are down-regulated, and D3 enzymes are up-regulated, so conversion rate from FT4 to FT3 is lowered and conversion rate from FT4 to rT3 is increased. As FT3 levels fall, the D2 enzymes are up-regulated, and the D3 enzymes are down-regulated, thus increasing FT4 to FT3 conversion and lowering FT4 to rT3 conversion.

Conversion from FT4 to FT3, and from FT4 to rT3, is regulated and variable. Conversion rate is different from person to person. Conversion rate also varies for an individual person during the day, and this conversion rate changes with the addition of thyroid medication.

I attach research references at the end of this article for those of you who wish to see even more detail.

The above is the background technical information. What is more interesting is how this information can be used and what it means for treatment.

What are the implications?
What happens if a patient adds more T4 medication when their TSH is not fully suppressed yet?

After an increase in T4 medication, the FT4 will accumulate to create a higher FT4 level over the next 4-8 weeks. Much of this FT4 change will occur during the first few weeks. TSH is likely to fall slightly. It may only be a small change but it is often significant. Most of the reduction in TSH will happen over the first weeks because that is when the biggest rise in FT4 will occur.

Until this change in TSH occurs, the patient will have more FT4, as a result of the increase in T4 medication, and this should produce a little more FT3. With a slight increase in FT3, the patient may feel an improvement in well-being. We know that FT3 is the active thyroid hormone, and that research has shown that FT3 is the only thyroid laboratory test result that rises when symptoms improve.

However, the lowering of TSH, and any increase in FT3, will tend to induce a reduction in the rate of conversion of FT4 to FT3 (due to the effect on down-regulation of the deiodinase enzymes described above). The production of T4 and T3 by the thyroid gland will also reduce due to the reduction of TSH. So, any initial improvement in the FT3 level will then reduce, and more of the FT4 will go into rT3 instead.

So, as a result of the increase in T4 medication, the conversion rate of FT4 to FT3 will often become lower, as the T4 medication increase begins to raise FT4. Any initial increase in FT3, may then be lost.

Consequently, after a few days, or a week of feeling better, the patient is often right back where they started and feeling poorly again.

Do you recognise that pattern?

For some patients, the regulation of conversion can act much faster. Even within hours of an increase in thyroid medication (especially T3), their conversion rate can lower. It is very patient specific. The person can either feel better, the same as they were before, or they can feel even more hypothyroid.

There are solutions and I will come to that in a moment.

Please do not make the mistake that the pituitary must know exactly what it is doing and will ensure that we have the perfect levels of FT4 and FT3, as this is simply not true. The pituitary gland is perfectly capable of lowering TSH, even when the person still does not have enough FT3. In actual fact, a healthy thyroid gland is highly involved in ensuring the person has the right level of FT3 for them. Once the thyroid is not functioning well, the pituitary gland cannot be relied upon to compensate for that. This is a common misunderstanding. The level of TSH is not infallible, as a healthy thyroid gland is critical to good balance of thyroid hormones in the body (homeostasis is how the thyroid researchers refer to this balance).

What happens if a patient adds some T3 medication?

The same mechanism occurs when a little T3 is added alongside T4 medication. But the results can be even more pronounced.

When a thyroid patient begins to add T3 to T4 medication, in most cases, the first thing that happens is that FT3 levels increase.

FT3 levels rise and the thyroid patient often feels better! This is not a surprise, as T3 is the biologically active thyroid hormone. This improvement can, in some cases, last for 2 to maybe 7 days. The improvement can be very quick and be more obvious than when T4 medication is increased, because the extra FT3 is immediate.

But the improvement is often not sustained. It is a top-up of T3 after all, so why should it not last?

The reason it frequently fails to last is due to the mechanism that I have explained above.

The lowering of TSH that comes with the increase in FT3, lowers the conversion rate of FT4 to FT3 (with more FT4 going into rT3). The extra FT3 alone, will also down-regulate conversion rate from FT4 to FT3. Consequently, for those patients who rely on some T4 medication (or some natural thyroid medication, or some T4 from their own thyroid gland), adding T3 medication can create an initially excellent result, which is then followed, after some time, by a lower conversion rate of FT4 to FT3. The circulating FT4 thyroid hormone begins to fail to convert to as much FT3 anymore. You have added extra T3, gained FT3, only to have lost the extra FT3 due to worsening conversion.

The net result is often a good improvement of symptoms, followed by a slow deterioration of symptoms, back to the situation they were in, prior to the added T3. This often happens over a period of a week or so. Note: for those thyroid patients who are adding only small doses of T3, the addition of the T3 might be met by an immediate down-regulation of conversion. This can leave the patient no better than they were before adding the T3 and in some cases they can be even more hypothyroid.

Some of you reading this may have added T3 thyroid medication and felt that increase in FT3, but then after some days, you may have found yourself back where you started in terms of symptoms.

This is a very frequent pattern.

For some patients, the worsening of FT4 to FT3 conversion can occur very quickly, and they can feel far more hypothyroid, without ever having experienced any benefit from the added T3.

This mechanism is important to be aware of and can make all the difference in getting thyroid hormone dosage correct for the person.

Unfortunately, all too often, a thyroid patient has persuaded their doctor to allow them to add some extra T3. When they go back and say that it has not made any difference, the doctor just tells them that they did not expect it to, or that the T3 just does not suit them! Frequently, the doctor takes this result and concludes that the person did not even need any extra T3. The T3 prescription may be stopped and the trial is over. This happens very frequently.

However, if adding some T3 results in a clear improvement that then disappears, one has to suspect the above mechanism is operating. If the person feels more hypothyroid quickly, and signs and symptoms also suggest they are more hypothyroid, then the mechanism described here has to be suspected.

In fact, I see this pattern as being very helpful!

This pattern of events is a huge clue that the patient does need higher FT3! So, it should be seen as encouraging and not disheartening.

What can be done if this pattern of feeling better, then worse again after a thyroid increase, happens to you?

Excluding other common problems may be helpful. Running the full iron panel is a good idea. Having a cortisol saliva test and an 8:00 am morning cortisol blood test is also sensible. Testing other things that might be low like B12, folate, vitamin D, etc. can uncover other important issues. See Article 2 in Chapter 10 on B12, as low B12 is a much misunderstood and important issue.

If the patient is on T4-Only medication (e.g., Synthroid or Levothyroxine), one approach is to continue to increase the T4. Eventually, TSH may get sufficiently low, that an increase of T4 begins to provide extra FT3. The success of this will depend on how well the patient converts FT4 to FT3, and whether the doctor is going to allow TSH to go low. I discuss the controversy around low TSH in Chapter 6.

If T3 medication has been added, a good way forward is to slowly increase the T3 content of the thyroid medication using 2-4 divided doses. This can frequently resolve problems.

Eventually, the addition of the T3 is sufficient to actually add and retain extra FT3. The T3 content may sometimes be T3 or NDT (depending on which is most appropriate).

It may also be VERY necessary to reduce the amount of T4-based medication that you are taking, whilst increasing the T3 medication. This can switch the balance to more T3, without having the same suppressive effect on TSH. Lowering the T4 medication, and increasing the T3 medication, can avoid any increase in rT3 (and the presence of more D3 deiodinase enzymes that actually block the effectiveness of the FT3).

When TSH is very low, or when the FT4 to FT3 conversion rate is as low as it is going to get, the mechanism described here ceases to operate. At this point, further additions of T3 begin to actually add FT3. However, if T4 has not been lowered, it is still possible for rT3 to increase substantially.

Sometimes, if the rT3 level of the patient gets very high (a marker of high D3 deiodinase enzyme levels, potentially blocking the effect of FT3), bigger reductions of T4 may be needed.

Sometimes, this lowering, or cutting, of T4 medication, may need to be VERY substantial. I have worked with thyroid patients who clearly have poor FT4 to FT3 conversion and high rT3, and I have had to suggest the T4 content of their medication be reduced by 50%. In some cases, it may need to be a 75% reduction. Patients can be very reluctant to do this. Doctors can be even more reluctant to do this. However, it is often the only way to improve and retain a higher level of FT3, without having rT3 get incredibly high.

It is all about getting the right balance of T4 and T3 medication for the individual thyroid patient.

Importantly, research has now shown that, when on thyroid treatment, a suppressed TSH is acceptable. It does not mean the person is hyperthyroid or thyrotoxic. A suppressed TSH in a thyroid patient under treatment with thyroid medication, is an entirely different situation to a patient who is not on thyroid medication. Unfortunately, many doctors and endocrinologists are still determined that TSH must be in range, even if this keeps the thyroid patient symptomatic and ill.

The Thyroid Patient's Manual covers both the mechanism described here and the research explaining that a suppressed TSH is safe when a patient is on thyroid medication (if there are no symptoms or signs of hyperthyroidism). I also wrote about the mechanism described here when I first released Recovering with T3, albeit far more briefly than covered in this article.

A simple analogy.

If any reader is struggling to take in the above information on the first read, this analogy might help. Imagine a large glass of water that is completely full to the brim, but not quite overflowing yet. If a golf ball is lowered into the glass and falls to the bottom, some of the water will spill over the top of the glass. The water that falls on the surface is displaced by the volume of the golf ball. The only easy way to add the golf ball, without spilling any water, would be to empty some of the water first.

In this analogy, the water is the FT4 and the golf ball is the FT3. The spilt water is the rT3 that is forced out due to the added golf ball (FT3). It is not possible to keep the existing amount of water and yet still add the golf ball, i.e., you often cannot get added FT3, without extra rT3, just by adding T3 to the existing dosage of T4 medication (if conversion is not excellent).

For those thyroid patients that do NOT have an excellent conversion of T4 to T3, their glass is already completely full and adding T3 to any current T4 dose is going to raise rT3 and lower the FT4 to FT3 conversion further. Lowering the T4 dose often makes the addition of T3 more feasible. This might well need to be repeated if more additional T3 is still needed. This is not a perfect analogy but it conveys the essence of the issue and the solution.

Note: MANY thyroid patients have poor FT4 to FT3 conversion.

2 + 2 does not always equal 4 with thyroid hormones.

Adding some T4, or even T3, medication to your existing dosage may not always increase your FT3 level.

However, knowledge is power! In this case, it helps to set expectations. It also helps patients and doctors to understand this response, and if it occurs, to know what the next steps need to be.

It can be a tricky balancing act, but knowing this at the outset should help greatly to get to a working dosage of thyroid medication that alleviates your symptoms - which is what we all want.

Note: Article 21 in this chapter, covers the specific issues associated with introducing T3, or using small doses of T3, which often have poor responses, due to the mechanism described above.

Additional research references:

Experiments have also been done with the livers and kidneys of rats that have been removed from their bodies. The livers and kidneys were kept alive and the experiments suggest that the addition of TSH can also affect conversion rate in these organs:

"Effect of thyrotropin on conversion of T4 to T3 in perfused rat liver" Ikeda, Takeuchi, Ito, Murakami, Mokuda, Tominaga, Mashiba. See: Life Sciences, Volume 38, Issue 20:1801-1806, 1986 http://www.ncbi.nlm.nih.gov/pubmed/3010024

and

"Effect of TSH on conversion of T4 to T3 in perfused rat kidney" Ikeda, Honda, Murakami, Kuno, Mokuda, Tokumori, Tominaga, Mashiba. See: Metabolism, Volume 34, Issue 11:1057-1060, 1985. http://www.ncbi.nlm.nih.gov/pubmed/4058310

Note: in these last two experiments, T4 medication was added to the rats' livers and kidneys. There was a control group of livers/kidneys in which no TSH was added and a group that had TSH added. Upon addition of extra TSH, the level of FT3 in this group increased, suggesting that TSH was affecting the deiodinase up-regulation. Liver and kidney tissues are not supposed to have TSH receptors within them, so more research in this area is required.

This paper highlights that D2 and D3 are expressed in a dynamic balance, in which the expression of one enzyme is regulated in coordination with that of the other, to tightly control intracellular FT3 levels, to provide the cell with what it thinks it requires at the time. So, FT3 level is definitely a factor in how the regulation of conversion is done. Adding T3 medication will change the FT3 content, and very often the FT4 to FT3 regulation, via the deiodinase enzymes, will adjust as a result:

"The deiodinases and the control of intracellular thyroid hormone signaling during cellular differentiation" Monica Dentice a, Alessandro Marsili b, AnnMarie Zavacki b, P Reed Larsen b, Domenico Salvatore a,c, See: Biochim Biophys Acta. 2013 Jul;1830(7):3937–3945. doi: 10.1016/j.bbagen.2012.05.007

URL:https://pmc.ncbi.nlm.nih.gov/articles/PMC3670672/

Note: there are many other research papers that prove that FT4 to FT3 conversion is variable and regulated.

Further research papers illustrating the way in which FT4 to FT3 conversion is not fixed but variable and regulated:

"Homeostatic equilibria between free thyroid hormones and pituitary thyrotropin are modulated by various influences including age, body mass index and treatment" Hoermann, Midgley, Giacobino, Eckl, Wahl, Dietrich, Larisch. See: Clin Endocrinol (Oxf) (2014) 81:907–915. doi:10.1111/cen.12527 https://www.researchgate.net/publication/263321383_Homeostatic_Equilibria_Between_Fre e_Thyroid_Hormones_and_Pituitary_Thyrotropin_Are_Modulated_By_Various_Influences_I ncluding_Age_Body_Mass_Index_and_Treatment

"Recent Advances in Thyroid Hormone Regulation: Toward a New Paradigm for Optimal Diagnosis and Treatment" Hoermann, Midgley, Larisch, Dietrich https://www.frontiersin.org/articles/10.3389/fendo.2017.00364/full

"Relational Stability in the Expression of Normality, Variation, and Control of Thyroid Function" Hoermann, Midgley, Larisch & Dietrich. https://www.frontiersin.org/articles/10.3389/fendo.2016.00142/full

"Relational stability of thyroid hormones in euthyroid subjects and patients with autoimmune thyroid disease" Hoermann, Midgley, Larisch, Dietrich. Eur Thyroid J. 2016;5:171-179. doi:10.1159/000447967 https://www.researchgate.net/publication/306267613_Relational_Stability_of_Thyroid_Hormones_in_Euthyroid_Subjects_and_Patients_with_Autoimmune_Thyroid_Disease

"Triiodothyronine secretion in early thyroid failure: The adaptive response of central feedforward control" Hoermann, Pekker, Midgley, Larisch, Dietrich. Eur J Clin Invest. 2020;50 doi:10.1111/eci.13192 https://pubmed.ncbi.nlm.nih.gov/31815292/

and finally:
"Effects of Thyrotropin on Peripheral Thyroid Hormone Metabolism and Serum Lipids" Beukhof, Massolt, Visser et al. Thyroid. 2018 Feb;28(2):168-174. doi: 10.1089/thy.2017.0330. Epub 2018 Feb 1. https://pubmed.ncbi.nlm.nih.gov/29316865/

16. SLOW RELEASE VERSUS PURE T3 (STANDARD T3/LIOTHYRONINE)

From time to time a thyroid patient may ask me whether slow release T3 or standard T3 (pure T3) should be used for T3 replacement. Slow-release T3 is sometimes referred to as sustained-release T3 or even as SRT3.

There are really two parts to this question:

1. Is standard T3 or slow-release T3 best in general for T3 replacement?
2. Which is best for the circadian T3 method (CT3M)?

Let me answer this by dealing with the general use of T3 separately from that of CT3M.

General Use of T3: Using T3 in the Daytime on Its Own or In Combination with T4 or NDT.

If only a small amount of extra T3 is required, some people can do well with slow-release T3, and others do better with standard T3, i.e., it would be a matter of trying the slow-release T3 and seeing how it worked.

For those people who need much more added T3 (without any T4 medication), there are two goals:

- To avoid causing hyperthyroidism in any of the different tissues of the body due to too much T3, i.e., tissue over-stimulation.
- To use enough T3 to overcome the cellular issues that have caused the problems in the first place. This requires enough T3 to reach the thyroid receptors in the cell nuclei so

181

that the genomic effect of T3 lasts for a long enough time to correct any hypothyroidism but is not too much to cause any hyperthyroidism symptoms. It does not matter whether the blood levels of T3 fluctuate – what matters is getting our cells to work well.

To achieve these two goals, different amounts of T3 may be needed at different times of the day. A lot of people using standard T3, need different sized divided doses at different times of the day. This is so that they receive only as much T3 at any given time as is required, to ensure that it lasts long enough until the next T3 dose, but without causing any signs of over-stimulation.

With slow-release T3 it can be difficult to provide enough T3 without either having too much or too little. It is difficult for most people to find a slow-release dosage that achieves these goals so that they remain euthyroid at most times with no evidence of hyperthyroidism.

Slow release T3 does not release a great deal of actual T3 during a period of one hour. So, for example, 20 mcg of slow-release T3 is far from equivalent of 20 mcg of standard T3 – in fact the experience of other patients would suggest something like 20 mcg of slow-release T3 might only be providing a few micrograms of T3 in an hour – perhaps even less than 5 mcg. This is why many patients on slow-release T3 are actually very under-dosed. However, if the patient cannot tolerate standard T3 for some reason that has not been determined, then slow release-T3 is an option.

In conclusion, some patients do find that slow-release T3 works for them, especially if they do not require very much T3. Others find that they have to have the slow-release T3 compounded differently a few times, in order to find the optimum release rate for them. This process can be quite expensive and time consuming to get right.

For the thyroid patient who simply wants to add a small amount of T3 to a mostly T4 based regime, slow-release T3 may work well though. However, in some cases, when other issues are present, only slow-release may be tolerable, even though finding the right dosage can be difficult.

T3 for Use in The Circadian T3 Method (CT3M).

For the CT3M, there is no question that standard T3, swallowed in one go, is the best way to implement it.

CT3M needs the entire circadian T3 dose to be absorbed as quickly as possible. We want the entire T3 dose to reach the pituitary gland, as fast as possible. We also want to be able to titrate the dose size and the timing of the CT3M dose in order to try to control cortisol levels with as much sensitivity as possible. Slow-release T3 would provide none of this. The CT3M definitely works better with standard T3. Can it work to some extent with slow-release T3? – yes. I have seen this happen. In those situations, when a patient cannot cope with standard release T3, a slow-release CT3M dose is still worth trying.

I hope this clarifies things for those that may not have been certain.

17. HOW TO GO ABOUT SWITCHING FROM ONE BRAND TO ANOTHER

This is a question that comes up occasionally from thyroid patients.

If someone is on one type of T3 (or even NDT), and it is being taken in several divided doses per day, but the patient needs to change brands for whatever reason, what is the best way to go about this?

Please do not wait until one type of medication runs out, before trying out the new brand! It is definitely a bad idea to accumulate any of a new brand, without testing it to see if it is going to work well. Also, swapping all doses at once is not advisable, as the brands may have different strengths and may even have unwanted side effects.

The advice I always give to thyroid patients is to pick the last dose of the day, and to swap this dose to the equivalent dose size in the new brand. Try this for a week or two, and fine-tune the new brand dose size until it really does perform as well as the current medication – in terms of signs and symptoms. If the new brand works well for the last dose of the day, then apply the same process, one by one, to your other T3 doses. If all goes well, and if you have plenty of your original brand left, then switch back to the original brand and dose sizes to use them up first as their expiry dates are likely to be earlier. Save your new brand with longer expiry dates for later, when your original medication runs out.

It is possible however, that the new medication might not work as well as the original brand. So, giving it at least a few weeks to assess it, is sensible. If the new brand is problematic (perhaps due to a binder or filler), then go back to your pharmacist, or doctor, and tell them quickly, so they can give you a different brand. This is why it is essential to begin testing any new brand quickly, even though you may have plenty of the original medication left. Waiting and using up the original whilst accumulating some of the newer brand of medication is not sensible, and would likely make your doctor and pharmacist upset, if you have to take back a lot of the new brand because you had delayed testing it.

The main thing to do is to start early, well before your old medication has run out.

18. A SMALL PERCENTAGE OF PATIENTS CANNOT COPE WITH ANY LEVOTHYROXINE

This article came out of a conversation with a thyroid patient who was still having some issues when on mostly T3 with a little T4 in the mix. She had improved greatly with the T3, but was not quite at the point she wanted to be.

I related my own story to her. I simply cannot cope with even small amounts of T4 medication, e.g., 5 mcg of T4 begins to make me feel ill after one week, with returning hypothyroid symptoms and signs. This is the case even when my T3 dosage is either kept the same, or lowered or increased. For me, even the smallest amount of T4 medication causes my T3 medication to not work well. This was not T4 brand dependent, as several different brands were tried. I mention this as some patients may react badly to a particular brand due to a filler or binder. This was not the case for me - it was just the T4 content itself.

This issue can also apply to any T4 produced by the thyroid. It does not have to be T4 thyroid medication. Some people simply cannot get well, until the thyroid gland stops making T4. This can often only happen when the patient takes T3 medication at a high enough level that prevents the thyroid gland from making further T4.

I have seen this type of situation many times before. It is very clear to me that some people simply cannot cope with anything but small amounts of T4, and in a few cases, any T4 at all makes them feel worse.

This does not apply to many thyroid patients, but for those who fall into this category, it is important to be aware of. It is also important for all those doctors and patients who push others into having some T4 in their mix, or using NDT, to realise that some patients simply CANNOT cope with T4.

The thyroid patient then asked me about FT3, FT4 and reverse T3 results. She wanted to know if the above issue could still be the case even if the numbers were all within the reference ranges and rT3 itself was not high. She said she was only taking some T4 in order to keep her doctor happy because he felt that everyone needs to have some T4. I told her that this can be the case, even with good results in the ranges.

Laboratory test results do not explain everything. In fact, having 'in range' lab results simply does not work for some people who have more complicated thyroid hormone metabolic issues. Lab ranges have been developed based on a huge number of people. Those patients who have unusual issues may not feel well when their results fit into the standard reference ranges. Lab test results show blood levels of thyroid hormones. They cannot show exactly how effective the active thyroid hormone T3 is at the nuclear thyroid receptors and the mitochondria – there is currently no blood test that can show this.

Everyone need to have enough T3 thyroid hormone, for them as an individual, working at the cell nuclei.

T4 does not work at the cell nuclei and it does very little. The main value of T4 is to be converted into T3. Only the T3 thyroid hormone binds to the nuclear thyroid receptors, as it is the active thyroid hormone. For example, those people with absolutely dreadful FT4 to FT3 conversion issues may find T4 leaves them woefully hypothyroid even when combined with T3. Atrophic thyroiditis (AT) is another example of a condition that can make the use of T4 extremely difficult, as it often causes highly variable conversion rates of FT4 to FT3, inducing swings from hypothyroidism to hyperthyroidism.

I explained to the thyroid patient that I did not know that this issue was definitely what was holding her back, simply that it could be.

I do believe that this issue is one of the reasons why a small number of people never fully recover until the very last vestiges of FT4 and rT3 clear out of their systems. I have seen this work successfully many times with thyroid patients on T3-Only therapy. It is not a common issue, but it does apply to some patients.

In my own case, over the past 30 years, I have tested whether I can cope with any T4 medication about ten times. I wanted to do this in case something had changed. Each time I have added even tiny amounts of T4 medication the same thing has happened. This is without reducing the T3 at all. When increasing amounts of T4 were used (with far less T3), I developed very high blood pressure and severe suicidal feelings. So, T4 medication has never worked for me - with any dosage or combination of T4 and T3.

Here is an extract from Chapter 10 in the Recovering with T3 book:

"ATTEMPTING TO USE T4 REPLACEMENT AGAIN

There have been occasions when I wanted to discover whether anything had changed in the way T4 worked in my body. However, whenever I have attempted to use T4 replacement therapy again, it still failed and I quickly became very ill.

T4 still does not suit me – even in small additional amounts to my T3, e.g., 12.5 mcg per day of T4 is not tolerated by me.

T4 in any quantity brings back my hypothyroid symptoms. I am healthy, fit, active and symptom-free whilst on T3 replacement therapy. However, sometimes people express views like, "everyone needs some T4". These types of views are stated from time to time, usually by doctors, but also, sometimes by thyroid patients. Unsurprisingly, the patients concerned are on some form of T4 based medication, and they think everyone else should be taking it too.

Sometimes this viewpoint is based on an old and not especially compelling piece of research that attempts to show that T3 cannot be used in the brain. Then they extrapolate from there that everyone needs T4. This is not the case. One of the big flaws in that type of argument is that people who are living well on T3 alone have not been studied for the very likely compensatory adjustments that the body makes when using T3 on its own.

The second big flaw is that more research is being found all the time to overturn old research. The 'brain requires T4 research' has just been proved wrong in fact. The new research is changing the entire understanding with its discovery of active transporters. There are T3 transporters and they are more active in adult life. So, circulating T3 is a source of T3 for the brain. It is definitely not dependent on T4 in adults. Older assumptions are being proven wrong all the time. This particular assumption had to be wrong anyway – as thousands of people on T3 replacement therapy are well and healthy.

I have used T3 replacement for over thirty years. I know many thyroid patients, who have recovered their health using T3 replacement and have been using it for a long time.

T3 replacement therapy can be a very effective, safe, long-term thyroid hormone treatment."

All of the above may seem a very heretical viewpoint to some thyroid patients who do very well on natural desiccated thyroid or a T4/T3 combination. Even those on only a little T3 and rely on their own thyroid for T4 and T3 may find the above to be far-fetched. All I can say is that I have lived my life in my own body and I know that the above is utterly true. I have also seen it in other thyroid patients who have near-miraculous recoveries when they are on T3-Only and have no T4 left in their systems.

We are not all the same. We have various issues. I am very pro-Levothyroxine (T4-Only) for those patients that convert it well to T3. T4/T3 combinations also work extremely well for many. This article is really just to make it clear how wide the spectrum of needs can actually be. I ask those who think the above is nonsense to try to be more open-minded and not just go on their own experience.

Some people cannot cope with ANY T4 in their system at all. It can be the thing that prevents them from recovering their health. Clearly, very poor conversion from FT4 to FT3 may be a factor for many in the same category. However, I do not rule out other more complicated problems, which may eventually become clear through research.

Finally, one big issue is that doctors and endocrinologists generally have strong views that FT4 levels need to be in range, and T3 medication is not needed. For them, having no T4 meds or having any T3 meds, is tantamount to having your window open at night and encouraging the Boogieman to come in. They cannot cope with the notion of not taking T4 or of taking T3. They have been taught their views in medical school and are usually very rigid in holding this view. This is why some thyroid patients, who feel much better on T3-Only medication, get told by their doctors that they need to have some T4 (even if they do not seem to tolerate T4 medication at all well).

Until medical training begins to acknowledge some of the newer research, the importance of T3, and that thyroid patients are not all the same, then patients will still keep facing archaic views that keep many of them sick.

In general, I still hold the view that T3-Only therapy is the treatment of last resort. I am very positive about the use of T4/Levothyroxine for a lot of thyroid patients who convert T4 well. T4/T3 combination therapy works extremely well for many patients. I just know that some thyroid patients need T3, with no T4 in order to recover.

19. BE PATIENT AND SYSTEMATIC WHEN CHANGING THYROID MEDICATION DOSAGE

During thyroid treatment, when either the medication type or the dosage is being adjusted, it is really important to use a systematic process and to expect that there will be some difficulties along the way.

It is extremely important to have a lot of patience in order to do this well and to find the best solution that fixes your symptoms.

Finding the right type and amount of thyroid medication can take some time and it can involve many small steps towards finding a dosage that works. Sometimes a change is made that makes someone feel worse and this has to then be undone. This should be expected. It is rarely a matter of looking at laboratory test results and simply picking the right solution out of thin air.

Working out what the right thyroid treatment is and finding the right dosage is a process of exploration that often has speed bumps along the way. I provide protocols for determining the right dosage of Levothyroxine (T4), Liothyronine (T3), T4/ T3, and Natural Desiccated Thyroid (NDT) in my book, *The Thyroid Patient's Manual*. I go into far more detail on T3 use, for those that are on mostly T3, or T3-Only, in my book, *Recovering with T3*. The protocols involve working through a process of making medication changes, and then measuring and assessing the response of the body to the changes. This process may have to be repeated many times until real improvement occurs.

I recommend the use of symptoms and signs to track changes in medication and doses. See Article 7 in this chapter.

Some thyroid patients who ask for support in finding the right choice of medication and doses are often **very anxious** and want to get some immediate improvement. Some of them have been looking for solutions for a long time and may have been given a lot of conflicting advice from different doctors, practitioners or other thyroid patients. In a few cases, the struggling thyroid patients may be on far too many medications including adrenal steroids, anti-depressants, and anti-anxiety drugs in addition to the thyroid medications. Often, some of these drugs are completely avoidable and are in fact, causing part of the problem and making it more difficult to adjust the thyroid medication properly.

When a thyroid patient is very anxious, it can be difficult for them to have the patience necessary to change the thyroid medication systematically and assess the response to the change objectively. Sometimes, the unfortunate thyroid patient wants to know that the change is going to work, even before it is made. That is simply not possible to know. Working on finding the right solution for any individual is a process and it takes time. It may involve several steps forward and then a step or two backwards. Even when someone has found an optimal dosage, this might not always remain right for them. The body changes and may require a different thyroid dosage at a later time, in which case more effort would be required to assess this.

The process of improving thyroid medication dosage requires a cool head and the willingness to collect daily data on the body's responses. In my view, basic signs like body temperature changes, blood pressure and heart rate changes are far more objective measures of real progress than just feelings. Some key symptoms like energy level, mental acuity and gut motility are also helpful and are easier to be objective about than other symptoms. This process is unlikely to be quick so, a lot of patience is needed. In some cases, it is critical to assess signs and symptoms frequently during the day in order to work out how thyroid medication doses are affecting the patient. Frequent measurement can show that a thyroid dose is too high, too low, too soon or too late.

I learned this myself the hard way when I was trying to recover from hypothyroidism around thirty years ago. I began using T3 in multi-doses and thought I could manage this using my symptoms. I failed utterly and found myself confused on too many occasions. I gave up trying to do it this way and began tracking signs and symptoms rigorously every day. Frequently, the signs (vitals) told a completely different story to what my feelings were telling me. There were also times when I needed to retrace my steps to a set of doses of T3 that I was using a few weeks earlier, and then try a different set of choices from that point onwards. T3-Only is harder to dose than other thyroid medications but the point still applies that being systematic and having patience is essential in all but the simplest of cases.

So, the worst combination I can think of is that of an anxious thyroid patient, who takes a cocktail of medications and supplements, and who is not being rigorous and systematic and lacks patience. In this situation, the person is likely to chop and change their plans far too often and will likely never find a good solution unless through pure luck. Luck tends not to happen that often in thyroid treatment!

The other way to look at this is to realise that most thyroid patients with medication or dosing issues often took many years to get to this stage. It is unreasonable to expect a quick solution to come without a lot of hard work and diligence.

In my own case, even when I was finally on T3-Only, it still took me three years to get onto the right dosage and a few more years beyond that to recover from ten years of severe ill-health. I only managed to do this by being very patient. I collected signs and symptoms every day and used them to guide me. I am not a naturally patient man – quite the opposite actually. So, this was hard for me. However, I realised that there was no other way that would work. There are no silver bullets when getting thyroid medication sorted. In my case, there were no books or any written work available to help me understand how to use the T3 thyroid hormone. My doctors had no clue how to use it either. I had to learn all of that as I went along. So, I learned the hard way that being patient and systematic was the only way to do it. I put all the lessons I have learned over the years into the pages of all three of my books.

Sometimes it is also important to get off some of the other drugs that thyroid patients may have had suggested to them along the way. Obviously, taking a doctor's advice about this is important.

There is a fable by Aesop, called "The Hare and the Tortoise". The two animals have a race but the hare gets too excited and runs around too much and gets distracted and makes mistakes. The Tortoise just plods on slowly, and systematically, with his goal in mind. In this fable, the tortoise wins the race!

Finding the right dosage and type(s) of thyroid medication for a thyroid patient can be like this Fable. The thyroid patient who is slow, patient and organised usually finds a working dosage of thyroid medication even if it takes a while – just like the Tortoise. The thyroid patient who makes quick changes, or does not analyse enough information (not just thyroid labs), or is not patient and organised, often gets very confused and goes around in circles without finding their solution – just like the Hare.

So, be prepared for a marathon and not a sprint. Use symptoms and signs as a key tool, as well as laboratory test results. Be calm. Anxiety and worry are not your friend. They get in the way of the ability to collect the right data and then to assess it objectively. My books also provide a lot of sensible guidance on how to go about adjusting thyroid medication in a safe, organised and effective way.

Above all, be very patient, slow, careful and systematic, even if this means you remain symptomatic for a little longer than you would like to be. Have expectations that a lot of hard work will almost certainly be needed and that setbacks will inevitably happen on the way. It is better to get there with small, slow steps than not get there at all. Be the tortoise!

20. WHY AVOIDING PANIC AND KNEE-JERK DOSAGE CHANGES IS SO IMPORTANT

Article 19 in this chapter talks about the need to be patient and systematic when managing thyroid treatment. This article goes one step further than that and discusses why avoiding large changes is critical and what problems can ensue if care is not taken.

As thyroid medication is being adjusted, sometimes one or more changes may be made that turn out to have been mistakes. This might mean that a type of thyroid medication has been added, or stopped. More frequently, it is due to an increase in thyroid medication or even a series of increases. Individual changes may have been quite small but collectively, over a few weeks, the overall change in thyroid medication may have been significant enough to now cause issues. The issues might have various symptoms which all add to the anxiety of the patient. They potentially include raised anxiety, tension, tremors, nervousness, sweating and signs that often include raised heart rate (tachycardia), and elevated BP. This is exactly the situation where the need to be patient and systematic is most needed. Unfortunately, it is often the situation when all thoughts of patience and systematic change just get forgotten.

I have been working with thyroid patients for well over fifteen years. In that time, I think rarely a month goes by when I do not get contacted by a thyroid patient who has abandoned patience and then caused more problems for themselves. The most typical situation is when a thyroid patient has been relatively stable and has been slowly adjusting their thyroid medication dosage. This applies to all types of thyroid medication, but medication that includes some T3 is usually the most common source of the problem that I am going to describe.

It may be that the thyroid patient has not realised, from signs and symptoms, that the last one or two dosage changes have not been good and that they have strayed into the territory of being over-stimulated. However, it can just take time for the cumulative effect of several small changes to begin to have an impact. Perhaps, at this stage of adjusting the thyroid medication, a far longer time interval between changes should have been used – I discuss the need for this in my books.

After the most recent thyroid dosage change, the signs and symptoms begin to worsen significantly and 'Boom!', panic sets in. This is absolutely the time that being calm and systematic is most needed.

What is required is:

- Any changes in medication dosage over recent weeks needs to be reviewed.
- The signs and symptoms that were present pre-change and post-change need to be looked at carefully, given the now far worse situation.
- Some change needs to be made to adjust the medication. However, this often only needs to be a retracement to the last successful dosage that the thyroid patient was on. In some cases, two or three small dosage changes may need to be undone.

- Typically, the size of the medication dosage reduction does not have to be large for the symptoms and signs to settle down in some hours or a day or so.

It is important to realise that, for the majority of thyroid patients, elevated heart rate, raised BP or even very uncomfortable symptoms are not dangerous at all, if they are only there for a short space of time.

However, what can sometimes happen is that the thyroid patient thinks that they must stop these symptoms and calm down the signs quickly. So, they may cut their thyroid medication dosage in half or even stop it. This is when things can go very wrong indeed.

A large change in what has been mainly a stable situation makes things very unstable. The sudden drop in FT3 level that often comes when any T3 content is lowered, will cause TSH to rise over the coming days. As TSH rises the cells make more D1 and D2 deiodinase enzymes so the conversion rate from any FT4 to FT3 begins to rise. If the thyroid patient is on any T4-based medication then the conversion rate is now in a state of flux and more FT3 is being generated. If the thyroid patient has some working thyroid tissue, the rising TSH begins to make the thyroid gland more active – this also makes the situation less stable.

So, at this point, the thyroid patient has made a large reduction in their thyroid dosage but this has introduced instability into the system, which is now continuing to occur. Every day following the reduction there can be a different situation and it can be incredibly confusing for the thyroid patient who was only really trying to get back to being stable once again. The thyroid patient may eventually become hypothyroid and think that they have now resolved the crisis. Sometimes, they try and add some of their thyroid medication back in. This can be even more confusing and stressful as they may find that it causes even higher heart rate, BP or worse symptoms than they had to begin with!

It is common for patients to have done something like this, and then one or two weeks later they contact me and are desperate for help, as they do not understand what is going on. They may say to me that they think they have become intolerant or allergic to T3 medication, whereas in actual fact, all they have really done is overreacted, made too big of a change and caused their own system to become highly unstable.

At this stage, when someone has already created an unstable situation, it is important that they get back on most of the medication that they were previously on. The total dosage may well need to be lower than when the symptoms and signs deteriorated, but not dramatically so. Having considered a suitable dosage, my main message is then to tell them to be patient and to wait for their own body to calm down and become stable once again.

Being patient and systematic is critically important when managing thyroid hormone dosage. This is especially true when things go very wrong and bad symptoms and signs begin to occur.

In Article 19 in this chapter, I refer to a famous fable by Aesop, called "The Hare and the Tortoise". The two animals have a race but the hare gets too excited and runs around too much and gets distracted and makes mistakes. The Tortoise just plods on slowly, and systematically, and wins the race. Being the tortoise and not the hare at the time when symptoms and signs have seriously deteriorated is a challenge but invariably it is the right thing to do.

Once a huge dosage change has been made, many aspects of the endocrine system relating to thyroid hormones become highly unstable and can make regaining stability once again a real challenge. This can take weeks to rectify. So, making a smaller adjustment and being patient will often result in the thyroid patient regaining some stability and alleviation of symptoms far faster and far more effectively.

21. SMALL T3 DOSES MAY NOT WORK AND CAN CAUSE WORSE SYMPTOMS

The content of this article is extremely relevant to those thyroid patients who plan on introducing some T3 into their treatment.

Working with so many thyroid patients over the past fifteen years has made me very aware of some of the pitfalls that can happen when someone introduces T3 doses. This is especially true when they already have T4 present in their system. The T4 may be there because they have some remaining thyroid function. However, it is more usually because they are already on some T4 medication but remain with many symptoms of hypothyroidism. They may also have low in the range FT3 and possibly high rT3. So, the patient or their physician, or practitioner, might decide to introduce some T3. I am also assuming that these patients have tested other hormones and nutrients before adding in any T3, and are addressing any issues. This basic testing is outlined in all my books, and it includes things like cortisol, iron, B12 etc.

When T3 is first being introduced, it is best to start with one or two doses of 5 mcg. If I am providing advice, then if the thyroid laboratory test results appear to suggest extremely poor conversion from FT4 to FT3, then I often encourage the patient to reduce the T4 content of their treatment at the same time as adding T3. Some very nervous patients, sometimes want to begin with even smaller doses than 5 mcg.

Whatever the starting T3 dose sizes are, the range of response to them can be quite varied by patient:

- In some cases, even small introductory doses of T3, do immediately benefit the thyroid patient. For many, this benefit can continue and the T3 dosage may be slowly titrated until an effective T3 dosage is achieved.

- More often in my experience, the thyroid patient may feel some immediate benefit which lasts for a few days. This can often be followed by a relapse to their previous symptoms. The patient may have felt elated with the response but is then deflated that it is not going to work. This type of response can even occur with T3 doses of 10 mcg or more, i.e., there is improvement but after some days this improvement vanishes. This is always an encouraging sign to me, as I understand it and know how to help the patient make progress.

- For some thyroid patients, small T3 doses like 5 mcg or 2.5 mcg may elicit no noticeable response at all in the symptoms or signs of the person.

- The last scenario is that, when the small doses of T3 are introduced, the thyroid patient's health further deteriorates. Even T3 doses of 5 mcg, 2.5 mcg or less, can cause this in some patients. Existing symptoms can worsen. New hypothyroid symptoms can appear. These thyroid patients often erroneously conclude that they are in some way allergic to T3, or will never be able to tolerate T3.

I have now introduced the type of response that can come when someone starts using T3 in small doses and why larger doses are often needed. Note: I understood the reason behind this issue, before I even wrote my Recovering with T3 book, which was released in 2011.

Here are a couple of extracts directly from Recovering with T3.
The first extract is from Chapter 14 in Recovering with T3 and it concerns the Lessons that I Learned on Divided Doses of T3:

"LESSON #7: WAVES OF T3

For each divided dose of T3, I discovered that there was definitely a 'threshold level' that had to be exceeded before any real benefit was experienced from the hormone. As I increased the dose beyond this threshold level, the effects were greater. If I exceeded the threshold too much, then I experienced symptoms of tissue over-stimulation. In the early years, my threshold level tended to be lower as the day progressed, this was due to some remaining issues with hypocortisolism, which eventually disappeared. So, later in the day I required lower doses of T3 to achieve the same effect. I often use a specific analogy to describe to other people how T3 appears to behave:

> 'Imagine a sandy beach, which is sheltered from the sea by large rocks. Only a wave that is large and powerful enough, is capable of striking the rocks and sending a spray of seawater over them, to drench the sand beyond.'

Each T3 divided dose is like a wave, the intra-cellular targets of T3 are akin to the beach and the rocks represent all the possible bio-chemical barriers that the T3 has to overcome. I do not believe that this is just some idle analogy. This is definitely how T3 replacement appears to feel and work within my own body."

The second extract is from later in the same chapter of Recovering with T3:

"I have also discovered that the contents of an individual T3 dose needs to be delivered at once. If I attempt to take 4 quarters of a single T3 divided dose spread over two hours then it is not effective at all. Lots of small doses of T3 do not work well. This fits well with the wave analogy above - you need a big enough 'wave' to be effective."

So, I have been aware of the potential for issues when introducing T3 and for using small doses of T3 for a very long time. In fact, this knowledge has really assisted me to help thyroid patients achieve safe and effective T3 or T3/T4 dosing strategies.

How the regulation of T4 to T3 conversion underlies the problems with introducing T3, and the use of small T3 doses

Thyroid patients who have some remaining thyroid function, or those already using T4 medication, will have some T4 in their systems. The conversion of FT4 to FT3 is not done at a fixed rate. The conversion rate is variable and regulated. It can vary from patient to patient, and it can vary throughout the day, even for the individual.

Conversion from FT4 to FT3 is performed by the D1 and D2 deiodinase enzymes. Conversion from FT4 to rT3 is performed by the D3 deiodinase enzymes. When the number of D1 or D2 enzymes increase, FT4 to FT3 conversion rate gets higher and FT3 rises. When the number of D1 or D2 enzymes decrease, FT4 to FT3 conversion rate lowers and FT3 can fall.

Similarly, the number of D3 deiodinase enzymes are regulated. When higher numbers of D3 exist, FT4 to rT3 conversion increases. With lower numbers of D3 enzymes, the FT4 to rT3 conversion rate lowers.

The cells in our body respond to the current situation and can regulate the conversion of FT4 to FT3 and FT4 to rT3. The clearance of thyroid hormones is also under regulation.

TSH is used by some of our cell types to regulate conversion from FT4 to FT3, and FT4 to rT3. The level of FT3 is also used by our cells to regulate conversion. So, a lowering of TSH, or an increase in FT3 will cause lower conversion from FT4 to FT3. Increasing TSH, or lowering FT3, will cause higher conversion from FT4 to FT3. A similar thing occurs with FT4 to rT3.

I explain the above in more detail in Article 15 within this chapter, so please refer to that for more technical details. Article 15 also has research references at the end that support the information that FT4 to FT3 conversion is variable and regulated.

Having introduced the mechanism involved, let me now explain what can happen when small T3 doses are used.

Doses that are as small as 2.5 mcg, or 5 mcg, can be especially problematic. When someone takes a T3 dose, not all of it will be absorbed from the small intestine to the bloodstream. Not all of this absorbed T3 will become Free T3 (FT3). Moreover, not all of the absorbed FT3 will make it to the cells and to the cell nuclei.

Therefore, very small doses of T3, will not provide very much extra FT3 to the cell nuclei. With tiny doses of 5 mcg or 2.5 mcg of T3, or less, you often do not know what the effect will be on the regulation of conversion rate of FT4 to FT3; whether it will result in more, the same or lower FT3 after the small T3 dose has been taken.

In some cases, a thyroid patient who may already feel very ill, might take a small T3 dose of 2.5 mcg or 5 mcg and the nett result may be that they end up with lower FT3 within hours of taking it.

I know of patients who were extremely hypothyroid to begin with, that felt even worse after the small dose was taken. Even 2.5 mcg doses of T3 can do this to some.

Now, whilst a very small number of thyroid patients actually seem to have genuine issues tolerating T3, most of the patients who react badly to small T3 doses, have actually simply become more hypothyroid. Elevated heart rate can also be caused due to the strain of lower FT3 on the heart – which can make the patient think that they are hyperthyroid!

In the vast majority of cases, the poor responses are related to the lowering of the existing FT4 to FT3 conversion rate due to taking the T3 dose. The T3 dose has been far too small to raise FT3 very much but the conversion rate has been down-regulated and the end result is worse FT4 to FT3 conversion than it was before taking the T3 dose.

What are the typical reactions of the patient who has tried taking small doses of T3 and had a poor response?

It is easier to deal with those patients who have some immediate improvement with introductory T3 doses. Even if this improvement vanishes within days, they may read my books, or talk to me and realise that this is actually an encouraging sign that T3 may well work for them. These patients will have seen the glimmer of hope that this is going to be the way forward for them. Reading my books will have explained how to proceed next - which is often to lower any T4 medication further and slowly increase the T3 dosage.

However, if the response of the patient is very bad indeed, the patient can, of course, be reluctant to explore the use of T3 again. Some patients can become more hypothyroid after taking small doses of T3. When FT3 levels fall, various symptoms can occur. If you review the range of symptoms associated with hypothyroidism that I describe in Article 2 in Chapter 3, then almost any of these might be induced. However, with lower FT3 levels, the cardiovascular system can be under more strain and this can raise heart rate. So, an elevated heart rate after a small T3 dose can appear to be the polar opposite of being more hypothyroid. The patient can think they are having a hyper or allergic response to the T3.

Some patients may continue to use very tiny T3 doses, because these do not seem to make their symptoms worse. I know of people who just end up using small doses such as 1 or 2 mcg of T3, just because they feel that this is all they can cope with. These patients may simply think that they are not able to tolerate T3, or they are allergic to it. Once they have this view, it can be very difficult to shift it.

What solutions are usually effective when a thyroid patient has experienced difficulty with small doses of T3?

For those who initially experienced some benefit which then quickly disappeared, a lot depends on whether they have read my work. These patients are unlikely to meet any doctors, endocrinologists or other practitioners who would explain that this is actually a good sign to them. As I explain in Article 15 in this chapter, and in my books, the solution for these people is usually to reduce their T4 medication a LOT, combined with slowly titrating the T3 dosage up. My Recovering with T3 book protocol can be used to manage the T3 dosing safely and effectively. Once the T4 medication is not high enough to convert to a lot of rT3, and the T4 medication cannot have a big impact on lowering FT3 levels through worse conversion, the T3 dosage can be raised enough to provide good FT3 levels. When FT3 is high enough from the T3 medication, then any lowering of FT4 to FT3 conversion will no longer make significant impact. The patient can get well.

However, for the thyroid patients who have been struggling to use anything other than the tiniest of doses without side effects, things can be far more difficult. The solution for these people is likely to be not only a reduction in the amount of T4 medication being used, but also an increase in the T3 doses to be used. Of course, when someone has had a bad response to 2.5 or 5 mcg of T3, the prospect of raising the T3 dose size usually makes them think that the response will be even worse.

The T4 medication would need to be reduced. This will be especially important if the FT4 was already high and/or rT3 was high. I would not want the FT4 to FT3 conversion to deteriorate significantly when more T3 was added. I also would not want FT4 to convert to more rT3. However, the patient may be too nervous to reduce the T4 medication, given that they are already feeling hypothyroid.

Larger doses of T3 would need to be used. The small doses, like 2.5 mcg or 5 mcg or even smaller ones, often fail their purpose. However, larger doses can often work really well. The reason for this is that with people whose regulation of conversion rate is poised at a point ready to deteriorate, it is important to have them take enough T3 to compensate for this. In this way, FT3 is at least maintained, and may actually be increased. Only by increasing FT3 for these people who have low FT3, and remain with thyroid symptoms on T4 medication, can symptoms be alleviated.

Even 7.5 mcg doses of T3 may actually be too small for some people. The threshold at which the T3 dose size becomes such that it actually adds extra FT3 will vary by person, and is dependent on how much T4 the person is on and how badly it is converting to FT3. The over-riding point is this. It should not be assumed that, because small doses are a problem, larger ones will not work. This is a mistake that many patients and doctors make. In fact, many doctors just end the trial of T3 because of a poor response to small doses of T3.

The two-pronged attack of increasing the T3 dose size, and reducing the T4 medication, is usually quite effective in this situation. It may be the only course of action that is actually going to work, if the patient is to recover.

However, any mention of this planned approach by myself, or in my books, or articles, can be extremely difficult for the thyroid patient. After all, they have only experienced poor results when adding T3 doses like 2.5 mcg or 5 mcg or even less. They have several hurdles to overcome:

- Firstly, there is the psychological issue to get over. These people believe they are intolerant or allergic in some way to T3. This is, of course, nonsense as T3 is a natural hormone and unless there is some filler or binder in the tablet, there is not going to be any allergy. In the majority of cases, the poor response occurs regardless of the brand of T3 and can even occur with compounded T3 with almost no extraneous compounds in it. This response may have even prompted the patient's doctor to begin suggesting that they have chronic fatigue syndrome or ME.

- Secondly, the patient may not understand the mechanism that is at work. I have now explained it here and in Article 15 in this chapter. Without an understanding of the mechanism at work, the patient will not understand why adding a small T3 dose has caused nothing but problems for them. If I am speaking to a thyroid patient, then I can explain it, and suggest one of my books or articles. But other than that, it is difficult to see how someone would take the necessary next steps, if they had not read my work, or talked to me.

- Thirdly, even when I have explained the actual reason why the patient can feel much worse after taking a small, or tiny, T3 dose, and I have outlined what the steps should be to move forward, they often remain too nervous to take those steps, as all their experience so far has been of having a poor response. They may still be frightened that larger doses will cause even worse symptoms. However, in the majority of cases, the opposite is true. Larger doses of T3 are actually the solution, when combined with less T4 medication.

Note: there are a few patients that seem to have a poor response to any form of standard T3, or even NDT. Sometimes, it is extremely difficult to ascertain why this is. One example is if mitochondrial disease is present. With mitochondrial problems the cells do not make enough adenosine triphosphate (ATP). ATP is cellular energy, needed by the cell nuclei. Taking T3 in the presence of low ATP can cause a range of bad reactions. For other patients, the problems may be due to a very fast clearance rate of T3. For these people, small doses of T3 may be cleared quickly leaving them hypothyroid, yet larger doses make them feel hyperthyroid. When patients do find that any form of standard T3 is far too difficult to use, and no root cause has been found, then trialling slow release T3 might be an option. However, this article is relevant to the vast majority who have had a poor response to small doses of T3.

Wrapping up

I have explained the types of symptoms and reactions that people can get when they first introduce T3, or add in small T3 doses. I have explained the mechanism behind this and why it can be so confusing if you do not understand how the regulation of the deiodinase enzymes works. This article, together with Article 15 in this chapter, explain the mechanism in enough detail for correct thyroid medication treatment to be applied.

I have also explained the particular issues with very small T3 doses and how these can make symptoms far worse, introduce new symptoms, or even appear to be causing hyperthyroid responses.

I finally cover the solutions that need to be applied to actually deal with the situation and introduce T3, without too many issues and with improvement to signs and symptoms. However, I also explain the particular issues faced by those patients who have experienced a bad response when using small doses of T3, or introducing T3.

I am hoping that this article helps some of the thyroid patients who may experience these problems with small doses of T3, or a physician or practitioner who is trying to assist them. Many patients have no issues with small T3 doses. But those that do experience issues often end up giving up the attempt to use T3. However, once the thyroid system is understood in a little more depth, then what appear to be incomprehensible responses, can actually become clear. After that, providing a better thyroid treatment is far easier.

Chapter 8

More Information on Cortisol

1. LOW CORTISOL OR HYPOCORTISOLISM OR ADRENAL FATIGUE?

I sometimes get asked whether the adrenals can recover from 'adrenal fatigue' over time, or whether adrenal cortex or hydrocortisone (HC) is required to 'support' them.

I do not believe in the idea that adrenals get weak, or sick, or damaged unless someone has an autoimmune disease that is attacking their adrenal glands, or a tumour, or an accident that damages them.

The adrenals themselves can easily be tested using a Synacthen Test (ACTH Stimulation Test). This test, amongst other cortisol tests, is discussed fully in Chapter 11 of my book, The Thyroid Patient's Manual. It is the definitive test for Addison's disease and it shows whether the adrenal glands are capable of responding to an effective signal from the pituitary gland. Adrenocorticotropic hormone (ACTH) is the signal that the pituitary puts out regularly, in pulses, to request that cortisol be produced by the adrenal glands. The Synacthen test reveals a baseline cortisol before the ACTH injection and then shows how cortisol rises in response to it. Most thyroid patients pass this test very easily and produce good levels of cortisol after the injection. This is because there is nothing wrong with their adrenal glands. There is no fatigue.

This is not to say, that cortisol cannot be low, because it can be. Often the baseline cortisol prior to the ACTH injection is too low. This will also show up in an 8-9:00 am morning blood cortisol test, and sometimes in a saliva cortisol test. However, the cause of this is usually hypothalamic-pituitary-adrenal axis (HPA axis) dysfunction and not that the adrenal glands are fatigued.

I do not believe in adrenal fatigue any longer. I have worked too much with thyroid researchers over the last few years, and seen patients respond well to treatment, to believe in adrenal fatigue.

I never use the term adrenal fatigue now. I use hypocortisolism or just low cortisol.

Let me be clear, YES, of course, low cortisol is a massive problem for many thyroid patients. This is NOT in question - it is just the cause of it, that I am discussing. The terminology also needs to be clearer.

The adrenal glands are incredibly simple organs. They keep making cortisol in as much quantity as someone needs, as long as there is enough ACTH from the pituitary, and enough cholesterol in the bloodstream. They can just go on and on. This is often why people with

Cushing's syndrome (incredibly high cortisol), keep having high cortisol for years, until they are diagnosed. Adding extra pregnenolone or progesterone, or some other supplement, is usually not going to make any difference to cortisol levels, as all the adrenals require is enough cholesterol and a decent level of ACTH stimulation.

The main cause for non-Addison's hypocortisolism (low cortisol) is hypothalamic-pituitary axis dysfunction – often of unknown origin, but sometimes because of low FT3.

The pituitary produces ACTH. It is the main signal to stimulate the adrenals to make cortisol, Dhea and to a much lower extent, aldosterone.

The pituitary converts FT4 to FT3 very efficiently within its own cells, if it makes the D2 deiodinase enzymes correctly. Gene defects with D2 (the DIO2 defect), can weaken this FT4 to FT3 conversion process.

The pituitary has been discovered to have the highest concentration of FT3 out of all the different tissue types in the body. The pituitary gland needs high FT3 levels in order to work correctly.

Thyroid patients who do not have enough FT3 will not be giving their pituitary the support that it requires to function normally.

Daytime dosing of thyroid meds often leads to low night time FT3 levels.

Some people also have poor FT4 to FT3 conversion, which can also lead to low FT3 levels.

A DIO2 gene defect may contribute to lower pituitary FT3 than the individual is supposed to have.

Loss of thyroid tissue, through Hashimoto's, or thyroidectomy, also loses a significant amount of conversion capability. Thyroid patients without a thyroid typically lose about 25% of their ability to make FT3 (mostly through conversion) - this conversion capability cannot be recovered.

I no longer think adrenals need to 'heal'.

In most cases of low cortisol, it is hypothalamic-pituitary-adrenal axis dysfunction that is the source of the issue. This can occur from prolonged stress, and also because of daytime dosing of thyroid medication. It can sometimes occur due to poor FT4 to FT3 conversion. The use of anti-anxiety medication or anti-depressants can also wreak havoc on the HPA axis and induce low cortisol. Sometimes, there are other issues, which may be very hard to get to the bottom of.

Fixing deficiencies or issues that influence FT4 to FT3 conversion like low iron, low vitamins, and low selenium can help the HPA axis. However, working on diet and supplements will not correct the issue, if there is a fundamental problem like thyroid tissue loss, or genetic defects that are actively impacting FT4 to FT3 conversion.

Sometimes, FT3 needs to be higher in order to support the pituitary gland more effectively. This might need to occur in the night, as this is when the pituitary begins to produce the highest level of ACTH during a 24-hour period. I created my Circadian T3 Method (CT3M), or protocol, specifically for this reason. CT3M can help to raise cortisol levels throughout the day. CT3M corrected my own extremely low cortisol levels. Thousands of thyroid patients have also used CT3M to correct their own low cortisol − without having to 'rest their adrenal glands,' or 'support' them with other medications or supplements.

Sometimes, there is no obvious reason for the low cortisol. However, I do believe it resides in the hypothalamic-pituitary area in the majority of cases. This clearly is not true for 100% of cases, but it is definitely true for the vast majority.

Trying to support the adrenal glands using adrenal cortex, in the hope that the adrenals will just get better, is not something I believe will work at all. Nor will using other supplements aimed at 'adrenal support'. The concept of supporting adrenals is not something I believe in any more. Resting something that is not fundamentally broken, is not a fix. Moreover, when adrenal cortex or HC is used, this will usually cause the pituitary gland to make even less ACTH and your own adrenal cortisol production will fall even lower. This makes it even harder to make a good recovery using your own body's capability.

If there is a clear reason for low cortisol like very low iron, or low B12, or some other health issue which can be addressed whilst using adrenal cortex, it can be helpful. Fixing some fundamental health issue which is interfering with cortisol production is, of course, a very good thing to do, and might ultimately be sufficient to restore cortisol levels. But just taking the cortex is not a solution to make the adrenals become healthy again. Resting the adrenals is very unlikely to be a solution on its own.

The two tests to rule out real adrenal organ issues are:

1. The ACTH Stimulation or Synacthen test. This tests whether the adrenals can respond to ACTH stimulation. If they do well, the adrenals are not the issue − most thyroid patients pass this.
2. The Insulin Tolerance Test. This tests if the pituitary is capable of responding to much lower blood sugar, and then produce enough ACTH. It will rule out proper hypopituitarism. However, it will not rule out less severe hypothalamic-pituitary dysfunction. Alternatively, a Metyrapone Test can be done, if the hospital supports this.

The above information is in ALL of my books. The cortisol tests are discussed in detail in The Thyroid Patient's Manual.

The term adrenal fatigue is discussed all over the Internet. It is even present in some cortisol saliva test companies' test results. In terms of cortisol saliva test results, I am one of the biggest fans of doing these, but they need to be done alongside an 8-9am morning blood cortisol test – see Article 4 in Chapter 8 for why this is. I am still an advocate for cortisol saliva testing, but the adrenal fatigue terminology is misleading.

When people talk of stages of adrenal fatigue, it simply means stages of failure to produce cortisol and Dhea (both of which are stimulated by ACTH). It is not just nomenclature, or giving things the right name (or wrong name in this case). The wrong name for something can imply issues that are misleading to the patients.

'Nursing the adrenals back to health' by supporting with adrenal glandulars, or adrenal cortex, is highly unlikely to fix the fundamental issue with low cortisol.

The best solution for hypocortisolism (low cortisol) is to fix the underlying cause. I have countless examples of thyroid patients I have worked with, who have clear test results for low cortisol, but they easily pass a Synacthen test. Their issues have definite roots in HPA axis dysfunction. Some have responded well to CT3M, as their FT3 levels were sub-optimal. In other cases, a deficiency was at the root cause.

An example of a deficiency that could cause low cortisol is low B12. I have even had cases where the patient was supplementing with B12, or even on hydroxy-cobalamin B12 injections but what they really needed was methyl-cobalamin injections. Some patients have methylation issues and cannot process inactive B12 into active B12. So, even excellent looking B12 test results did not show the problem. Providing the correct type of B12, and the right co-factors, corrected the low cortisol. See Article 2 in Chapter 10 for more details on B12.

I realise that a lot of these comments may cause consternation, but I believe them to be true. I have done my own research over 35 years, and I have spoken with very clever thyroid and cortisol researchers. I have also benefitted from working with many thyroid patients who have had extremely low cortisol. Hopefully, this article will help some of you.

2. HIGH CORTISOL SYMPTOMS – HIGH BP & CHEST PAIN

It is worth being aware of one particular effect that high cortisol can have on the human body.

High cortisol can cause raised blood pressure. This short article explains one reason for this.

High cortisol can cause chest pains and symptoms like angina.

High cortisol makes the body more sensitive to the effects of adrenaline and noradrenaline, which in turn, causes vasoconstriction and reduced blood flow.

Cortisol is also an antidiuretic and causes the body to retain sodium. Both these effects can raise blood pressure (which can be a symptom of high cortisol).

So high/raised cortisol can make the body respond more to normal levels of adrenaline and noradrenaline and can, therefore, cause vasoconstriction, which in turn can cause chest pains (which can mimic angina).

Here is an article on this: https://breakingmuscle.com/health-medicine/the-ups-and-downs-of-cortisol-what-you-need-to-know

3. T3 THYROID HORMONE AND CORTISOL RELATIONSHIPS

I have been asked many times to explain my views on the relationship of the T3 thyroid hormone to cortisol. This is an easy question to ask, but an extremely complex one to answer fully, in order to provide a good enough understanding for the person to be able to make really good decisions.

My books are definitely the best source of information that I have to offer to thyroid patients about the relationships between T3 and cortisol.

I write about this topic extensively in all three of my books: The Thyroid Patient's Manual, Recovering with T3 and The CT3M Handbook.

However, this article provides supplementary information on the important relationships between T3 thyroid hormone and cortisol. I have put them in bullet point form for greater clarity.

Some important T3 thyroid hormone and cortisol relationships:

1. Cortisol and T3 are partners. T3 and cortisol both need to be at good levels. Cortisol increases T3-effect, and T3 increases cortisol-effect. They are in a partnership within the cells. They both work at the mitochondria and at the cell nuclei, and are essential in the production of proteins, amongst other things. In addition, one of cortisol's roles is gluconeogenesis. This converts stored sugars into available sugar in the bloodstream in between meals. Glucose (blood sugar) is needed by the mitochondria in order to produce cellular energy (ATP). Assessing glucose levels is an indirect way of assessing cortisol levels. It is not the most definitive way, but it can help when trying to get cortisol optimal. Note: adrenaline also mediates gluconeogenesis.

2. The pituitary gland controls cortisol production via the Adrenocorticotropic Hormone (ACTH). ACTH stimulates the adrenal glands to produce both cortisol and Dhea. Without enough ACTH, cortisol production by the adrenals will be too low.

3. Studies show that the pituitary gland needs more FT3 than any other organ in the body. The pituitary basically runs using FT3 as its fuel. This makes the pituitary vulnerable to not

working well if FT3 is low. This is fundamentally why low cortisol is so prevalent amongst thyroid patients. Many thyroid patients are on treatments that do not give them sufficiently good FT3 levels. It is such an obvious conclusion. Poorly treated hypothyroidism (low FT3 levels), often results in low cortisol.

4. Adrenal fatigue is a myth. Adrenals do not usually get 'tired' or 'overworked" unless they are damaged by disease or autoimmune attack - i.e., Addison's disease. Usually, the issue is the lack of enough pituitary signal (ACTH).

5. The pituitary can fail to produce sufficient ACTH signal to the adrenal glands because of hypopituitarism (which can be tested for), or simply because it is not receiving enough FT3 thyroid hormone (see point 3 above). Many other issues can cause the hypothalamic-pituitary (HP) system to fail to regulate the adrenal glands with sufficient ACTH at all times during the day.

6. FT3 is more likely to stimulate cortisol production than FT4. FT3 helps to keep cortisol levels up as it stimulates the hypothalamic-pituitary system more than FT4. This latter point is why thyroid medications that contain T3 often help to keep cortisol levels higher.

7. Low cortisol is very common in thyroid patients, as many have lower FT3 levels than they had when they were well (for reasons I have discussed in my books and in various other articles).

8. Cortisol is not required for FT3 to be able to enter the cells. FT3 enters our cells through transporter molecules and these do not require cortisol to function. Therefore, there is no evidence that low cortisol causes T3 'pooling', or 'build-up', or inability to enter our cells. In fact, new research as of 2021, proves the opposite is true; high levels of cortisol actually inhibit T3 transport into the cells, whereas low cortisol levels do not.

9. Low cortisol causes FT3 to work less effectively within the cells. This is because FT3 and cortisol are partners within our cells. High cortisol also causes problems and can reduce the effectiveness of FT3 within the cells, hence thyroid patients with high cortisol often complain of feeling hypothyroid, even when they appear to have reasonable FT3 levels.

10. When patients try to raise FT3 levels in the presence of low cortisol, they may find that the body compensates for low cortisol by producing more adrenaline. This can cause anxiety, rapid heart rate, the feeling of heart palpitations etc. This is usually the adrenaline response rather than a direct issue with the T3. Very often, it is the low cortisol that is at the root, but it can be caused by other factors.

11. When cortisol is low, taking daytime T3 is often enough to correct it. However, it sometimes needs a night-time dose of T3. See my Circadian T3 Method (CT3M) protocol in the Recovering with T3 book. CT3M is also covered to some extent in The Thyroid Patient's Manual and in detail in The CT3M Handbook.

12. Cortisol dysfunction patterns are numerous. Often there is low cortisol in the morning, rising to high cortisol in the evening, due to the pituitary being very slow to catch up. Sometimes there is low cortisol all day. Sometimes there is high cortisol due to the strain of low FT3 and high rT3. In many cases, if the person is hypothyroid, getting the FT3 levels up, without high rT3, can help. Sometimes it needs CT3M. CT3M can help with many patterns of cortisol dysfunction - not just low morning cortisol.

13. Low cortisol is a serious issue for thyroid patients. It is important to rule out Addison's disease by having the appropriate ACTH Stimulation test done (also known as a Synacthen test). This can only be done under the supervision of a qualified endocrinologist. Addison's disease can be life-threatening and any thyroid patient with low cortisol needs to have this tested and ruled out.

14. If Addison's disease is diagnosed, then cortisol will need to be replaced and this is likely to be a lifelong requirement. This should be done under the supervision of an experienced endocrinologist. There are many alternative medications and approaches to cortisol replacement. If one solution does not work, another may be tried. Some endocrinologists are far more experienced with various solutions for cortisol replacement than others. So, finding a specialist who is knowledgeable and experienced is very important when cortisol replacement is needed.

15. Some Addison's disease patients are finding that when cortisol replacement is needed, only a cortisol pump replaces cortisol in a physiological way. See Article 17 in this chapter for more information on cortisol pumps. Replacement with cortisol is a serious step and it needs an extremely competent endocrinologist to help with this.

16. Hypopituitarism can result in an insufficient ACTH signal to the adrenal glands. This can also be tested for (see Chapter 11 in The Thyroid Patient's Manual book for some of the possible tests). There are various tests for hypopituitarism and these can also be organised by a competent endocrinologist. If hypopituitarism is present then replacement of cortisol is also likely - see points 13 and 14.

17. However, most causes of low cortisol are not as serious as Addison's disease or hypopituitarism. Correcting hypothyroidism may frequently resolve any low cortisol issues. Hence the need to be aware of the potential connections between T3 and cortisol. Sometimes another deficiency or issue is behind the low cortisol problem, e.g., prolonged stress, low iron, low B12.

18. Many thyroid patients who have low cortisol, or have the symptoms of low cortisol, are often persuaded to try to raise cortisol by various methods. Some are told that herbs known as Adrenal Adaptogens will work. However, these usually lower cortisol levels (herbs do not have brains – herbs cannot work out whether to raise or lower cortisol for the individual). Some patients are persuaded by doctors, or other patients, to try to use either hydrocortisone (bio-identical cortisol) or adrenal cortex extract from animals. These types of approaches are a mistake if the problems are really connected to low T3 levels, or some other issue that needs to be addressed, e.g., low B12, low iron etc. I would always want to explore other solutions for low cortisol before resorting to any form of cortisol replacement, as this switches off, or down-regulates, the individual's own cortisol production ability.

19. The effects on temperature, BP, and heart rate, of cortisol and T3 can be far more complex than the simple explanations that are often used on Internet websites and forums. Low body temperature may occur if either T3 is low or cortisol is low. However, if cortisol is very low for the person, then adrenaline may be produced to compensate and raise blood sugar, and this might actually raise temperature to a better level. In that last case, the adrenaline might cause a high heart rate and elevated BP. It is never as simple as people think. High BP can come from high cortisol, excess adrenaline from very low cortisol, or too much T3. This is why understanding the thyroid system and how it works with cortisol etc. is so important. I have tried to explain this as best I can in both The Thyroid Patient's Manual and in Recovering with T3. These are just examples. Reading the books will help more.

20. If cortisol is low, and if the thyroid treatment is not optimal, then adjusting the thyroid treatment can work wonders. Improving FT3 levels in the daytime can improve cortisol levels. This often involves increasing the amount of T3 in the treatment. Sometimes, both FT4 and rT3 need to be lowered, in order to allow FT3 to work better. Improving daytime FT3 levels are often enough but some people with low cortisol that is due to low FT3 may need more help than this. In some cases, the FT4 and rT3 really need to be reduced a lot. In some cases, my CT3M protocol needs to be used.

I have five articles that cover the various relationships of thyroid hormone, cortisol and sex hormones. They include Article 3 (this one), 4, 5 and 6 in Chapter 8, along with Article 7 in Chapter 10. They have helped me to assist many thyroid patients.

Finally, I emphasise again that, The Thyroid Patient's Manual is a good starting point to learn about the thyroid hormone and cortisol systems. Recovering with T3 is also excellent and covers the safe use of T3, and of CT3M, if it is required. This book has numerous supplementary articles which add further detail and explanations.

I would advise against relying mainly on Internet forums. Building a more comprehensive knowledge base is always the best thing to do. Once you understand how the important systems of the body actually work, it is then possible to make sense of things. Hence, I recommend reading my books. Clearly, finding a knowledgeable doctor, or endocrinologist, that you can work well with can be very important to regaining your health. Be prepared to switch doctors, or keep looking for someone who you can work with, and who listens to you. This can help a great deal.

4. INCONSISTENT FREE SALIVA AND BLOOD CORTISOL TEST RESULTS

This article may help to explain why sometimes we might see an inconsistency between the result for an 8:00 am morning cortisol blood test, compared to the free cortisol measured in a cortisol saliva test. An inconsistency between the two types of tests, can provide additional information. This is why I always prefer both tests to be run.

It is very important to realise that cortisol saliva testing and cortisol blood testing measure entirely different things. A cortisol blood test measures the total cortisol contained in the blood, i.e., both the free/unbound cortisol and the cortisol bound to protein (cortisol binding globulin or CBG). A cortisol saliva test only measures the free cortisol. A cortisol blood test result might be high or low in the range compared to cortisol measured in saliva.

Clearly, every situation is different, and the entire history and situation with an individual needs to be taken into account.

The link below explains that the amount of cortisol produced and the amount of free cortisol available can be very different in some scenarios. Measuring both allows for insight into the rate of cortisol clearance/metabolism, and what might be behind any inconsistencies between the two types of cortisol testing.

Here are two examples:

1. Higher levels of metabolised cortisol (compared to free cortisol) are often seen in obesity where adipose tissue is likely pulling cortisol from its binding protein (cortisol binding globulin or CBG), and allowing for metabolism and clearance. The adrenal glands have to keep up with this cortisol sequestering and excretion, so cortisol production is often quite high (as seen in an 8:00-9:00 am morning cortisol test, or in the levels of metabolized cortisol if using the Dutch test). This insight is quite helpful for those looking to lose belly fat and suspect cortisol/stress is a major factor. These patients are often misdiagnosed, as having low cortisol production when only free cortisol in saliva is measured. However, if blood cortisol is tested and found to be high, combined with low saliva cortisol, then the obesity may well be the cause and this can be worked on.

    Increased cortisol clearance (and low free cortisol in saliva and urine) may also be seen in hyperthyroidism, and is suspected to be part of the chronic fatigue story as well.

2. In patients with low thyroid (low FT3 specifically), the opposite pattern is often seen. When the thyroid slows down, or if there is peripheral hypothyroidism, where free T3 cannot get into the cells, the clearance (or metabolism) of cortisol through the liver slows down. As a result, free cortisol (measured in a saliva test), starts to increase and may show up elevated. In this case, 8:00-9:00 am morning blood cortisol may well still be low, even though salivary cortisol appears high. Note: this is a pattern I have seen multiple times with thyroid patients. It is useful to know, as assuming on-going tissue-level hypothyroidism may be the best way to go forward when low/normal blood cortisol and high saliva cortisol is seen. Simply assuming that the saliva test is correct and the blood test is not, is often the incorrect assumption. In these cases, it can be helpful to raise the T3 dosing. If cortisol in blood at 8:00-9:00 am is low, then introducing a CT3M dose can sometimes be very helpful – even if free cortisol (saliva cortisol) is high. See Recovering with T3 for more information on CT3M.

Here is the link:
https://dutchtest.com/2017/09/25/metabolized-versus-free-cortisol-understanding-the-difference/

The bottom line is that I am a great believer in testing both free cortisol in saliva, and total cortisol in blood at 8:00-9:00 am, as you get the whole picture. Relying on free saliva cortisol only is not sensible. There can be inconsistent results between blood cortisol testing and saliva cortisol testing and this needs to be assessed properly.

Using the same test laboratory all the time is equally important if you want to see how cortisol has changed after making any adjustments to your regime. Different labs can have extremely different test results.

It is also possible that a lot of patients who have apparently high cortisol from a saliva test are being given guidance to lower the free cortisol with adaptogens, when what they really need to do is to fix the tissue hypothyroidism with more thyroid hormone. In some cases, the person might have low total cortisol (a blood test at 8:00 am or 9:00 am will show this). In this case, raising total cortisol with CT3M might also help.

Other causes of inconsistent blood cortisol and saliva cortisol test results:

- The use of topical natural progesterone creams can corrupt the results in many saliva testing labs. The progesterone molecule is so similar to cortisol that many labs cannot distinguish between the two and show higher cortisol as a result. Even stopping the cream/gel a few days before might not stop this as it sits in the tissues. It might need 1-2 weeks without any progesterone cream, in order to do a saliva cortisol test. I realise in some cases that this will not be feasible.

- The use of any hydrocortisone (HC) cream can do the same and inflate cortisol saliva test results.

- Those patients on oral estrogen replacement can have much higher cortisol in blood tests, than in saliva tests. The reason for this is that oestrogen increases cortisol binding globulin (CBG) and falsely elevates any cortisol blood test. So, patients who need to do a cortisol blood test or a Synacthen test (ACTH Stimulation test) need to be off estrogen replacement for 8 weeks prior to the test. The oral oestrogen replacement tends to leave the free cortisol levels the same but blood cortisol levels can be much higher than normal. Note: transdermal estrogen replacement does not affect CBG. See: https://pubmed.ncbi.nlm.nih.gov/17492949/

  I believe that this is because the hypothalamic-pituitary system (HP system) uses free cortisol as its input. Oral estrogen replacement raises CBG, thus binding more of the free cortisol to protein. The HP system then responds by requesting the adrenals to make more cortisol to compensate for higher CBG. The net result is that cortisol blood tests can show falsely inflated cortisol levels. Meanwhile, the free cortisol in saliva tests remains unaffected. Note: the same thing can occur in those women with unusually high estrogen levels.

This is personal opinion that follows on from this last point:

1. In the case of a patient, who is taking oral estrogen, or has high estrogen, this can raise CBG a lot. If this person is already struggling to get sufficient hypothalamic-pituitary-adrenal axis response (either ACTH is too low from the pituitary, or the adrenals themselves are struggling to make enough cortisol), then I believe it is entirely possible for the free cortisol to drop and for the blood cortisol to not rise. In this case, the patient could end up with lower cortisol due to the estrogen intake or high estrogen.

2. I also think it is entirely feasible for topical/transdermal estrogen replacement to have the same effect, if estrogen levels in the blood are raised a lot, due to good absorption of the transdermal estrogen. Transdermal estrogen does not go immediately through the liver. However, any significant rise in blood estrogen level will still flow through the liver and could raise CBG. Therefore, there is still the potential for either higher blood cortisol, or even lower free cortisol levels, as suggested in the previous point 1.

So, if my take on this is correct, then any form of estrogen replacement, or elevated estrogen levels, has the potential to cause: higher blood cortisol but no change to saliva/free cortisol OR no change to blood cortisol but lower saliva/free cortisol. This would be due to increased CBG due to the estrogen replacement.

- Gene mutations can lower cortisol binding globulin, thus increasing free cortisol but lowering total cortisol.

What about consistent 8-9 am morning blood cortisol and saliva cortisol?

This is a lot more straightforward. It was not what the article was about, but saying a little is important for completeness.

If both saliva cortisol and blood cortisol are LOW, this is often due to the patient still being hypothyroid and low in FT3. Very often more T3 is needed (sometimes with less T4) and also CT3M may be required to boost cortisol. Of course, if cortisol is extremely low then ruling out Addison's (via a Synacthen test), and hypopituitarism (via an insulin tolerance test or metyrapone test) may be needed.

If both saliva cortisol and blood cortisol are HIGH, you would need to exclude hyperthyroidism and other factors that could be causing stress in the body – chemical imbalances, low/high nutrients, infections etc.

I have five articles that cover the various relationships of thyroid hormone, cortisol and sex hormones. They include Article 3, 4 (this one), 5 and 6 in Chapter 8, along with Article 7 in Chapter 10. They have helped me to assist many thyroid patients.

5. SEX HORMONES AND CORTISOL RELATIONSHIPS & THYROID HORMONES

I was not going to write this article. However, there are so many differing views expressed on the Internet, on other peoples' websites and by some doctors who practice in this area, that I felt that I ought to write something. It will at least give me a simple way to answer future questions.

Note: this article is mostly related to women, as the interaction between sex hormones and cortisol has the most relevance for women.

I use the terms estrogen and estradiol (which is the main estrogen hormone) somewhat interchangeably. In the UK and parts of Europe 'estrogen' is called 'oestrogen', and 'estradiol' is called 'oestradiol'.

Is there a relationship between estradiol and cortisol?

I will deal with this in two parts: higher estradiol and then lower estradiol.

Can high levels of estradiol lower cortisol?

Estrogen does not 'control' or 'suppress' cortisol. The effect is far milder than that. However, if estradiol (the main estrogen) is raised significantly, it does tend to reduce cortisol production, as well as impact cortisol activity in the tissues. This is why more women than men tend to have trouble with hypocortisolism and autoimmune diseases.

'Estrogen dominance', where estradiol is not matched to enough progesterone, can have the same effect, and cause a tendency towards lower than ideal cortisol. It can also lead to autoimmune conditions, like Hashimoto's. There is a useful post from Izabella Wentz on estrogen dominance and the connection to Hashimoto's that I will provide at the end of this article.

Sex Hormones and Thyroid hormones.

This is not the focus of this article but it is worth including, as sex hormones can affect the levels of Thyroid Binding Globulin (TBG).

It is also possible for increases in estrogen levels (as a result of HRT or some other imbalance), to reduce free thyroid hormone levels. There is research that shows that higher levels of estrogen can increase TBG. TBG binds to T4 and T3 and limits the bio-availability of both, i.e., it lowers free levels of both T4 and T3. So, increasing estrogen as a result of HRT, can result in both FT4 and FT3 levels becoming lower (due to higher TBG). So, it is possible that someone who is increasing their HRT may need to increase the dosage of their thyroid medication. If estrogen dominance begins to become an issue, then this may do the same thing, and FT3 and FT4 may reduce. Cortisol can also be affected if increases in estrogen lower FT3. Cortisol production is highly dependent on good FT3 levels, because the pituitary gland requires a healthy FT3 level to function well and produce adequate ACTH. The bottom line is that thyroid hormone dosage might need to be increased during the use of estrogen or if estrogen dominance becomes an issue:

See: https://www.nejm.org/doi/full/10.1056/nejm200106073442302

There is also some evidence that increases in progesterone levels can lower TBG. This could result in an increase in free thyroid hormone. This research article suggests FT4 can increase but FT3 might not. However, they have not considered the possibility that an increase in FT4 might lower TSH which in turn can lower conversion to FT3. For someone with already low TSH, an increase in progesterone might increase both FT4 and FT3.

See: https://onlinelibrary.wiley.com/doi/10.1111/cen.12128

There is also some scant evidence that increases in progesterone levels speed up the conversion of FT4 into FT3. Some practitioners believe adequate progesterone is important for optimal thyroid function. However, I have been unable to find any research that indicates that progesterone does actually increase the active hormone FT3 – so I would not pin your hopes on this.

Note: I also found some research and supporting evidence that indicate that increases in androgen levels (like dhea and testosterone) decreases TBG, improves T4 to T3 conversion and lowers TSH. Consequently, men and women who are taking testosterone or dhea may see higher free T3 levels, and may need to reduce thyroid replacement as a result. There are a lot of articles that suggest this. See: https://pubmed.ncbi.nlm.nih.gov/19942152/

There is also evidence that high free testosterone levels tend to displace cortisol from cortisol binding globulin (CBG) and so raising free testosterone can raise free cortisol levels. Lowering free testosterone can lower free cortisol.

What about low estradiol levels and high cortisol?

Conversely, low estradiol does not cause high cortisol. Women in menopause, with almost no estrogen in their bodies, do not normally have high cortisol levels. However, they often do have slightly improved cortisol levels and tissue effects compared to when they were menstruating. So, for many women with insufficient cortisol or chronic inflammation, menopause can often bring some improvements.

What should someone with high cortisol do?

A person who has very high cortisol levels needs an evaluation for Cushing's syndrome or Cushing's disease (a type of Cushing's syndrome caused by a pituitary tumour that over-secretes

ACTH). If there is no tumour, their cortisol levels may be an appropriate response to stress or other diseases. If no other condition can be found, one form of treatment often recommended is to take sublingual DHEA to counteract and balance the high cortisol (as long as they do not already have high DHEA).

What kind of dose of sublingual DHEA can a woman with high cortisol and low DHEA take? For most women, 5-6.25 mg, or 12.5 mg (1/2 of a 25 mg tab) is a good dose often used by doctors who regularly treat high cortisol and sex hormone imbalances. Higher doses could be used if DHEA is very low, but this would need expert advice. Some women can take the higher amount without getting adverse symptoms, e.g., acne or hirsutism. However, good advice would be needed.

How can estradiol replacement affect blood cortisol tests and saliva cortisol tests?

Those patients on oral estrogen replacement can have higher blood cortisol than saliva cortisol. This is because oral estrogen increases cortisol binding globulin (CBG) and falsely elevates any blood cortisol. So, patients who need to do a cortisol blood test, or a Synacthen test (ACTH Stimulation test), need to be off estrogen replacement for 8 weeks prior to the test. The oral estrogen replacement tends to leave the free cortisol levels the same, but blood cortisol levels can be much higher than normal. Note: transdermal bio-identical estrogen replacement does not affect CBG. See: https://pubmed.ncbi.nlm.nih.gov/17492949/

I believe that this is because the hypothalamic-pituitary-adrenal axis (HPA), uses free cortisol as its input. Oral estrogen replacement raises CBG, thus binding more of the free cortisol to protein. The HPA responds by requesting the adrenals to make more cortisol to compensate for higher CBG. The net result is that all cortisol blood tests can show falsely inflated cortisol levels. Whilst the free cortisol in saliva tests remains unaffected. Note: the same thing will occur in those women with unusually high natural estrogen levels.

Note: in the cases of those women who may have a poor HPA response and struggle to raise cortisol, then estrogen replacement or estrogen dominance might simply lower blood cortisol and free cortisol. This particular point is my own thinking based on how I understand the HPA system to work.

Finally, what about the ideas of 'progesterone steal' or 'pregnenolone steal'?

There are various ideas promoted on websites all over the Internet. This one is the idea that a woman will see a huge drop in progesterone in order to meet cortisol demand. This is stated, in various places on the Internet, to be due to the pregnenolone that is made from cholesterol being used to make cortisol, thus leaving insufficient pregnenolone for progesterone production. I commit this idea to the category of 'Internet Myths', along with some other ideas, and I will attempt to explain this here. These are not entirely my own ideas by the way. I base this on several things: some articles, and also discussions with thyroid and sex hormone doctors who do research in this area. Note: there are no published actual research studies on 'progesterone steal' - likely because it does not really exist. There are of course many internet opinion pieces - but these are not actual research studies.

The structure of the adrenal glands is the same in men and in women – this includes the pathways to cortisol production.

Women's progesterone levels are usually much higher than men's, but only when they are cycling and getting ovarian progesterone production.

When a woman is cycling, the adrenal progesterone production is a tiny percentage of overall progesterone production volume. Both the adrenal cortisol production pathways and adrenal progesterone production pathways are independent. Cortisol levels can be increased due to stress and never require any reduction in the rate of production of progesterone. Plus, the ovarian progesterone production is independent and constitutes the majority of a woman's progesterone. Dr Fiona McCulloch writes about this. She says that a stress response itself can affect the hypothalamic-pituitary axis and down-regulate both LH and FSH thus leaving sex hormones lower than they ought to be: https://drfionand.com/pregnenolone-steal-closer-look-popular-concept/

Here is another doctor posting who dismisses the 'progesterone steal' or 'pregnenolone steal' concept. She also states that a stress response is really the cause of a downgrade in the hypothalamic-pituitary control of sex hormones: https://www.drkateld.com/blog/is-the-cortisol-steal-real-how-stress-messes-up-your-hormones

Note: any extreme stress, or poor response to stress, and a lowering of sex hormone levels as a response is nothing to do with the concept of 'progesterone steal'- it is just a stress response that can happen in some women. Neither progesterone, nor pregnenolone, are being 'stolen' to make cortisol.

Note also: supplementing with extra pregnenolone is extremely unlikely to fix things, regardless of what is written on various Internet sites. This is because it is not a lack of pregnenolone that is causing lower progesterone, or estrogen – it is the stress response. So, let me leave the cycling woman to one side, as the concept of 'progesterone steal' just will not fit.

When cycles are finished and the estrogen and progesterone levels fall, it is the small background production of these hormones by the adrenals that continues. This background production of progesterone and estrogen is the same level as in men - because men and women share the same physiology of the adrenals. There is no difference in the structure and the pathways.

Healthy men (and women) of any age continue to have good cortisol levels and are able to increase cortisol production in times of stress. This does not involve any decrease in progesterone in the bloodstream. Men also require progesterone and estrogen, but at a much lower level than cycling women. Any intermediate step through progesterone is entirely internal to the adrenal glands. The physiologies of men and post-menopausal women, in regard to cortisol and progesterone, are exactly the same in terms of producing the cortisol and progesterone.

The major source of raw material for cortisol is cholesterol. There is no need at all to lower blood progesterone, or consume the pregnenolone used for making progesterone, in order to make cortisol, even if cortisol has to rise to meet a stress demand. As long as there is enough cholesterol in the diet, there is a good enough ACTH signal from the pituitary to request cortisol production. Moreover, as long as the adrenal glands are not damaged due to Addison's disease, or other disease or tumours, then progesterone levels will not drop due to cortisol being produced, (or struggling to be produced), at the right level. However, as the two doctors above have acknowledged, changes in the hypothalamic-pituitary system due to stress could still see lower progesterone and/or estrogen levels. Any extreme stress could still see progesterone or estrogen fall, but only if the ovaries are still contributing a little of these sex hormones. The pituitary LH and FSH signals have no effect on adrenal production of progesterone or estrogen.

So, the argument that a woman has low progesterone because the adrenals are using pregnenolone destined for progesterone, or limiting progesterone production in favour of making cortisol, is incorrect and misleading. Progesterone can of course be too low for a woman. This can be a very big issue, as progesterone is essential in order to balance estrogen. But there can be many reasons for low progesterone.

It is also worth noting that the amount of background adrenal progesterone and estrogen production between different people can vary substantially. This might not be obvious until cycles finish and the ovarian production stops. Some women go through menopause and find they have excellent post-menopausal levels of estrogen and progesterone, because their adrenal production was always good. Whilst others find that their progesterone and/or estrogen levels are far too low post-menopause and that this causes symptoms. These can often only be corrected using bio-identical hormone replacement.

Many women can have very low progesterone but excellent cortisol levels (because the cortisol production pathway begins with cholesterol). Moreover, stringent dieting, and the low cholesterol that can result, can often be the worst thing for patients, and this can result in both low cortisol and low progesterone.

So, the entire idea that someone with low progesterone has this due to the adrenals trying to produce cortisol is a flawed concept. I consign 'progesterone steal' and 'pregnenolone steal' to the 'Internet Myth bin'.

Note: none of the above takes away from the need to have progesterone at a good healthy post-menopausal level and to have it balanced to the right level of estrogen in post-menopausal women.

Fixing a low progesterone level, especially one that is not balanced against the estrogen level, is a good thing and will often lead to the patient feeling far healthier.

Note: I do have a whole chapter on sex hormones in my book, The Thyroid Patient's Manual.

I have included five articles that cover the various relationships of thyroid hormone, cortisol and sex hormones. They include Article 3, 4 and 5 (this one), and 6 in Chapter 8, along with Article 7 in Chapter 10. They have helped me to assist many thyroid patients.

Here is Izabella Wentz's estrogen dominance post:

https://thyroidpharmacist.com/articles/estrogen-dominance-as-a-hashimotos-trigger/

6. HIGH & LOW CORTISOL EFFECTS ON THYROID HORMONE & AN INTERNET MYTH

Higher cortisol levels reduce TSH (through the effect on the hypothalamic-pituitary system). A reduced TSH does two things:

1. For those patients with working thyroid tissue, lower TSH will decrease thyroid hormone production.
2. Lower TSH also reduces FT4 to FT3 conversion, resulting in less FT3 (active thyroid hormone)

Lower cortisol levels increase TSH. An increased TSH does two things:

1. For those patients with working thyroid tissue, higher TSH will increase thyroid hormone production.
2. Higher TSH also increases FT4 to FT3 conversion, resulting in even more FT3. Studies have found that in severe cortisol deficiency, the TSH and FT3 are often high. Cortisol (HC) supplementation in these people, normalises the TSH and FT3.

We know that cortisol and T3 are both required to increase mitochondrial energy production. So, a lack of cortisol is likely to reduce T3's effectiveness in the mitochondria. But there are probably other mechanisms at work, yet to be discovered.

FT3 and cortisol both need to be at good levels. Cortisol increases T3-effect, and T3 increases cortisol-effect - they are in a partnership within the cells. T3 helps to keep cortisol levels up as it stimulates the hypothalamic-pituitary system more than T4. This latter point is why thyroid medications that contain T3 help to keep cortisol levels higher. Low cortisol is very common in thyroid patients, as many have lower FT3 levels than they had when they were well (for reasons I have discussed in my books and in various other articles). For all the reasons above, it should be clear that with low cortisol, T3 does not work as effectively as it should. High cortisol also causes problems and can reduce the effectiveness of FT3 within the cells, hence thyroid patients with high cortisol often complain of feeling hypothyroid even when they appear to have reasonable FT3 levels. High cortisol can also increase thyroid binding globulin (TBG) which can reduce the FT3 and FT4 levels.

However, I know of no evidence whatsoever that FT3 is less able to enter cells when cortisol is low. That would require low cortisol to affect the T3 transporter molecules in the cells' membranes. There is no evidence that low cortisol does this, and I do not know of any researchers who believe this (and I have spoken to some about this specifically). I stated this clearly in the first edition of Recovering with T3. I said that cortisol was not required to allow FT3 to enter the cells.

If someone comes to me and says that their FT3 level seems quite good or high, but they are still not feeling well, it simply means that there is another problem that needs to be resolved. If low cortisol is behind the problems, it can result in slightly higher FT3 due to the mechanism that I have described above.

The bottom line is that a high FT3 on a T3 combination treatment is not unusual, but this does not mean the FT3 is not getting into the cells ('pooling' as some people call it). The FT3 is still getting into the cells. The issue is simply that having enough FT3 is no guarantee that metabolism is going to work correctly. Many other things also need to be right, including the cortisol level, as T3 and cortisol work synergistically.

As I stated in the opening paragraph here, low cortisol does have some effect on raising TSH, which also increases FT4 to FT3 conversion. So, people whose cortisol is low may get a small amount of extra FT3 from this. But their cellular FT3 will also be a little higher too. It is not that the FT3 cannot reach the cells.

When someone is still not feeling well, and their FT3 levels look good to high, it could be assumed that FT3 is not getting into the cells. There are many reasons for metabolic rate not to be correct, including low cortisol.

However, low cortisol does not prevent the entry of FT3 into the cells. The 'pooling' concept may scare some patients to rush into cortisol supplementation because many thyroid patients have come to associate this word with low cortisol issues. Yet, there can be many reasons for thyroid treatment not working. Yes, these need to be resolved. However, the reason for thyroid treatment not working is not always low cortisol.

A good FT3 level does not mean the FT3 is not available within the cells – it will be. I have written about many reasons for thyroid treatment not working properly in my book, The Thyroid Patient's Manual.

If someone is on too much thyroid hormone treatment, but it is not working well, and the issue that fixes the problem is resolved, they can feel hyper-thyroid. This is not a sudden rush of

FT3 into the cells – the FT3 is already there! It is simply that they were taking too much thyroid hormone, to begin with. The issue that has been resolved has simply allowed the biologically active T3 to do its job.

It is important not to rush into using synthetic cortisol (HC or adrenal glandulars), as soon as thyroid treatment is not working and the FT3 level appears to be good, or even high. Cortisol needs to be tested fully (via a cortisol saliva test and an 8:00 am morning cortisol test), and other vitamins and minerals also need testing – see The Thyroid Patient's Manual for details on these.

The word 'Pooling' is sometimes used on the Internet. However, there is no evidence to support this idea. It is just another Internet myth that has been spread for too long. What is always important to focus on, is what is stopping a treatment working, fixing it, and getting the treatment to be successful.

To make matters even clearer, there is new research, as of 2021, that has actually tested whether hydrocortisone has an inhibitory effect on T3 transport into cells. They discovered that LOW doses of hydrocortisone do not inhibit T3 transport into cells via the MCT8 transporter, but HIGH levels do inhibit T3 transport into the cells. Also, Dexamethasone, a steroid that also activates cortisol's receptors, is more potent than hydrocortisone as an MCT8 transport inhibitor.

These recent research findings confirm that the 'pooling' idea is incorrect. The research is saying that high cortisol levels actually prevent some level of T3 transport into the cells and that low levels of cortisol do not do this. See Cosmo et al, 2021: "Dexamethasone and Some Commonly Used Drugs Inhibit MCT8-mediated T3 Transport in Vitro." This might go some way to explaining why some patients with low cortisol do not respond well to hydrocortisone, as it might inhibit FT3 entry into the cells.

I have five articles that cover the various relationships of thyroid hormone, cortisol and sex hormones. They include Article 3, 4, 5 and 6 (this one) in Chapter 8, along with Article 7 in Chapter 10. They have helped me to assist many thyroid patients.

7. WHY I NEEDED TO CREATE CT3M AND WHY IT CAN BE SO HELPFUL

CT3M stands for Circadian T3 Method.

I created this approach nearly thirty years ago, in order to raise my cortisol from a desperately low level to a healthy level.

It requires no use of hydrocortisone or adrenal glandulars to do this. It just uses T3 thyroid medication (Liothyronine). For some people, it can also work with natural desiccated thyroid (NDT).

Let me explain how I came to create the Circadian T3 Method (CT3M).

I had been on T3-Only (with no T4 medication at all), for about 6 or 9 months and felt better in many ways. However, my low cortisol was still an issue.

Low cortisol showed up in my 8:00 am morning blood test. On a 24-hour urinary cortisol collection, my total and free daily cortisol levels were almost at the bottom of the reference ranges. I had low cortisol all day long.

However, I had passed a Synacthen test (ACTH Stimulation test), so my adrenals themselves were healthy. This latter situation is quite common with many thyroid patients, and I will return to this point later.

In terms of low cortisol symptoms, my main ones were fatigue, low blood pressure, passing out (fainting) and weight loss. I was so weak that I was virtually housebound, and had to spend a lot of my time lying down. The passing out instances became quite frequent and were linked to low blood pressure.

For part of this time, I was struggling at work. Several times, I woke up in a corridor, being looked at by worried colleagues.

My weight loss was severe. I had gone down from 170 pounds (12 stones or 76 kg) to 110 pounds (just under 8 stones or 50 kg), i.e. I had lost about 35% of my body weight. In contrast to most cases of poorly treated hypothyroidism, which causes weight gain, severe low cortisol can cause severe weight loss. I looked extremely ill.

I had been reading endocrinology books for a while and was aware of the pattern of FT3 over 24 hours, and the pattern of cortisol over 24 hours. Here are two charts showing these. These charts are straight out of medical literature, and this knowledge has been around for a very long time:

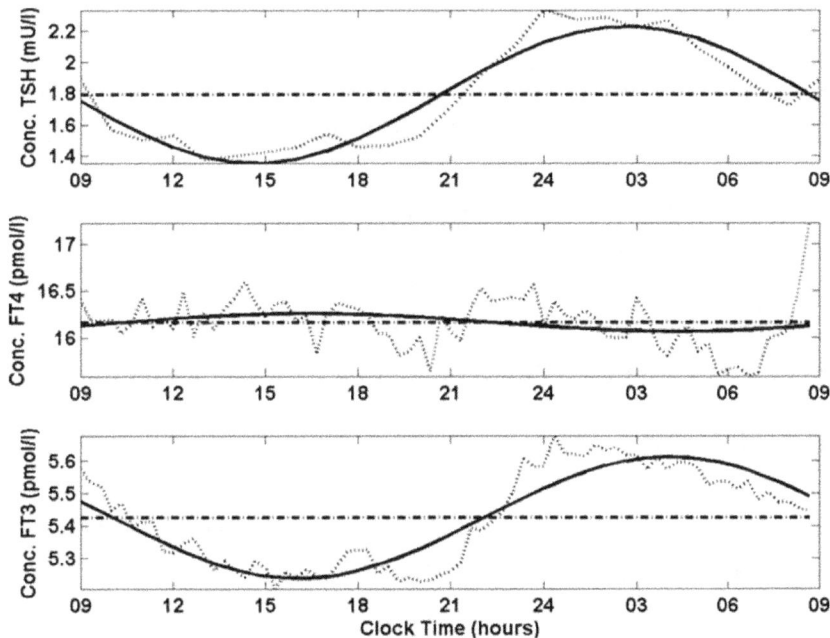

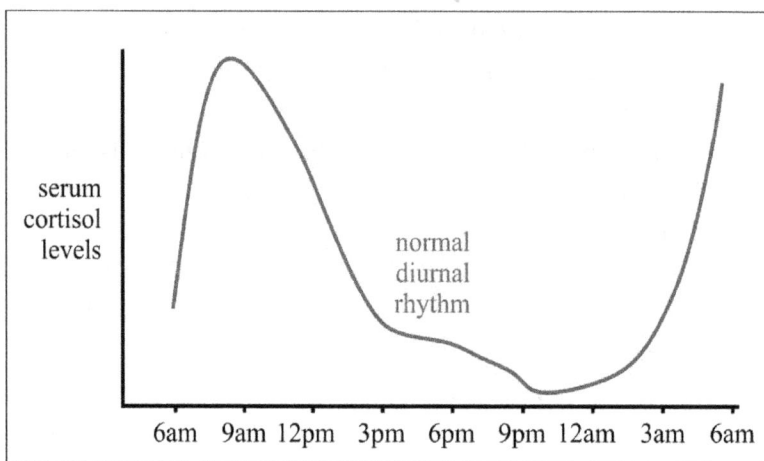

TSH is known to have larger and more frequent pulses in the night, and can be seen to peak around 3:00 am in the morning. TSH is at its lowest in the afternoon.

FT3 peaks an hour or two after TSH peaks. It is also at its lowest in the middle of the day.

FT3 peaks in the night following the high point of TSH for two reasons:

TSH drives a healthy thyroid gland to produce more T3 and more T4. We also know there is a connection between the TSH level and the rate of conversion of FT4 to FT3. When TSH is higher, the conversion rate of FT4 to FT3 increases. When TSH is lower, the conversion rate is lower. So, a high TSH in the night not only requests more T4 and T3 production from the thyroid gland, but it also increases the conversion rate of FT4 to FT3. Hence, FT3 increases in the middle of the night. In actual fact, TSH affects the regulation of the number of deiodinase enzymes being produced – which is why it affects the conversion rate of FT4 to FT3.

It should be immediately obvious that there is not a huge variation in FT4 – it reduces slightly when there is more conversion to FT3, and it increases slightly when the conversion rate to FT3 reduces.

So, I knew all of this information already at this stage of my attempt to recover from hypothyroidism.

Looking at the cortisol rhythm, it is easy to see that cortisol begins rising around 3:00 am and climbs to a peak between 7:00 am and 9:00 am in most people. This is to get us primed-up and ready to start the day. After this, cortisol normally declines steadily during the day, until the cycle repeats itself.

I knew my cortisol was very low and I was searching for an answer.

I was on T3-Only medication. At that time, I took 3 daily doses. One when I awoke in the morning, one around lunchtime and one in the late afternoon/early evening.

It occurred to me that, just like other thyroid patients, I was taking daytime thyroid medication. This tends to suppress the TSH, and the action of the thyroid gland (if someone still had a functioning thyroid gland at all).

The second thing that taking daytime thyroid medications tends to do, is to achieve good levels of thyroid hormone (FT3) in the daytime, but this FT3 is going to be lower during the night because we do not keep receiving the medication during the night. The use of daytime thyroid medication is not a physiological replacement pattern at all. People on thyroid medication tend to have a lower TSH than healthy people have. Plus, the normal, healthy pattern of FT3 is far less likely to occur. I had worked this much out but still had not understood why my cortisol was so desperately low.

Then, one night, I just woke up around 3:00 am and I had the answer. I had seen the connection. Part of the answer lay in the two charts and their relationship.

We know from research that the pituitary gland has the highest concentration of FT3 in the body (more than any other organ or body tissue). The pituitary makes its own D2 deiodinase enzyme and uses it to convert the FT4 flowing through it to extra FT3. Much of this FT3 remains within the pituitary in order to keep its own FT3 levels high. The pituitary gland runs on FT3, like a car runs on fuel!

The answer I had been searching for, lay deep within the pituitary gland. If the pituitary was not receiving (or being able to create) the level of FT3 that it used to have, how could it function normally?

A person with lower FT3 levels than they had when they were healthy could easily have pituitary dysfunction. In this case, one of the pituitary hormones, like ACTH, could be lower than it used to be when the person was healthy. ACTH is the signal that drives the adrenal glands to make cortisol and Dhea. The adrenals usually perform well, if they have enough cholesterol and an adequate ACTH signal. But without enough FT3 the pituitary is unlikely to be able to function ideally.

By the time I got up the following morning, I had the entire hypothesis worked out. I had low FT3 in the night time! This could be causing poor pituitary function and lower than adequate ACTH, thus low cortisol. I just had to test this hypothesis.

The following night I set my alarm to take my first T3 dose about 2 hours prior to my normal 'get out of bed' time. I took it that coming night and I did feel a LOT better during the next day. So, the next night I took it 3 hours before the time I usually got up. I felt better again! I was on to something here. This finally made sense.

I waited a couple of weeks to ensure that the improvement held – it did. I was elated. I went to see my family doctor. I explained it all – in fact, I bombarded her with science and evidence. I then asked her if she would support me by allowing me to do multiple 24-hour urinary cortisol collections. She agreed! So, this started a 6-month long experiment.

I went back to daytime only dosing for a week and then did a 24-hour urinary cortisol collection. I then moved the first dose to 30 minutes before getting up and waited a week and then did another cortisol collection.

I repeated this process about 8 times. The last 2-3 tests were done by moving the first dose a full hour earlier. It was amazing that my doctor supported me. However, I had been sick for so long and medically retired by my company at this stage and I was still extremely ill – so I think she was desperate for an answer too.

The results were incredible!

Every time I moved the first dose earlier by 30 minutes, both total and free cortisol levels rose. I tested it to about 6 hours before getting up – to mirror the rise in natural FT3 rhythm. Once I got to about 4-5 hours prior to getting up there was no further benefit in taking it earlier, and it actually started to reduce the cortisol level beyond that. However, the correlation between the time the T3 was taken, and both free and total cortisol levels, was virtually linear. The earlier the dose, the more cortisol. It supported my hypothesis totally.

I began referring to the approach as the Circadian T3 Method or just CT3M.

The optimal time for my CT3M dose appeared to be about 4 hours before I got up in the morning. I got an immediate benefit from CT3M and it enabled me to begin to function quite well again. I even began to exercise, and I started on the long road to recover my fitness. Over the following few years, my cortisol slowly improved. I have been using CT3M for many years now. If I try to not use it, my cortisol levels lower and I feel unwell.

I have also discovered that I have both copies of the DIO1 and DIO2 gene defects. DIO2 can impact the production of effective D2 enzymes. Thus, this could also have impacted my pituitary and its ability to convert FT4 to FT3, when on T4 and NDT medication. By the time I was on T3-Only during the daytime, it was the strictly daytime use of T3-Only that was the issue.

I published Recovering with T3 in 2011. The majority of this book is about the safe and effective use of T3-Only and the protocol for doing that. Only a small part of the book introduced CT3M and its potential benefits to those with low cortisol. It included a protocol for starting CT3M, and determining the correct CT3M dose size and timing.

In 2013, I published The CT3M Handbook, with more information on using CT3M. I have worked with thousands of thyroid patients now. Many of them have also improved their cortisol levels using CT3M. Some have regained their lives in dramatic ways through using

CT3M. It can work with NDT in some cases, but T3 works best. However, a T3 CT3M dose and daytime NDT is something that thyroid patients opt for quite often.

In 2018, I published The Thyroid Patient's Manual, which also explains how so many thyroid patients appear to have low cortisol. It also refers to CT3M but in slightly less detail than the other books.

These books now form a series, which deals with recovering from hypothyroidism: The Recovering from Hypothyroidism series.

I recommend reading them in this order: The Thyroid Patient's Manual first, Recovering with T3 second, followed by The CT3M Handbook for those that need more information on CT3M.

I no longer believe in the concept of Adrenal Fatigue. I do not believe that the adrenals get tired at all. If they could get tired, those with Cushing's disease would not be able to have super-high cortisol levels for years. I actually believe that most cases of low cortisol are caused by hypothalamic-pituitary dysfunction and the lower-than-normal ACTH signal that goes with this.

Sometimes, there is no known cause for hypothalamic-pituitary dysfunction, but stress could well be a factor. In some cases, the low cortisol is due to the way we use thyroid meds and the fact that this is not physiological. In these cases, CT3M can bring about profound improvements in cortisol levels throughout the day. Results with many thyroid patients have shown how worthwhile a trial of CT3M can be.

It is a shame that so many thyroid patients who are taking T4, NDT or T3 medication are sometimes persuaded to use hydrocortisone or adrenal glandulars to 'top-up' their cortisol levels. This often does not work well, as the added cortisol in these medications usually causes the pituitary gland to produce even less ACTH, and the patient's own adrenals produce less cortisol. This frequently leads to the dependence on a full replacement dose of cortisol, and the issues associated with this (needing to carry stress doses, needing to carry some kind of medical bracelet or medallion in case of emergency hospitalisation etc.).

CT3M is often worth a trial first before going down these routes. In many cases, CT3M raises cortisol throughout the day. In some cases, it does not work well, depending on the severity/nature of the hypothalamic-pituitary axis issue. In a few cases, the issue is actual adrenal damage - but this is far rarer.

Note: CT3M can help low cortisol throughout the day and can even help dysfunctional patterns of cortisol with some highs and lows in the pattern.

So, this is a little more background on CT3M. It explains how I came to create it and why it can be so amazingly helpful.

I believe that the connection between T3 thyroid hormone and cortisol ought to be part of mainstream endocrinology. I also think that CT3M ought to be in the 'toolbox' of every endocrinologist or doctor who is dealing with thyroid and cortisol issues.

See this very old video recording that I made about CT3M (I apologise for the quality but it is the only one I made on CT3M in detail): https://youtu.be/gGs6po4D-YI

8. THE FLAWED CONCEPT OF 'RESTING ADRENALS'

So much is written on the Internet by thyroid patients, and thyroid patient groups, about the idea of 'resting the adrenal glands.'

This concept is based on the idea that when a thyroid patient is suffering from low cortisol, their adrenal glands are the root cause. It is based on the idea that adrenal glands get tired and exhausted due to stress or some other reason.

The way in which this 'rest' is proposed by some thyroid patient groups and some doctors is often to suggest the thyroid patient uses hydrocortisone (HC) or adrenal glandulars. The idea is to 'take the strain off the adrenal glands' and 'rest them'. It is based on the idea of 'adrenal fatigue', i.e., the adrenal glands have got tired of making cortisol, and that this is why the thyroid patient has low cortisol.

I no longer believe in 'adrenal fatigue'.

The adrenals are very simple glands with ample capability of producing high levels of cortisol, indefinitely.

In the majority of people, all the adrenal glands require is a good ACTH signal from the pituitary and adequate cholesterol. ACTH stands for adrenocorticotropic hormone, and it stimulates the adrenal glands to make more cortisol and DHEA.

The above goes a long way to explaining why people with Cushing's syndrome can go for years and years with extremely high cortisol levels. Their adrenal glands never get 'fatigued' because undamaged adrenals do not get fatigued.

I believe the majority of cases of low cortisol are due to hypothalamic-pituitary dysfunction (HP dysfunction) and the lower level of ACTH that results from it.

Some people do have Addison's disease of course, which can usually be discovered via an ACTH Stimulation test (Synacthen test). Addison's disease is caused by adrenal tissue destruction, often through an auto-immune attack. It requires hydrocortisone (HC) replacement for life. With Addison's disease, the thyroid patient would have a very low 8-9 am morning blood cortisol and probably very low free cortisol throughout the day (seen in a 4-point saliva test of cortisol).

But for the typical thyroid patient with low cortisol, it is likely to be HP dysfunction causing the low cortisol. Many things can cause this, e.g., prolonged stress, toxicity etc. The result is the same – low cortisol.

Sometimes the cause for the HP dysfunction cannot be discovered and the patient may require some HC or adrenal glandular support.

However, it is often caused because the thyroid patient no longer has a working thyroid gland, and no longer has a normal 24-hour cycle of thyroid hormones, i.e., because they are on thyroid medication.

Why Can the Use of Thyroid Medication Cause HP Dysfunction?

The pituitary has the highest concentration of Free T3 (FT3) in the body. It makes its own D2 deiodinase enzymes. It converts around 80% of the FT4 present in its cells to FT3, and it keeps most of this FT3 inside itself. The pituitary gland 'runs on T3' for fuel.

The pituitary gland needs a good supply of FT3 to function well. If anything lowers FT3, e.g., an FT4 to FT3 conversion problem, the pituitary may suffer, and ACTH could be lower.

With lower ACTH, comes low cortisol. This has to happen. Cortisol cannot be made by the adrenal glands without enough of an ACTH signal (and enough cholesterol – which comes from the diet).

By the way, lower pregnenolone, or progesterone, is not going to be a problem in making cortisol. Cortisol is made in adequate amounts if there is enough of an ACTH signal and enough cholesterol (and most people have enough cholesterol).

What can cause a lower level of T3 in the pituitary gland?

Factors include Hashimoto's thyroiditis, thyroidectomy, a DIO1 and especially a DIO2 enzyme defect (which affects the internal pituitary conversion of T4 to T3), or anything else which lowers FT3 levels.

Taking thyroid medication only during the daytime is also likely to lead to lower levels of FT3 by the night time when the pituitary begins to produce a lot more ACTH.

Treating HP dysfunction with levothyroxine or Synthroid is often not going to work. It needs extra FT3 to bring the system back to normal. In some cases, it needs T3-Only.

'Resting the adrenals' with steroids is an Internet myth and a fallacy. The adrenals will not miraculously recover through 'rest', as there is usually nothing wrong with the adrenals themselves. It needs a better, smarter approach.

Using more T3, and the Circadian T3 Method (CT3M) can often help resolve the HP-dysfunction and raise cortisol levels back to normal.

For those who want to dig deeper into CT3M, please read Recovering with T3.

A companion book, The CT3M Handbook, is also available if you need even more information on CT3M.

9. CAN T3 THERAPY STRESS THE ADRENAL GLANDS?

This is a question I have heard many times. Here is an answer that hopefully will deal with this: NO!

The language of 'stress the adrenals', or 'adrenal fatigue' or 'weak adrenals' is the language that you see all over the Internet. It is flawed, and out of date. Unfortunately, it is a type of expression that continues to get spread around from patient to patient.

Thyroid patients get advice like, "You need to take hydrocortisone (HC) to rest your adrenals", or "You have adrenal fatigue, so use adrenal glandulars until they are less tired" or "You may have weak adrenals, that is why you have low cortisol", and other such rubbish.

Let me attempt to be very clear:

1. The adrenals do not get 'stressed'. They are simple, robust organs that rarely have any issues. If they become issues at all, it is usually due to an autoimmune condition that eventually develops into Addison's disease. All the adrenals need is cholesterol and enough ACTH signal from the pituitary. This is why thyroid patients with low cortisol often pass a Synacthen (ACTH Stimulation) Test very easily. This brings me to point 2.

2. Hypocortisolism (low cortisol), does exist of course. This is usually due to the hypothalamic-pituitary axis not working. Often, this is due to far too little FT3 during the night and in the daytime, as the pituitary effectively 'runs on' FT3.

3. FT3 actually stimulates the pituitary-hypothalamic system more than any other form of thyroid hormone. So, for low cortisol, raising FT3 is a great solution in many cases. T3 therapy does this more effectively than other thyroid treatments.

Note: If T3 is used and the hypothalamic-pituitary system cannot respond, adrenaline can get produced. This feels like a high heart rate and anxiety etc. This can happen in a few situations, e.g., through the use of long-term anti-anxiety drugs, or anti-depressants. Lyme disease can also cause this. But if it does happen, it is still NOT the adrenals getting stressed. They cannot get stressed. It is the hypothalamic-pituitary system which is failing to respond correctly.

In most thyroid patients, the adrenals are capable of working well. It is simply that the hypothalamic-pituitary system is not working well. In these cases, persevering with some T3 can sometimes correct this over time. The use of Low Dose Naltrexone (LDN) can also help sometimes. See Article 16 in this chapter for more information on LDN. Obviously, addressing any other significant issues is essential.

I cover this further in my books The Thyroid Patient's Manual in Chapters 5 and 7, and in Recovering with T3 in Chapter 16 and in The CT3M Handbook.

10. INTERPRETATION OF SIGNS IN THE CT3M (TEMP, BP, HR)

This article assumes that the thyroid patient has low cortisol, but that there is no Addison's disease or hypopituitarism. It is designed for the simplest case of someone who responds straightforwardly to the Circadian T3 Method (CT3M).

Essential Tests.

Thyroid patients should not attempt to use the CT3M unless they know, with confidence, that they have low cortisol.

Many thyroid patients who have been ill for some time and have not simply bounced back from thyroid treatment will indeed have low cortisol. It is also common for patients with Hashimoto's thyroiditis to have less than ideal cortisol levels. Even so, low cortisol should be confirmed by laboratory testing. This can only be achieved, with confidence, if a 24-hour cortisol saliva test and an 8:00am or 9:00 am morning cortisol blood test have both been done. In addition, serum iron, serum ferritin and transferrin saturation % should also have been tested. Ideally, B12, folate and vitamin D will also be tested. Iron and cortisol must be tested prior to starting to use CT3M. Starting CT3M without adequate testing may waste a significant amount of time and cause incorrect actions to be taken.

There must also be no Addison's disease or hypopituitarism, as neither of these conditions will respond to the CT3M. If there are any issues with blood sugar balance, e.g., diabetes, pre-diabetes or insulin resistance, these also have the potential to get in the way.

General Observations.

High and low cortisol can both cause thyroid hormones to be rendered less effective. High cortisol can block the effect of thyroid hormone and low cortisol will reduce the flow of glucose from the bloodstream to the cells and also make thyroid hormone less effective (due to the adverse effect on ATP production and because thyroid hormone works synergistically with cortisol). Why mention this? Well, it means that when applying the CT3M, it is very easy to be confused if you do not know if cortisol is high or low. Guessing about cortisol is not a good idea.

If cortisol is very low and the circadian dose is increased or moved earlier, this can cause a worsening of symptoms and signs. So, at times, there may be a need for trial and error and careful thinking. The guidelines in this article are really just a starting place and will not cover all cases and all patients' needs. It is often better to discuss the symptoms and signs that are being experienced with your doctor or other thyroid patients to get more input.

It is also important to start with low levels of daytime thyroid medication to avoid problems. If a thyroid patient has found out about the CT3M but is already on a high T3 dosage, e.g., 80-120 mcg of T3, but they report low body temperatures and feeling cold and tired, they almost certainly have more than enough thyroid hormone. The symptoms and signs could be due to low cortisol, or the high level of T3 that is somehow causing problems.

I have seen symptoms and signs that suggest hypothyroidism that have been caused by excess T3. The problems then get worse when someone like this begins to use the CT3M, as all this excess thyroid hormone may begin to become effective. As a result, we often see body temperature, blood pressure, and heart rate all shoot up dramatically, as well as other symptoms that suggest hyperthyroidism.

Problems can also ensue if a patient reduces their daytime T3 dosage, whilst already doing the CT3M, as this can also make more of the thyroid hormone effective and balanced with the cortisol availability. To avoid these issues, it helps to start with low daytime doses of thyroid medication (T3 or natural desiccated thyroid) to reduce the risk of this happening.

So, with all of the above in mind let us make some simple and general observations.

General Guidelines on Signs in The Circadian T3 Method (CT3M):

Lowered BP, Temps, and HR over the day often indicate low T3. This may be accompanied by a greater sense of pain, (if you have muscle or joint pain issues), tiredness, lack of motivation, brain fog, and anxiety. The full list of hypo symptoms is extensive.

Higher BP, Temps, and HR over the day, often indicate too much T3. This may be accompanied by shakiness, wired anxiety, agitation, weakness, spacey feeling, brain fog, muscle tightness (pain in neck, headache) and/or feeling physically overheated, among a host of other symptoms, which can indicate too much T3.

Note: Too much T3 can manifest with higher systolic (top number) BP, with diastolic perhaps remaining the same or only slightly raised. Too much T3 usually raises the heart rate and makes someone feel warmer (but this depends on whether there is enough cortisol and iron etc.). Anxiety and a feeling of tension/stress can also be caused by too much T3, as can diarrhoea. See the 'Recovering with T3' book for more information on the effect of excessive or too little thyroid hormone.

Temperature Guidelines:

Lower than normal temps < 98.4F average, is indicative of low thyroid hormone levels, and >99F average, is indicative of high thyroid. Temps may start the day lower, but average should be 98.4 – 98.6F.

Basal temps below 97.8F can be indicative of hypothyroidism, but basal temperature is not the best indicator. Note: Basal temp is the body temperature taken first thing when you awake, before getting out of bed. It should be averaged over a 3-5-day period and can be as low as 97.4 without being indicative of hypothyroidism.

Taking Temps: We need to assess the success of the circadian dose. So, taking the temperature within the first hour after rising is essential. A mid or late morning and mid/late afternoon and evening reading are also useful.

Repeating these at the same times each day is important so that a comparison can be made and any trends spotted (the same applies to heart rate and blood pressure readings. Several days of readings may be needed to draw any real conclusion.

For natural desiccated thyroid users, taking an average daytime temperature, i.e., averaging the morning, afternoon and evening body temperatures may be more helpful.

For T3 users: Temperatures should be taken within the first hour of rising and then in between each T3 dose and just before the next dose is taken as well as some time in the evening. Taking temperature in between each dose provides information on whether the previous dose was effective. Taking the temperature just before each dose is taken, provides information on whether the dose that is about to be taken is actually needed yet or not (if the vital signs are still good then maybe the dose should be delayed). No averaging of these temperatures for T3 users should be done, as each T3 dose should be assessed in terms of its effect on body temperature.

Note: Temps can drop if you are very relaxed, sleepy (taking a nap), without being low T3. Everyone has had this experience, but when you get up and do something, temps rise again. At least one other symptom of either hyper or hypo should go along with the temp fluctuation before using temp as a dosing guideline.

Heart Rate Guidelines:

Heart Rates <60 (less than 60) and >90 (more than 90) BPM, are often indicative of low and high thyroid respectively, but there are individual variations. Anything below 66 is suspicious of hypo, unless you are an athlete and very fit, in which case you can have a much lower than normal HR without symptoms. Normal HR for an average person is in the 70-80 range. Exceptions to this rule: High HR or high normal, with lower temp and BP may be an indication of hypo. (HR should fall and BP and temps may rise after dosing)

Low HR or low normal, but raised BP, and lower temps, may be an indication of hypo. (HR should rise, BP may lower a bit, and temps may rise after dosing)

High HR, with raised BP may be an indication of adrenaline production due to low cortisol. In this case, temps may be low, normal or even high. In this case, the heart rate is often well above 90 and the BP much higher than normal.

Feeling as if the heart is pounding with normal BP, HR (beats per minute) and temp, could indicate you need electrolytes such as magnesium/potassium /calcium or any combo of those. A fast, pounding heart rate can be low sodium. A slow pounding heart with low (or raised) BP and (low) temps could indicate low T3. A pounding heart can also be the effect of adrenaline due to low cortisol (this is often accompanied by raised BP but it depends on how low the cortisol is and how high the adrenaline is).

Note: The late Dr John Lowe said if all vitals seem normal, a mild pounding sensation, could be a sign of adequate thyroid, as thyroid patients are not used to the normal healthy heart beat

Other Observations:

One patient's experience with dosing: "I am finding that if I wake with my temperature lower than 97.6 and it does not get to 98.4 by 1:00 pm (for a couple days in a row), I need to add a little (2.5 at a time) to the CT3M dose the next day, or to my 10:00 am dose. I try to get the temp up to (no less than) 98.4 by 2:00. My temps, BP and HR all seem to line out great if I go by this timing of temp readings".

In addition to all the above it is very important to look at trends and changes that have occurred due to thyroid medication dosage changes.

Often the most important information is, in fact, to be found by assessing a number of different changes in circadian dose or daytime thyroid medication dosage that has caused changes in symptoms and signs to occur.

Very often just looking at heart rate, temps and BP alone, at any given time, will not be enough to assess what should be done to improve adrenal function and symptoms and signs. It is the overall assessment, over a number of dosage changes, that will reveal a clearer picture of what is occurring.

Finally, repeating laboratory testing of cortisol and iron and other nutrients may also be required to provide sufficient insight into what is happening with thyroid hormone and cortisol levels.

11. THE CT3M CAN IMPROVE CORTISOL THROUGHOUT THE DAY

The Circadian T3 Method (CT3M) is a means of improving cortisol levels for thyroid patients. I originally created it because I had incredibly low cortisol throughout the day. CT3M successfully raised my cortisol at all points of the day. I have been using CT3M for nearly thirty years and continue to be well.

This article was prompted by me seeing a comment that CT3M only works to improve low morning cortisol. This is not true.

Many thyroid patients end up using hydrocortisone (HC) or adrenal glandulars in order to help improve their cortisol levels. Unfortunately, this often causes the thyroid patients to produce even less of their own cortisol and makes them dependent on yet another medication. In many cases, the use of HC or adrenal glandulars makes little difference and can even make some patients feel worse.

So, what is the real truth?

CT3M can work incredibly well for many thyroid patients. It is capable of raising morning, afternoon and evening cortisol levels back to normal.

Sometimes, a dysfunctional cortisol pattern like very low morning cortisol, followed by high cortisol the rest of the day, can also be corrected, simply by getting the cortisol production to be higher in the morning.

The most common cause of low cortisol in thyroid patients is, in fact, dysfunction of the hypothalamic-pituitary system. Frequently, this is due to low FT3 levels in that system. So, correcting this, using CT3M, can fix the root cause of the problem.

Many dysfunctional cortisol patterns can be addressed by the use of CT3M. It is definitely worth trying if the thyroid patient has low cortisol across the day, low morning cortisol followed by high cortisol or simply low morning cortisol.

CT3M does not always work in every single case, but it works for many thyroid patients. CT3M frequently results in better cortisol levels throughout the day. This is why I continue to tell thyroid patients that CT3M is worth trying before the use of HC, or adrenal glandulars, is attempted. If CT3M is successful, it can make the thyroid patient feel really well, as their own cortisol production begins to work, as nature intended it to do.

CT3M has now helped thousands of thyroid patients raise their cortisol levels, or be able to wean off the use of hydrocortisone or adrenal glandulars.

For the best, most reliable information on CT3M please read the Recovering with T3 book and The CT3M Handbook.

12. WHY THE CT3M NEEDS BOTH TIME AND DOSE SIZE ADJUSTMENTS

People frequently ask me about the difference between adjusting the time of the CT3M dose in the Circadian T3 Method (CT3M) and adjusting the size of the CT3M dose.

I have been asked why do we not just start at a time four hours before we get up and then adjust the dose size.

Why does the time have to be adjusted (titrated) as well as the circadian dose size?

Why must it be done the way I have written about in my books, 'Recovering with T3' and 'The CT3M Handbook'.

The majority of people with low cortisol have it as a consequence of hypothyroidism, although it may have been made worse by issues such as immune system stresses, overall health issues, or personal stress.

However, in many people, the low cortisol occurs due to low free T3 levels that have been present for too long. The results that have been seen using the CT3M prove that this is the case.

The vast majority of people suffering from low cortisol issues easily pass an ACTH stimulation test (Synacthen test). So, their adrenal glands are fundamentally quite healthy, i.e., there is no Addison's disease present.

I believe that only those with proven Addison's disease or hypopituitarism really require hydrocortisone (HC) or adrenal glandulars. A large number of patients using these medications would be better off if they had tried the Circadian T3 Method (CT3M) first. I also do not believe that adrenals get 'fatigued' and need to be 'rested'.

I believe that low FT3 is the real reason for a great many thyroid patients having low cortisol.

I also believe that it is the direct effect of raising the FT3 level in the pituitary gland that makes CT3M work. The pituitary is responsible for the ACTH signal to the adrenal glands. I believe, in many cases, it is low FT3 within the pituitary gland that causes a low ACTH signal and, hence, low cortisol.

Right, let me discuss the Time vs. Dose Size Adjustment question.

These two adjustment methods are quite different.

Adjusting the Time of the Circadian Dose of T3 Containing Medication.

The adjustment of the time of the circadian dose provides a gentle change of FT3 level to the pituitary gland. A later T3 dose means slightly less FT3 arrives inside the pituitary and we get less response. An earlier T3 dose allows slightly more FT3 within the pituitary cells. Once the T3 dose being used is big enough, then the time changes provide a seemingly linear improvement in cortisol level for those patients that have relatively undamaged adrenal glands (and most have quite healthy adrenals – even those who have been encouraged to use adrenal steroids).

Once the circadian dose is at the 1.5 hours before waking time and the dose is high enough (often 15 mcg of T3 or 1.5 grains of natural thyroid), the response by even moving the CT3M dose 15-30 minutes earlier is often quite noticeable.

The CT3M dose may be moved back as far as 4 hours before waking time (and even in rare circumstances a little further e.g., 5 hours). Doing this often sees a more powerful response from CT3M.

Consequently, adjusting the time of the CT3M dose is the fine-tuning dial in the CT3M.

Adjusting the Circadian Dose Size in the CT3M.

T3 acts like a wave. This is described in my book, Recovering with T3:

"For each divided dose of T3, I discovered that there was definitely a 'threshold level' that had to be exceeded before any real benefit was experienced from the hormone. As I increased the dose beyond this threshold level then the effects were greater. If I exceeded the threshold too much then I experienced symptoms of tissue over-stimulation. My threshold level tended to be lower as the day progressed. So, later in the day, I required lower doses of T3 to achieve the same effect. This perception may be due in part to some cumulative effect of the previous doses of T3 but the interaction with other hormones, which reduce in level during the day, may also be relevant.

I often use a specific analogy to describe to other people how T3 appears to behave:

Imagine a sandy beach, which is sheltered from the sea by large rocks. Only a wave that is large and powerful enough is capable of striking the rocks and sending a spray of seawater over them to drench the sand beyond."

The way this works is that as you increase the circadian dose the size of that wave increases and significantly more FT3 becomes available to the cells (including the pituitary gland, which we are trying to encourage to work properly).

Adjusting the size of the CT3M dose by even 2.5 micrograms can produce a profoundly different effect.

Consequently, adjusting the size of the circadian dose is the rough-tuning dial on our cortisol production in the CT3M.

We need both Time and Dose Size Adjustments.

For the CT3M to work properly we need a rough adjustment and we need fine-tuning.

It is too easy to cause too much cortisol to be generated in some people and in others, their system takes longer to recover and we need to have a CT3M dose that is as good as it can be without over-straining the system.

So, the process works quite well. I suggest using it, rather than trying to short cut it.

In summary, the typical steps are:

1. The circadian dose size is adjusted so that it begins to work starting typically at around 1.5-hours (possibly 2 hours) before someone gets up in the morning. Moving the CT3M dose back as far as 4 hours before your average 'get up time' is also possible. This should be done slowly though, allowing time to evaluate after any change.
2. Then the time of the circadian dose is adjusted.
3. Once an optimal time is found then the circadian dose size may be titrated once again.
4. Once this circadian dose size appears to be about right then the time adjustment is our friend again and we can subtly adjust our cortisol output (as well as other adrenal hormones).

It is a little iterative, with time allowed after each small change, but there is no way around that.

13. MORE ON THE CIRCADIAN T3 METHOD (CT3M) TIME AND DOSE SIZE CHANGES

Over the years I have had discussions with people who wanted to know how much to increase the circadian dose when taken at one and a half hours before getting up, before moving the circadian dose earlier in time. I hope this article helps to clarify this.

In the Circadian T3 Method (CT3M) the adjustment of circadian dose timing and dose size are both necessary.

A change to the time the circadian dose is taken provides a gentle change of FT3 level to the pituitary, in order to help it to provide the adrenal glands with the right level of ACTH. A later T3 dose ensures slightly less FT3 arrives inside the pituitary cells and usually produces a lower response from the adrenal glands. An earlier T3 dose allows slightly more FT3 and may produce a larger response.

A change to the size of the circadian dose can produce very large effects as even small increases of 2.5 micrograms of T3-containing medication can increase FT3 levels in the cells.

Ideally, only enough T3-containing medication will be used but it will be taken early enough in the cycle of cortisol production that it will fully support the pituitary and the adrenal glands.

The CT3M process begins by finding the smallest circadian dose size that has some positive effect on symptoms or signs taken at one and a half hours before getting up.

This initial dose does not have to fully resolve symptoms - it only needs some detectable benefit.

Once the initial circadian dose is large enough to produce some effect then timing changes to the dose provide a smoother change in adrenal function. Adjusting the time of the circadian dose is the fine-tuning dial on cortisol in the CT3M.

Hence it is better to find the smallest circadian dose that appears to have some positive effect at one and a half hours before getting up, and then adjust the time of the dose to find the optimal time to take it. Only once the optimal time is found should the circadian dose be increased to discover the best dose size.

If the circadian dose is increased too much when taken at one and a half hours before getting up, then when the circadian dose is taken earlier, it can be far too potent.

Consequently, thyroid patients have found that using a circadian dose of 10, 12.5 or 15 micrograms at one and half hours before getting up is often a good starting point before adjusting the time of the circadian dose.

The initial circadian dose size does not need to resolve all symptoms, it only needs to be seen to have some positive effects. Hence, only a small increase in this starting circadian dose may be necessary from a starting dose of 10 micrograms of T3-containing medication. Some sensitive thyroid patients may need to begin with an even lower dose of T3 medication, less than the 10 micrograms suggested.

As already stated, increasing the circadian dose by even 2.5 micrograms can produce a very strong result. Consequently, adjusting the size of the circadian dose may be viewed as the rough-tuning dial on our cortisol level in the CT3M.

The optimal time to take the circadian dose is frequently somewhere between two and a half and four hours before the individual gets up in the morning, although there are exceptions to this with some people doing well at only one and a half hours before rising. Once the ideal time has been found to take the circadian dose then the circadian dose size may be increased further. After this, further fine-tuning of both time and size of the circadian dose may be performed if needed, based on symptoms and signs.

Therefore, within the CT3M, both time and dose size adjustments are required to tailor the necessary T3 support for good cortisol production.

14. MORE RESEARCH ON THE IMPORTANCE OF T3 TO CORTISOL PRODUCTION

Here is are two research articles that provides more scientific support for using T3 to support cortisol and for my Circadian T3 Method (CT3M).

T3 is critical to the way that the pituitary gland functions. Without adequate FT3, the pituitary is susceptible to dysfunction, and the anterior pituitary hormones may be affected. These hormones include adrenocorticotropic hormone (ACTH) that drives both cortisol and Dhea production in the adrenal glands.

This is another piece of data that supports the CT3M protocol I developed in Recovering with T3:

"Disruption of the Pituitary Circadian Clock Induced by Hypothyroidism and
Hyperthyroidism: Consequences on Daily Pituitary Hormone Expression Profiles."
Bargi-Souza P, Peliciari-Garcia RA, Nunes MT.
Thyroid. 2019 Apr;29(4):502-512.
doi: 10.1089/thy.2018.0578. Epub 2019 Mar 13.
https://www.ncbi.nlm.nih.gov/pubmed/30747053

Here is additional research that supports CT3M. This is a 1978 piece of research that confirms that TSH and FT3 peak in the night. This knowledge is important and it is partly what supports my CT3M optional protocol. We also know that the pituitary has the highest concentration of FT3 in the body and that it is the pituitary that begins to drive cortisol levels up in the latter part of the night. Keeping FT3 levels up during that part of the night is important. This happens normally in healthy people, but often it does not in thyroid patients on daytime thyroid medication. Any loss of thyroid tissue (through Hashimoto's or thyroidectomy) also makes things worse as this loses a significant amount of FT4 to FT3 conversion capability. Any DIO1 and DIO2 gene defects might also be a big factor as they can impact conversion capability.

Here is the research paper:
"Circadian and 30 Minutes Variations in Serum TSH and Thyroid Hormones in Normal Subjects."
Jorgan Weeke and Hans Jorgan G. Gundersen.
EJE Clinical and Translational Endocrinology.
DOI: https://doi.org/10.1530/acta.0.0890659
https://eje.bioscientifica.com/view/journals/eje/89/3/acta_89_3_024.xml

15. THE CIRCADIAN T3 METHOD AND WEANING ADRENAL STEROIDS

Observations on Weaning Adrenal Hormone Medications Like Hydrocortisone (HC) and Florinef.

This is based on the experience that patients have had with weaning adrenal steroids when applying the Circadian T3 Method (CT3M). These are not recommendations. They are merely a collection of experiences that have been gathered by thyroid patients in the process of reducing and stopping the use of adrenal steroids like hydrocortisone and florinef.

These observations only apply to those patients who have no fundamental adrenal damage (Addison's disease) and no hypopituitarism. It is also extremely important that any weaning of adrenal steroids is done under the supervision of a qualified medical practitioner.

When applying the CT3M, adrenal hormones need to be weaned in order to allow the adrenals to receive an adequate request from the body to make adrenal hormones. For cortisol, this request comes in the form of ACTH from the pituitary. For aldosterone, the request arrives by more subtle routes from the nervous system. However, all forms of adrenal hormones, in synthetic or adrenal glandular form, are 'the lullaby that sings the adrenals to sleep'. Whilst these adrenal hormones are being taken, the CT3M will not work and the adrenals themselves will not recover.

There is a myth that by taking adrenal hormones the adrenal glands will be rested, and then these steroids may be weaned slowly and the patient's adrenals will have recovered.

This recovery hardly ever happens. Thyroid patients frequently find themselves fighting continued ill health and unable to stop the use of these steroids. Consequently, the CT3M should be offered as the first-choice treatment before any adrenal steroids are considered.

If a thyroid patient is already on adrenal hormones when the CT3M is applied, then the following approach for weaning these adrenal steroids has been seen to be successful:

APPROACH TO WEANING ADRENAL STEROIDS STEP BY STEP:

If a thyroid patient is already on adrenal hormones when CT3M is applied, the approach described here for weaning off them, has been seen to be successful. It is based on the experience of many thyroid patients, but it should also be carried out with the support of the patient's own personal physician:

1. No adrenal steroids should be taken within the main cortisol production window (i.e. the last four hours of sleep). Consequently, the first dose of any adrenal medication should be taken no earlier than when the thyroid patient gets up in the morning (ideally, at least an hour or two later). This is to give the HP system and the adrenal glands a chance to respond to the CT3M dose.

2. **Florinef weaning.** All Florinef (which is the synthetic equivalent of aldosterone), and all slow potassium, should be weaned first. This is before any attempt is made to reduce cortisol-containing medication (hydrocortisone or prednisolone). Florinef affects blood pressure too much to be left in place, as the CT3M dose is titrated. High blood pressure may result if CT3M is applied without weaning Florinef at the same time.

3. Thyroid patients have found that Florinef should be weaned in stages, with a small fraction of the Florinef being removed at a time, as CT3M is applied. Florinef depresses potassium, and if someone is taking slow-release potassium, this needs to be reduced at the same time that the Florinef is weaned.

4. Good results have been seen when Florinef is weaned by quarter tablet reductions, sometimes reducing by a half a tablet every week (1 tablet is 0.1mg of Florinef). Slow potassium should be weaned in proportion. For example, for someone on half a tablet of Florinef and 16 MEQ of slow-K, they may wean to a quarter of a tablet of Florinef and at the same time reduce their slow-K to 8 MEQ (MEQ stands for milliequivalent). If the Florinef remains too high when CT3M is applied, it will raise blood pressure very quickly after taking it. By tracking symptoms and signs, it should be possible to manage the weaning process as CT3M is applied.

5. CT3M may be started, and the CT3M dose adjusted (i.e., dose time and size), as the Florinef and any potassium medication is fully weaned. This may need the support of the patient's doctor. At the very least, the patient's own medical practitioner should be

aware of this process and be available to support the patient. Once a CT3M dose has been found that seems to help, many patients have found it useful not to change that dose during the weaning of adrenal steroids, as too many changes can be confusing and unnecessary.

6. If high blood pressure is present during the weaning of Florinef, the weaning of hydrocortisone (HC) or any cortisol containing medication, should be started at the same time (see points 7 - 10). In this case, the first HC dose should be the focus of weaning (points 8 - 9).

7. **Hydrocortisone weaning.** Once all Florinef and any slow potassium are weaned, the next task is to remove cortisol-containing medication, such as hydrocortisone (HC). HC depresses potassium, and this is another reason to wean all slow potassium before any HC is reduced.

8. HC is normally taken in divided doses during the day. The following three approaches have been seen to work well:

a) The first HC dose of the day (which must not be taken during the last four hours of sleep), is delayed or pushed forward in time. Ideally, the delay should be for as long as feels comfortably possible. If the delay is long enough for the second HC dose to be due, this first HC dose may be dropped completely. This may occur immediately if the response to CT3M is good. If the first HC dose is still needed before the second HC dose is due, the first HC dose is trimmed by at least 2.5 mg.

b) An alternative is to begin by weaning the first HC dose of the day and, at the same time, move this trimmed-HC dose to later in the day. Every day or two, the first dose of HC may be moved an hour or so later. It should be trimmed by at least 2.5 mg each day if possible. Eventually, the first HC dose will be close to the second HC dose, and may be dropped totally.

c) The third approach to weaning HC is to delay the first HC dose by as much as is comfortable, and to delay all the other HC doses by the same amount of time. In this approach, the last HC dose of the day will end up being later in the day, and will be reduced by at least 2.5 mg every time the movement of the doses occur. This approach may be relevant if the thyroid patient appears to need both the first and second HC doses to remain at the same levels for a little longer whilst the CT3M dose is adjusted.

9. By moving the first dose of HC to a later time, this creates more time during which the adrenal glands are required to support the patient's body on their own (with no suppressive effect from HC via any lowering of ACTH from the pituitary). This movement later in time of the first dose of HC, and the frequent cutting of it by 2.5 mg, really allows the adrenal glands freedom to work correctly. As the HC weaning progresses, the CT3M dose is adjusted further if needed.

10. Once the first HC dose has been moved and effectively dropped, the remaining doses of HC may be weaned by 2.5 mg (or more) each day. Eventually, when there is only 10mg of HC adrenal medication being used, it may be stopped completely.

11. **General Observations on weaning of adrenal steroids.** It is worth pointing out that sometimes, during the weaning of steroids, when a dose of HC or Florinef (or adrenal glandulars if these are being used) is taken, this may produce very marked adverse symptoms. An example of this might be extreme nausea following a dose of HC or Florinef. When noticeably adverse symptoms occur, this may also provide excellent information suggesting that the adrenal steroid dose is ready to be weaned further.

12. CT3M should be enabling the better HP system response and therefore improved ACTH. ACTH stimulates cortisol, DHEA and androstenedione production strongly. ACTH also has some effect on aldosterone. So, improvement in all of these hormones may have occurred. However, further titration of the CT3M dose may be required. In some cases, when no steroid medication is being used, the response to the CT3M dose may be too potent because of the suppressive effect that the steroids were previously having on the adrenal glands.

13. Following the process of slow weaning and stopping all adrenal steroids, if symptoms and signs are not normal and do not suggest good adrenal function, CT3M should be re-started. This means restarting with a low dose of T3 (possibly 10-micrograms) or NDT (1 grain), 1.5 hours before the time that the thyroid patient gets up. Adjusting the CT3M dose fully, with no steroids present, often resolves any remaining issues. This may need to be repeated over time as the adrenal glands improve their production. It is important to allow several days in between each change to the CT3M dose to ensure the effects can be assessed.

14. This weaning process does not need to take months and months - four to six weeks is often sufficient. However, cortisol levels may not fully recover immediately, and a CT3M dose may need to be found that supports the HP system without over-stressing it. Over time the HP system should improve the production of ACTH, which should improve cortisol, and potentially other adrenal hormones. It is advisable to re-take a twenty-four-hour cortisol saliva test from time to time. In some cases, the CT3M dose of T3 may need to be fine-tuned further. If there is any doubt over what is going on, a re-start of CT3M may be required.

The process outlined above is based on the experience of many thyroid patients who have applied CT3M and, at the same time, successfully weaned themselves from adrenal steroids.

For those patients using adrenal glandulars, these may be treated more like the HC weaning part of the above process, with the first adrenal glandular dose being weaned first.

The above process appears to work well, but inevitably it may not be a smooth process because of the powerful nature of adrenal steroids. Having good support in place while this is happening is essential.

It is very important to be aware that, even after all steroids have been weaned, the adrenal glands may take a considerable amount of time (weeks or months) to fully recover their ability and that during this time more adjustment may be required to the circadian dose.

However, being completely off adrenal steroids and using the CT3M is a very effective way to enable the thyroid patients' adrenal gland function to fully return (in the cases where there is no Addison's disease or hypopituitarism).

As stated at the start, this is not a set of recommendations and thyroid patients should consult their own medical practitioner if they are considering weaning adrenal steroids.

16. LOW DOSE NALTREXONE AND THE CORTISOL CONNECTION

Here is another article about a drug called low dose naltrexone (LDN) and its use in lowering autoimmune reactions - see Article 11 in Chapter 10.

I have personally tried LDN and found that it had some positive effects and some negative ones. I have also talked to many patients who have used LDN themselves.

Some patients using LDN experience lower autoimmune reactions (which is obviously good). Others can experience alterations in other neurotransmitters (like serotonin and dopamine balance – which may be good or bad).

Importantly, some thyroid patients appear to have improved hypothalamic pituitary adrenal (HPA) axis response. This can mean that some thyroid patients experience improved cortisol levels. I have definitely seen cortisol levels improve in some people when they begin to use LDN.

LDN is not a guaranteed way of improving Hashimoto's or cortisol. It can have unpredictable results. It can be very helpful for some people, do nothing for others, and make some feel emotional and cause problems in dosing thyroid hormones.

However, LDN is a useful tool in the toolbox.

It is one approach that I recommend leaving until the last, after other things have been tried, as it can have unpredictable results.

I prefer to see autoimmune issues addressed through diet, supplements, toxicity removal, the correction of nutrient imbalances, and the good and sensible use of a thyroid hormone treatment that the thyroid patient requires.

As I mentioned above, I have personally tried to use LDN. My own experience is that LDN is definitely potent. It caused emotional changes that were not good in my case. I have witnessed this in others too. LDN did raise my cortisol levels, but the other side effects were not acceptable to me.

Some people may not experience any side effects. However, my experience with LDN is not extensive and I have not made a large study of it. So, my experience is anecdotal.

So, anyone considering LDN use should do their own research.

Circadian T3 Method (CT3M) and LDN.

I believe that there is potential in the combination of the CT3M and LDN for those people who really have very low cortisol and cannot improve it sufficiently using CT3M alone.

More will be discovered about the connection between LDN and cortisol over time but considerably more research is needed.

17. COULD CORTISOL PUMPS HELP THOSE WHO CANNOT TOLERATE HC

My main aim has always been to provide information that can help thyroid patients recover from hypothyroidism as fast as possible. The majority of my written material is about the correct use of thyroid hormones. However, because so many thyroid patients have low cortisol problems, I also deal with the treatment of low cortisol in my books.

To correct very low cortisol levels, I created the Circadian T3 Method (CT3M). I first wrote about CT3M in my book, Recovering with T3. Since then, CT3M has helped thousands of thyroid patients correct their low cortisol levels. My books and other articles contain a great deal of information about CT3M and low cortisol.

In some patients, the use of Low Dose Naltrexone (LDN) can also be helpful in raising cortisol levels.

However, in some low cortisol patients, there is simply no choice for them other than to use the steroid hydrocortisone (bio-identical cortisol) or an adrenal glandular that contains cortisol.

Many patients do well on hydrocortisone (HC) tablets, particularly if they have someone who is very capable working with them to get the dosing right. However, some patients have problems getting their HC doses and timings correct. For instance, some need a bedtime dose; some individuals must avoid a bedtime dose. Some do best with one large HC dose in the morning, and some need 2 to 4 doses spread out (in just the right amounts and timing). It can be a lot of work to try and get the HC to work well.

However, inevitably there are patients with low cortisol that appear to never do well on HC or adrenal glandulars. They may try to change the doses over months and years but they still remain very ill.

This is not really a surprise. Oral HC doses are quite large and do not represent what a healthy body actually does, i.e., tablets do not provide the drip feed of cortisol on an on-going basis which the body is designed to do. The bottom line is that taking oral HC is not as physiological.

Insulin pumps have been around for a while. Over recent years this type of pump technology has started to be used to deliver cortisol. The Cortisol Pump has started to be used. In the UK, one of the pioneers of cortisol pump technology, and treatment, is Professor Peter Hindmarsh.

Cortisol pumps deliver cortisol in a programmable manner, which makes it possible to more closely mimic what a healthy person's cortisol levels would actually look like. Cortisol blood levels from a cortisol pump are maintained at more natural, physiological levels than taking oral HC. The natural 24-hour circadian rhythm of cortisol can also be reproduced.

I believe that, for those patients who cannot fully recover using my CT3M protocol, or LDN, or using HC or adrenal glandulars, the cortisol pump technology might prove helpful.

There are two cortisol pumps that I am currently aware of:
- The Crono P that delivers cortisol in pulses over 24 hours.
- The Medtronic Pump that delivers cortisol continuously and can be tuned to replicate the natural pattern of cortisol over 24 hours.

This is an extract from an email I received very recently from someone who was kind enough to update me on his progress:

"For the past 3 years, I have been extremely ill with low cortisol symptoms. The symptoms are exactly the same as you describe in your books (hell on earth) and that's putting it mildly. Six months ago, I discovered the cortisol pump and my life has changed so dramatically that I find it incredible. In fact, I would say I am functioning at 90% of my old self.

What I have discovered is that cortisol has to be dosed per circadian rhythm just like thyroid hormone. Oral steroids and current treatment practices are wrong. You cannot wake up and then take your first dose of hydrocortisone (HC), as this is completely against the way the body works. The other major problem with oral steroids is you cannot micro-dose with them as the body does.

With an insulin pump, you can micro-dose as low as 0.1 mg of cortisol.

I only take 7.55 mg of cortisol a day between 3:00 am and 11:00 am along with 1.5 grains of NDT in the morning and 5 mcg of Cytomel (T3) at 2:00 pm. With cortisol, it is not about the milligrams, it is about the distribution of the drug. I honestly believe that almost everyone on oral steroids is most likely over-dosing even on low doses like 20 mg because they are taking it the wrong way, which in turn makes the body need even more to feel somewhat normal.

Anyway, I thought you would be interested in how well the pump can work. I am amazed by this technology and the fact that nobody really knows about it. This needs to be taken seriously by doctors. In fact, my doctor is so impressed by this that he wants to put more of his patients on the pump."

For those patients who cannot correct their low cortisol through the improvement of T3 levels, CT3M, or the use of oral HC, the cortisol pump technology offers a potentially excellent solution.

Because cortisol pumps use micro-doses of HC, the cost of hydrocortisone is significantly less than the cost when taking it in tablet form. Note: that the person above only requires a little over 7 milligrams of cortisol per day, which is a relatively tiny amount compared to oral HC dosing. However, there is the initial outlay for the pump itself to be paid for, and expert help needs to be found to set it up.

This obviously raises the question over why low cortisol issues have occurred.

Some researchers are starting to consider whether the paraventricular nucleus of the hypothalamus (PVN) could be behind the low cortisol issues, i.e., a Hypothalamic-Pituitary (HP) system issue.

Others researchers believe that the reason HC medication does not work in some patients is due to chronic infections. For such people, the non-physiological ups and downs with tablets make them worse, and any decline in cortisol from a higher level increases their immune reaction to the infection and makes them worse. Clearly, in these cases eradicating the chronic infection is critical but sometimes this can be very difficult. Cortisol pumps appear to work more effectively in these cases.

It also makes me wonder whether chronic fatigue syndrome, which has so many overlapping symptoms with low cortisol, could also be an HP system issue, and whether some CFS patients with low cortisol could also benefit from cortisol pumps.

It can be quite difficult to begin using a cortisol pump and it definitely requires a great deal of analysis and set up work with support from a knowledgeable medical professional. In the USA, a 24-hour blood draw is done to see how well the individual is absorbing and excreting the medication and the set-up is based on that. In Canada, typically, a morning and evening blood cortisol test is done. I understand that there are target levels of cortisol. The pumps are then adjusted until the targets are achieved and the patient responds symptomatically.

In the UK, I believe that endocrinologists will only assist those patients who have had a diagnosis of Addison's disease (via a failed Synacthen Test) to obtain and set up a cortisol pump. The person who wrote to me above uses a Medtronic insulin pump. Currently, Medtronic will sell anybody a pump as long as they have a reference letter from a doctor (a prescription is not needed). However, there are online groups who are devoted to assisting patients to obtain cortisol pumps.

This is a link I was given about one low cortisol sufferer. It is her story of how a cortisol pump helped her get her life back:

https://cortisolmusings.wordpress.com/2020/06/10/4-years-with-the-cortisol-pump/

Interestingly, the idea behind cortisol pump delivery of micro doses of HC has also been pioneered with oral HC. This article by a patient explains this:

https://www.pituitary.org.uk/news/2017/08/hydrocortisone-regime--gail's-story/

As I mentioned at the start, my own work is aimed at returning thyroid patients to good health and good cortisol levels without ever resorting to the use of oral steroids. However, in some cases, medications like HC just have to be used. For some of these low cortisol patients (and potentially some CFS patients), cortisol pumps might offer a great solution.

I am not currently planning to write more about cortisol pumps, as using hydrocortisone is not one of my main focus areas. This article contains just about all I know about the technology. However, I felt that I ought to share it, as it may be that some readers ultimately find that a cortisol pump is the best solution for them.

I hope this also serves to explain to readers that I am not fundamentally against using cortisol medications when there is no other possible solution. I just prefer to find simpler and more natural ways and be certain that cortisol meds are actually necessary before people take that path.

18. T4 MEDICATION IN THE EVENING MAY LOWER CORTISOL IN POOR CONVERTERS

This article is based on working with thyroid patients who have some level of cortisol dysregulation. Usually, this dysregulation is sub-optimal cortisol, that has been seen in an 8:00-9:00 am morning cortisol blood test, or in a saliva cortisol test. In some cases, the patients have simply described their symptoms to me, which have invariably included finding that getting up and functioning well in the morning is incredibly difficult. The term that is often used to describe how they feel in the morning is 'dragging'. Often the patient does not start to feel better until the afternoon or evening.

For those patients with clearly sub-optimal cortisol, I usually recommend trying my CT3M protocol using T3. Even if they are on T4 or NDT medication in the daytime, a T3 CT3M dose can still be effective in improving cortisol.

For those patients who have not yet tested cortisol, I encourage them to actually test it properly in blood and saliva. It is always best to get actual test data when cortisol is concerned, as attempting to diagnose low cortisol just on symptoms can be difficult. For some patients, getting the right tests done can be problematic because of their situation or location. For these patients, a trial of CT3M can actually be the only viable diagnostic available.

In the majority of cases of low cortisol, I tend not to suggest much in the way of changes to the daytime dosing strategy of the patient. However, the exception to this is for poor converters of T4 to T3. When thyroid patients have an FT4 level which is much higher in the reference range than their FT3 result, it is usually because these patients are poor converters. They may also have a high in the reference range rT3 result, which would tend to confirm this situation. The reasons for being a poor converter are many. They include thyroid tissue damage, and genetic defects, which I discuss in other articles. But there are many other potential causes. Whilst some causes of poor conversion might respond to intervention, there are some that will not and the only thing to be done is to manage the situation. Often this requires less T4 medication and added T3 medication.

Having introduced the basic background let me talk about the very specific situation that prompted me to write this article. Some poor converters of T4, may be taking their T4, or NDT, in the evening or at bedtime. It is actually quite common practice for T4 meds to be taken at bedtime and many thyroid patients are convinced it makes them feel better. However, I believe these people are invariably fairly good converters of T4 to T3.

For the poor converter of T4 to T3, a bedtime dose of T4 can be the worst thing to be using. The reason for this is that by the time the T4 absorbs from the gut and gets to peak levels in the bloodstream, it will be the middle of the night. This is the time that the pituitary gland begins to slowly raise ACTH to stimulate the adrenal glands to produce more cortisol. The pituitary will begin to crank up ACTH so that in the last hour or two prior to getting up, the thyroid patient ought to have good cortisol levels. As I explain in my books, and other articles, the pituitary gland is known to have the highest concentration of FT3 compared to all our organs and glands. It 'runs on FT3'.

When a poor converter of T4 to T3, uses an evening or bedtime dose of T4, they are basically risking the situation where rT3 is rising higher, and FT3 might even fall. As I have explained elsewhere, the T4 dose could lower TSH slightly, which will down-regulate FT4 to FT3 conversion. As conversion is down-regulated, FT3 could lower and rT3 could rise. This is entirely the opposite situation to that of using a T3 CT3M dose. For poor converters of T4 to T3, a bedtime dose of T4 (or NDT), may well have an 'anti-cortisol effect'.

Now, this article is based on working with thyroid patients. It is not based, on a published research study, so I cannot provide any peer-viewed published papers. However, what I can say is that I know of thyroid patients who have had either clear low cortisol results, or obvious low cortisol symptoms, who have provided me with good evidence for what I have written here. They have simply changed the time that they take their T4 medication from the evening to the morning, and have immediately felt far better. This is without any other dosage changes at all. It is also possible that, if a thyroid patient was on a T3 CT3M dose, then the bedtime dose of T4 might be totally counterproductive.

Clearly, this article is only relevant to poor converters of T4 to T3, and to those that also have sub-optimal cortisol, or low cortisol symptoms. But for this subset of patients, it is worth them considering whether any bedtime dosing of T4-based medication might in fact be contributing to their low cortisol.

Chapter 9

Useful Research Papers & Summaries

1. TIME FOR A REASSESSMENT OF THE TREATMENT OF HYPOTHYROIDISM

This is a great new article from thyroid researchers that points the way to a better way of thyroid treatment, which is more focused on relieving patient symptoms.

The article shows the massive flaws in the previous research that has concluded T4/T3 therapy offers no clear benefit.

It points out the many flaws in relying on TSH and other lab tests alone as a means of assessing whether thyroid patients are adequately treated. It concludes with references to the increasing rate of patient complaints about the non-relief of symptoms.

I asked one of the co-authors for a summary of the article. Here are Dr John Midgley's own words on it:

"Hi Paul,

Yes, it has a year since first submitted. A long haul indeed but got there in the end.

This paper describes the history of thyroid function testing and therapy. It shows how the original therapeutic use of desiccated thyroid extract (DTE) was superseded by T4 monotherapy. It demonstrates that there was no formal clinical trial to compare effectiveness at the time. The principal reason was the inconsistency of DTE content at the time of change. However, nowadays DTE is carefully controlled by accepted chemical/physical methods. There has been no trial comparing DTE and T4 until about 2013.

The first milestones in the detection of dysfunction and therapy control were the development of tests to measure first total T4 and T3, and an initially insensitive TSH followed 15 years later by free T4 (FT4) and free T3 (FT3) tests + a sensitive TSH which could simultaneously detect hypo and hyperthyroidism. Historically Total T3 / FT3 was only used for diagnosing hyperthyroidism, for which it is still used today. Total T4 / T4 was found to be unsatisfactory for controlling T4 monotherapy because often the Total T4 or FT4 was above the healthy reference range. Sensitive TSH was found to be far more sensitive in detecting primary hypo and hyperthyroidism.

However, because the simple idea took hold that a lost thyroid meant lost T4 which could be fully substituted by oral hormone without further complication, the use of TSH as a therapy control was extended to patients on T4. We now know this is incorrect.

247

The thyroid makes both T4 and T3 so that the T3 in the body comes from a combination of direct thyroid production and body T4 conversion to T3. If the thyroid is lost, the whole system is severely altered.

In some cases, T4 only therapy cannot make up for the T4 + T3 the thyroid originally made so that no matter how much T4 is given, the body's conversion cannot make up for the T3 directly made by the working gland. It is these patients who need T3 in some form direct as oral therapy.

Finally, we all have our unique healthy combination of TSH, FT4 and FT3. They together define our health state and cannot be separated. Classical statistical analysis has in fact separated the parameters when studying a population. This is called univariate statistics. However, to get the proper picture, bivariate or trivariate analysis is need to keep the three parameters together for an individual in any group. This has implications for the value of TSH as a satisfactory control of therapy.

Finally, the results from randomised clinical trials, as to the efficacy and suitability of combined T4/T3 therapy, are severely compromised by including all patients, whether satisfied or dissatisfied, with T4 monotherapy in the analysis. The significant minority of patients that prefer combination therapy get swamped out and lost. This is an example of a statistical error called Simpson's paradox. All trials so far fall under this problem and are therefore of no use. We provide ways to avoid this problem in future trials.

In short, therefore, the use of TSH in monitoring thyroid hormone therapy is highly unsatisfactory and should be replaced by triple FT4/FT3/TSH measurement + the presentation symptoms of the patient (which should have a primary role). Unthinking automatic biochemical definition of treatment success independent of the patient must cease, i.e., the laboratory test result focus must cease. Individuality is the decision-maker for optimum therapeutic outcomes.

Best Wishes

John"

Note: The loss of the thyroid in the above summary includes both thyroidectomy and Hashimoto's thyroiditis, which destroys thyroid tissue.

Here's the information on the actual research article:

"Time for a reassessment of the treatment of hypothyroidism" John E. M. Midgley, Anthony D. Toft, Rolf Larisch, Johannes W. Dietrich & Rudolf Hoermann.

BMC Endocrine Disorders volume 19, Article number: 37 (2019) https://bmcendocrdisord.biomedcentral.com/articles/10.1186/s12902-019-0365-4

2. TRIIODOTHYRONINE (T3) SECRETION IN EARLY THYROID FAILURE

Here is a very important research article, which explains how a failing thyroid gland makes more T3 to compensate for damage within its tissues.

In one of the co-authors own words, "The paper shows that during the course of thyroid decline from the start, increases in TSH resulting from the shortfall of T4 production has a stimulatory effect on thyroid direct T3 production, to make up as far as possible the shortfall in corporeal T4-T3 conversion caused by lack of enough T4. The feed-forward TSH-T3 stimulation in the gland can go on for a long time, whereby at the end game when the gland finally dies, the T3 produced by the thyroid is greater than T4-T3 conversion in the body (because of the gross lack of T4). This can mean that the body tries to keep as stable as possible regarding T3 production until the thyroid is totally lost and this then enters an entirely new phase. It can be round about now when the patient feels hypo strongly."

The Importance of The Thyroid Gland.

It should be clear from the above description, and from the article, how important the thyroid gland actually is. It compensates for damage to itself so much that it can mask this for a long time. The article explains why so many patients that suffer from Hashimoto's thyroiditis feel well for such a long time, due to the extra conversion from T4 to T3 that the thyroid is capable of. Towards the end of the progression of Hashimoto's, when thyroid tissue damage has become very significant, severe symptoms can suddenly begin to appear. Lab testing at this stage often shows very high TSH, and very low FT4 and FT3 levels. This is exactly what happened to me. In the case of thyroidectomy patients, they are thrown into the state of thyroid tissue loss immediately, so getting their FT3 levels back up to a healthy level is very important (obviously the right level is very individual).

Please enjoy this very important research study:

"Triiodothyronine Secretion in Early Thyroid Failure: The Adaptive Response of Central Feedforward Control" Rudolf Hoermann, Mark Pekker, John Edward M Midgley, Rolf Larisch Johannes W. Dietrich December 2019 European Journal of Clinical Investigation DOI: 10.1111/eci.13192 https://pubmed.ncbi.nlm.nih.gov/31815292/

Note: In one place in the article, it states:
"Whereby at the end game when the gland finally dies, the T3 produced by the thyroid is greater than T4-T3 conversion in the body (because of the gross lack of T4)".

What the authors mean by this is that, just before the thyroid gland finally dies, the T3 produced by the thyroid is greater than T4-T3 conversion in the body (because of the gross lack of T4). After this point, the gland fails catastrophically and T3 levels plummet leaving the thyroid patient with low T3 and T4 levels.

In the words of another of the co-authors:

"Our data reveal that 1) there is a strong rescue mechanism based on direct thyroidal T3 secretion and activated on demand, and 2) this does not depend on conversion/ deiodinases and may explain 3) why experimental animals deficient in all three deiodinases, but with an intact thyroid were reported to survive and live well (they are not hypothyroid.). The thyroid gland and its massive ability to contribute T3 is crucial."

The article is saying that in a declining T3 environment (not a euthyroid healthy state) the central role of the thyroid gland is paramount in maintaining healthy T3 levels. This is through the gland's ability to shift as much of its ability as possible into making T3. Furthermore, this is not controlled by TSH.

It is as another of the author's says, "Strong T3-protective mechanisms of the control system emerge with declining thyroid function when glandular T3 secretion becomes increasingly influential over conversion efficiency."

They also conclude that this shows, once again, that the influence of TSH is being overestimated and the reliance on it to determine whether someone is properly treated, or not, is flawed.

It is very interesting and explains why so many of the Hashimoto's patients are not aware of the problem until the symptoms suddenly get severe.

3. TREATMENT NEEDS TO BE TAILORED TO THE INDIVIDUAL

Here is a published article that refers to a collection of pertinent research papers that have been written over the last few years.

The papers point the way to a new, and better, way of managing thyroid treatment.

My book, The Thyroid Patient's Manual, is consistent with this thyroid research.

Here is the link to the research article:

https://www.researchgate.net/publication/326984710_Homeostasis_and_Allostasis_of_Thyroid_Function

You can use the link provided to download the .pdf file containing the research papers.

One of the researchers Dr John Midgely summarises the conclusions with these words: "This collection is a large part of our work that shows:

1. The individual nature of thyroid function parameters (i.e., each person occupying their own narrow range within the much wider general population range).
2. The incorrectness of using the healthy TSH normal range as a diagnostic for therapy.
3. The effects of non-thyroidal illness on thyroid parameters.
4. The important role of direct T3 production by the thyroid as a controller of T4-T3 conversion by the rest of the body.
5. The absolute need to monitor FT3 in therapy.
6. The collapse of the control system when all thyroid activity is lost and the resulting fundamental change in T4-T3-TSH relationships.
7. Because of individuality in thyroid parameters and response to treatment, the need to go back to patient symptom presentation as a key part of diagnosis and treatment."

The overall implication is that patients need to be treated as individuals. The present approach of viewing laboratory test results as either being in or out of the normal range does not work well for patients. The paper also urges a serious examination of combined T4/T3 therapy in suitable patients.

This research is incredibly important and illustrates that the approach currently being used is failing thyroid patients.

4. SOME PATIENTS DO NEED T3 IN THEIR TREATMENT

This is another useful research article. One of the researchers is a previous president of the American Thyroid Association. So, this paper ought to be taken on board by sceptical doctors and endocrinologists.

The research study compares T4, with T4/T3 and NDT treatments.

It definitely concludes that some patients do need T3 in their treatment in order to feel well and recover from hypothyroidism.

The paper may help some readers in their discussions with their doctors and endocrinologists to obtain better thyroid treatment.

We need more research focused on those patients who have to use T3 in order to feel well.

I still hope for more open-minded thyroid treatment within my lifetime. In the meantime, my books are a great resource that any reader can use. The books are very practical and will give you the tools you need in order to find your own way back to good health.

Here are the details about the paper:

"Comparative Effectiveness of Levothyroxine, Desiccated Thyroid Extract, and Levothyroxine + Liothyronine in Hypothyroidism"

Mohamed K M Shakir, Daniel I Brooks, Elizabeth A McAninch, Tatiana L Fonseca, Vinh Q Mai, Antonio C Bianco, Thanh D Hoang

The Journal of Clinical Endocrinology & Metabolism, dgab478, https://doi.org/10.1210/clinem/dgab478

Published: 29 June 2021

Here is the link to the paper:

https://academic.oup.com/jcem/advance-article/doi/10.1210/clinem/dgab478/631

5. ONLY CHANGES IN FT3 TRACK SYMPTOMS DURING TREATMENT

Only improvements in FT3, track symptom improvement during treatment.

This is a fairly recent and terrific piece of research that clearly places FT3 centre stage. It is the most useful lab test to measure, as it correlates to symptoms more than the other thyroid laboratory test results.

Moreover, the research shows that in T4-monotherapy, many patients did not find symptomatic relief until FT3 was elevated in the range, and TSH was suppressed.

The research findings are especially relevant to those patients on either T4 monotherapy or a T3/T4 combination who are still struggling with some hypothyroid symptoms.

Clearly, other issues should be ruled out (cortisol, iron etc.). However, when symptoms remain, it is always very important to focus on the symptoms themselves, and the signs (like body temperature) and the FT3 level, plus reverse T3.

FT3 is the most important thyroid lab level, as only changes in FT3 correlate to symptom changes in patients. If FT3 stays the same and FT4 goes up, this is unlikely to result in symptom improvement. Likewise, if FT3 goes up but FT4 and reverse T3 also go up, this may also be unlikely to result in symptom improvement.

We usually want to see better levels of FT3 without any significant increase in reverse T3. Changes in FT4 level are far less significant. Even having FT4 at the bottom of the lab range (or lower) is unimportant, as long as FT3 is at a good level and the patient's symptoms are improving.

Here is the research article:

"Symptomatic Relief is Related to Serum Free Triiodothyronine Concentrations during Follow-up in Levothyroxine-Treated Patients with Differentiated Thyroid Cancer"

Rolf Larisch, John E M Midgley, Johannes W Dietrich, Rudolf Hoermann

Exp Clin Endocrinol Diabetes 2018; 126(09): 546-552

DOI: 10.1055/s-0043-125064

https://www.thieme-connect.de/DOI/DOI?10.1055/s-0043-125064

All the information in this article is contained within my book, The Thyroid Patient's Manual. The book is a 'manual' that includes many critical pieces of information that all thyroid patients require. It was written based on my thirty-plus years of researching thyroid disease, and the best possible approaches to dealing with hypothyroidism.

6. FT4 AND FT3 INDIVIDUAL RANGES ARE LESS THAN HALF AS WIDE AS POPULATION RANGES

The FT4 and FT3 ranges for individual people are less than half as wide as the large laboratory test population ranges. The research suggests that individual person laboratory ranges for FT4 and FT3 are more like 38% as wide as the lab ranges that endocrinologists and doctors are using to determine if thyroid treatment is correct. So, they are closer to one third the width of the actual lab ranges for FT4 and FT3 – and often in the higher part of the range for FT3.

Simply having FT4 and FT3 levels 'in range' is absolutely no guarantee of a thyroid patient feeling well. However, most doctors and endocrinologists appear to be happy as long as FT4 and FT3 are somewhere in the range – no matter how low.

I sometimes say, "The laboratory test ranges for FT4 and FT3 are the size of a barn door! Simply throwing a ball and hitting the barn door anywhere at all, is not hitting the target. You need to throw the ball and land within a circle drawn on the barn door. That circle is likely to be around about 38% the size of the total barn door – nearer to one third the size of the barn door. If you do not hit within the circle, you have missed your target!"

Here is the article:

"Narrow Individual Variations in Serum T4 and T3 in Normal Subjects: A Clue to the Understanding of Subclinical Thyroid Disease" Stig Andersen, Klaus Michael Pedersen, Niels Henrik Bruun, Peter Laurberg. The Journal of Clinical Endocrinology & Metabolism, Volume 87, Issue 3, 1 March 2002, Pages 1068–1072.

See:

https://doi.org/10.1210/jcem.87.3.8165

and (just in case one link breaks at some point):

https://academic.oup.com/jcem/article/87/3/1068/2846746

You also have to be aware of what Normal Ranges actually are. Normal refers to the statistical distribution. This is a technical term, sometimes referred to as 'Normal', sometimes as 'Gaussian' and sometimes as a 'Bell Curve'. It means that the shape of the results from a large population fit this particular distribution.

What it DOES NOT mean is that, if you have a result that falls within it, then you are Normal or Healthy – that is entirely the Wrong Conclusion. Sadly, many doctors and endocrinologists appear to either have forgotten this or did not know it to begin with.

This research paper explains that the 'normal range' is Not a range, and being just somewhere in this range does not mean you are Normal: ncbi.nlm.nih.gov/pmc/articles/PMC6352401

7. FLAWED CLINICAL TRIALS & CURRENT TREATMENT MISTAKES

This paper clearly points out the design flaws in previous T4/T3 research studies. The previous studies found little or no benefit of combination therapy over T4 monotherapy but there were large flaws in the design of all of them.

It also points out the problems with using TSH or FT4 and their reference ranges to manage thyroid treatment.

The paper lays out what a good clinical trial has to do to be unbiased and not flawed.

It points to a better way to manage thyroid treatment that is more focused on the patient, and on the patient's response to treatment.

It finally puts a bullet into the incorrect conclusion that T3 does not have a benefit. This conclusion is held as gospel by so many doctors and endocrinologists.

My book, The Thyroid Patient's Manual, is highly consistent with the new paradigm of thyroid treatment that the authors believe is absolutely necessary in order to relieve patient symptoms.

The following text comes directly from Dr Midgley, who is a co-author of the new research paper:

"The essential problem is that the implications of our physiological studies are lethal to the acceptability of randomized clinical trials. This is as true of comparing T4 only v T4/T3 combination responses, or TSH, FT4, and osteoporosis, or TSH, FT4, and atrial fibrillation.

The paper by Fisher et al is a complete rejection of the validity of most medical clinical trials based on RCTs (Randomised Crossover Trials), in whatever discipline. I cannot emphasise enough how great a paper, Fisher's is. Our paper in the Journal of Thyroid Research follows exactly the same path in thyroidology, and draws exactly the same conclusions.

It follows that no longer can one link parameters such as TSH and FT4 to osteoporosis and atrial fibrillation in a generalised fashion. The whole corpus of so-called 'knowledge' on which these conclusions rest is essentially swept away – there is no other conclusion, however strongly objectors may complain.

All thinking based on these trials has to be completely revisited.

The new paradigm is a return to individualised diagnosis and treatment, and not assessing patients by their placement within or without a particular reference range.

Thyroid diagnosis can no longer be a parameter-based acceptance of normal ranges but the examination of the particular and unique position that a patient occupies, perhaps in some cases outside the range, and their individual presentation. No longer simple biochemistry, but real medicine is needed. This conclusion has only gradually emerged as the disjoint between physiological and clinical trial implications has become clear."

This is a short excerpt from the paper by Fisher et al.:

"That is, even in the best-case scenario, we should not think of a correlation in group data as an estimate that generalizes to any given individual in the population. Stated bluntly, this implies that the temptation to use aggregate estimates to draw inferences at the basic unit of social and psychological organization—the person—is far less accurate or valid than it may appear in the literature. Indeed, even the best-case scenario is quite alarming: Only 68% of all individual correlational values fall within a range that would be predicted by group data to cover 99.7% of all possible correlations—a discrepancy of nearly 32%. The worst-case scenario is clearly dire: It is plausible that inattention to nonergodicity and a lack of group-to-individual generalizability threaten the veracity of countless studies, conclusions, and best-practice recommendations."

A strong statement indeed!

NB Ergodicity is a term that states that variability within an individual is equivalent to that within a group. Non-ergodicity occurs when this does not happen, as in thyroid clinical trials.

Here are the relevant research papers (the second one needs to be paid for, but on accessing the link you can read the abstract and get a good sense of the nature of the paper):

"Lessons from Randomised Clinical Trials for Triiodothyronine Treatment of Hypothyroidism: Have They Achieved Their Objectives?" Journal of Thyroid Research. Research Article | Open Access Volume 2018 | Article ID 3239197 | 9 pages https://doi.org/10.1155/2018/3239197 Rudolf Hoermann, John E. M. Midgley, Rolf Larisch, and Johannes W. Dietrich. https://www.hindawi.com/journals/jtr/2018/3239197/

and

"Lack of group-to-individual generalizability is a threat to human subjects research" Aaron J. Fisher, John D. Medaglia, and Bertus F. Jeronimus PNAS July 3, 2018 115 (27) E6106-E6115; first published June 18, 2018 https://doi.org/10.1073/pnas.1711978115
http://www.pnas.org/content/115/27/E6106

8. SUCCESSFUL PREGNANCY OF WOMAN ON T3-ONLY THROUGHOUT

This is a paper that supports everything I have ever written on the safe experience women have had throughout pregnancy when on T3-Only replacement therapy.

It is consistent with the information I provide on Page 147 in Chapter 18 of The Thyroid Patient's Manual.

Here is the research article:

"Normal neurodevelopment of children from a mother treated with only Liothyronine (T3) during pregnancy – a case report"
Sidrah Khan & Trevor Wheatley Endocrine Abstracts (2016) 44 EP105 DOI: 10.1530/endoabs.44.EP105E
https://www.endocrine-abstracts.org/ea/0044/ea0044EP105

The woman concerned had very low FT4 during her pregnancy and there were no developmental issues with the foetus or baby at all.

This paper shows that T3 crosses the placenta and provides the foetus with adequate thyroid hormone for the first 20 weeks, after which, the foetus is self-sustaining.

One further research paper, dating back to 2006, shows that both T3 and T4 cross the placenta via the MCT8 transporter throughout pregnancy. I will provide a link to the abstract and the full paper below. The evidence is there, from practical experience and from research, that T3 does indeed cross the placenta during pregnancy, and that those women on T3-Only or T3-Mostly treatments, do not have to reduce or stop their T3 and replace it with T4 medication.

Here is the abstract followed by the link to the full paper:

https://pubmed.ncbi.nlm.nih.gov/16731778/
https://joe.bioscientifica.com/view/journals/joe/189/3/1890465.xml

It supports what I have been saying for many years about the misinformation and twisting of small pieces of research that often leads to people being frightened of T3-Only therapy.

There is no need to be frightened, as T3-Only therapy (if it is required) replaces the function of T4 without any adverse consequences. There is plenty of anecdotal evidence of women who have had successful pregnancies using T3-Only throughout the entire pregnancy, from conception to birth.

Dr John C. Lowe also had many women patients who had successful pregnancies whilst on T3-Only.

Over the past ten years, there have been doctors and patients who have argued that only T4 can cross certain systems. The blood-brain barrier and central nervous system were being mentioned for a long time, as areas that only T4 could access. This has been shown to be totally false due to the discovery of active transporters (see the article later in the Chapter).

I believe any other claims that T3 cannot replace the function of T4, will also be proven, in time, to be false. There is already enough evidence from people who live healthy lives over many years on T3-Only, that I am certain of this.

As I mention on page 147 of The Thyroid Patient's Manual, anyone who is still concerned about needing some T4, could take some during the first 20 weeks of pregnancy. However, after that time, the foetus is self-sustaining with its own thyroid hormones. The foetus begins to make its own thyroid hormones after 12 weeks but does not need any at all from the mother after 18-20 weeks. However, T4 is not really needed, as from practical experience of women who take T3-Only, the T3 must cross the placenta during the early stages of pregnancy.

9. T4/T3 STUDY SHOWED EXCELLENT LONG-TERM OUTCOMES

Here is a research study published in 2018, that shows excellent long-term outcomes for thyroid patients on T4/T3 combination therapy:

"Effects of Long-Term Combination LT4 and LT3 Therapy for Improving Hypothyroidism and Overall Quality of Life"
Anam Tariq, Yijin Wert, Pramil Cheriyath, and Renu Joshi.
South Med J. 2018 Jun; 111(6): 363–369.
Published online 2018 Jun 1.
doi: 10.14423/SMJ.0000000000000823
https://www.ncbi.nlm.nih.gov/pmc/articles/PMC5965938/

Yet again, this points the way to more enlightened treatment.

10. T4 IS NOT NEEDED IN THE BRAIN – RESEARCH BACKS UP PATIENT EXPERIENCE

This is an article that finally proves that thyroid patients do NOT need to take some T4 medication in order to make their brain function properly!

I have been told too many times that 'research shows that our brain and central nervous system can only use T4'. I have always known this view to be incorrect and finally, this research paper backs me up!

There are large numbers of people, just like me, who are fit and healthy on T3-Only. I have zero T4 in my body and I am healthy, can certainly think clearly and have no central nervous system issues!

We also have studies that prove that there are no negative effects from long term use of T3-Only.

This new research that proves that adults use T3 in the brain and central nervous system, can finally draw the curtain closed on the false belief that all thyroid patients should be taking some T4 medication.

This new research is changing the entire understanding of how the body compensates and alters how it operates with thyroid hormones. It reveals the discovery of 'active transporters'.

There are active T3 transporters and these are more active in adult life. This mechanism is now known to explain how T3 passes easily into the brain and central nervous system.

So, circulating T3 is a source of T3 for the brain which is, therefore, not exclusively dependent on T4 as previously believed.

This change of belief in transport, rather than diffusion, is relatively new, and more transporters are being discovered. I have spoken with many thyroid researchers who believe our understanding of how thyroid hormones work within the body may continue to be revised as this area of research is expanded and reveals more.

So, the people who say we cannot live without some T4, need to reassess their views – and keep quiet!

Here is the research paper:

"Thyroid Hormone Action: Astrocyte–Neuron Communication"
Beatriz Morte and Juan Bernal Front Endocrinol (Lausanne). 2014; 5: 82.
Published online 2014 May 30. Prepublished online 2014 Apr 22.
doi: 10.3389/fendo.2014.00082
https://www.ncbi.nlm.nih.gov/pmc/articles/PMC4038973/

11. T3 AND INSULIN – ANOTHER BENEFIT OF T3

A 2016 research study by the Endocrine Society showed that the thyroid hormone T3 controls and regulates the release of insulin, suggesting that low thyroid function could raise the risk of developing type 2 diabetes, especially in people with pre-diabetes.

This should really not be surprising at all as T3 is the active thyroid hormone. T3 is the only real thyroid hormone and it alone is able to bind to the thyroid receptors in the nucleus of every single cell. T3 enables all our cells to work at the correct rate and perform their proper function. Every major function in the body is regulated by the T3 thyroid hormone. Therefore, having low free T3 (FT3) levels is going to impact people in many different ways.

This is yet another reason for ensuring that FT3 is tested during thyroid treatment. Testing TSH, or even TSH and FT4, will not reveal whether FT3 is adequate or not. Someone can have perfectly 'normal looking' TSH and FT4, yet still have low FT3.

It is also possible that someone can have other issues that stops the proper function of even good levels of FT3. So, testing other things is also important. Cortisol for instance has to be at a healthy level and not high or low. High reverse T3 (rT3) can be an indicator that T3 is not as effective as it should be. See my book, The Thyroid Patient's Manual, for more information on what additional tests to run and how to assess the results.

Here is a link to the article:

https://www.diabetes.co.uk/in-depth/can-abnormal-thyroid-function-affect-the-course-of-diabetes-2/

Also, this article is interesting. It suggests that a low Free T3 level increases mortality rates in diabetic patients:

https://www.sciencedirect.com/science/article/abs/pii/S0168822723005740

Here is a piece of research that helps to provide another reason why T3 helps some thyroid patients struggling with blood sugar issues. T3 appears to improve insulin sensitivity and can reduce or stop insulin resistance:

"Thyroid hormone potentiates insulin signaling and attenuates hyperglycemia and insulin resistance in a mouse model of type 2 diabetes"

Br J Pharmacol. 2011 Feb; 162(3): 597–610. doi: 10.1111/j.1476-5381.2010.01056.x

Yi Lin and Zhongjie Sun

http://www.ncbi.nlm.nih.gov/pmc/articles/PMC3041250/

12. 20-YEAR RESEARCH STUDY DISMISSES REASONS FOR NOT PRESCRIBING T3

Here is a 20-year observational piece of research.

It confirms that T3 has no adverse effects on the heart and bones.

This disproves two of the major reasons that doctors use to avoid prescribing T3. The risk to the heart and to bone loss are the two most common reasons (excuses) used to avoid prescribing T3 to patients. It is common for me to hear from thyroid patients that their doctor does not want them on any T3 because it will cause a heart attack or heart issues. Thyroid patients are often old that T3 will cause bone loss too.

There is a minor reference in the report to psychological side effects of T3-Only treatment, but I believe that this is likely to be due to one of two factors:

1. Incorrect dosing of T3 – see the Recovering with T3 book for how to use T3 safely and effectively.

2. Other issues. Patients who are eventually given T3-Only or T3-Mostly therapy, often have other issues by this stage. See my book, The Thyroid Patient's Manual, if you need more help with the exclusion or resolution of any of these other issues.

This study is very useful and it throws out the argument that has been used in the past about T3 causing heart issues and bone loss, which many of us have known was not true anyway.

Here is the article:

"Safety review of liothyronine use: a 20-year observational follow-up study"
Enrique Soto-Pedre & Graham Leese
Endocrine Abstracts (2015) 38 OC5.6 | DOI: 10.1530/endoabs.38.OC5.6
http://www.endocrine-abstracts.org/ea/0038/ea0038OC5.6.htm

13. CANCER – SCIENTISTS POINT FINGER AT T4 AND REVERSE T3

Research has shown that T4 and reverse T3 (rT3), both act on receptors on the cell wall called Integrin $\alpha v\beta 3$ (these receptors are also referred to as 'Integrin alpha-v beta-3 receptors', or as 'Vitronectin receptors'). Through these receptors, T4 and rT3 can cause many types of cancers to grow.

However, T3 may come to the rescue.

In a clinical study, cancer patients who were dying had their survival extended by the addition of T3 thyroid hormone, which significantly reduced their circulating T4 and rT3 levels.

Aleck Herbergs and Paul J. Davis are at the forefront of this type of research. Hercbergs and Davis et al. call this therapy "euthyroid hypothyroxinemia".

By using T3 in this way, the research team maintained or increased FT3, whilst lowering both FT4 and rT3. This is exactly the same method that thyroid patients use with T3 therapy when they find that they cannot get well on T4.

In 2019, the research team published a review of their therapy and the history of it:

Hercbergs, A. (2019). Clinical Implications and Impact of Discovery of the Thyroid Hormone Receptor on Integrin αvβ3–A Review. *Frontiers in Endocrinology, 10.* Here is the link to the research paper:

https://doi.org/10.3389/fendo.2019.00565

Here is an article that a fellow thyroid patient advocate wrote about this. You will find far more detail here:

https://thyroidpatients.ca/2020/02/05/cancer-scientists-point-finger-at-t4-rt3-hormones/

If only the medical profession and endocrinologists would see the numerous benefits of using the biologically active hormone T3, for those patients who require it!

14. CANCER – T3 IS PROTECTIVE AGAINST CANCER

This is a research study that implies that, when FT4 and FT3 are at a healthy level, they are protective of health. FT3 and FT4 tend to protect against many sources of mortality, including cardiovascular-related mortality.

In particular, good FT3 levels protect against cancer. By 'good levels', I do not just mean in range – I mean at the right place in the reference range for the individual so that signs and symptoms are made healthy.

Here is the research study:

"Thyroid hormones and mortality risk in euthyroid individuals: the Kangbuk Samsung health study."

Zhang Y, Chang Y, Ryu S, Cho J, Lee WY, Rhee EJ, Kwon MJ, Pastor-Barriuso R, Rampal S, Han WK, Shin H, Guallar E. J Clin Endocrinol Metab. 2014; 99(7):2467-2476.
https://www.researchgate.net/publication/261441377_Thyroid_Hormones_and_Mortality_Risk_in_Euthyroid_Individuals_The_Kangbuk_Samsung_Health_Study

The implications of this are pretty clear.

1. Those who are on T3, T4/T3, and NDT treatment, have good levels of FT3 and feel properly treated (no symptoms), are in a lower risk situation with regard to developing cancer.

2. Those thyroid patients who are on T4 therapy but who are not converting well enough and have remaining symptoms, are likely to have too low an FT3 level and are more at risk of health issues.

The sooner the entire medical profession wises up to this the better. Keeping thyroid patients healthier will reduce future health issues. This is not only important for the patients but ultimately, this would save health services a lot of money.

All thyroid patients deserve good health!

Far too much emphasis is placed on keeping everyone on the same, simplistic T4 treatment (also the cheapest) without considering the long-term costs of other conditions that could potentially be avoided. Cancer, especially, is a very expensive condition to treat.

It is only right to provide a variety of therapies and put the effort into finding the one that works for the individual.

Here is another article that supports the cancer-protective effect of T3:

"The thyroid triodothyronine reinvigorates dendritic cells and potentiates anti-tumor immunity."

Vanina A., et al. Oncoimmunology 5.1 (2016): e1064579. doi: 10.1080/2162402X.2015.1064579.

Here is the abstract (but there are .pdfs: https://pubmed.ncbi.nlm.nih.gov/26942081/

15. CANCER - STUDY SUGGESTS LONG-TERM LEVOTHYROXINE USE ASSOCIATED WITH CANCER

I would urge everyone to read this entire article and the full content of the study prior to considering the implications. The research I am referring to will not apply to everyone on Levothyroxine.

Many thyroid patients will do just fine on Levothyroxine and never have any issues. So, it is important to put this in that context.

Having said that, I believe that relevant information needs to be available to thyroid patients so that they can make informed decisions regarding their own health.

This is a recently published study. The research showed that levothyroxine use was associated with a significantly increased risk of cancer, particularly brain, skin, pancreatic, and female breast cancers.

Levothyroxine, also known as T4, and brand names such as Synthroid, is the main medication prescribed by endocrinologists and doctors in the treatment of hypothyroidism. The prevailing endocrinology view is that Levothyroxine always works and that TSH can be used to assess the adequacy of the treatment. There are many research papers that show that these views are flawed. This new paper adds more evidence.

This research study was very large and included 601,733 cases of cancer and 2,406,932 controls. So, this was not a small number of people being studied. It needs to be taken very seriously.

The researchers recommend more work to understand the biological reasons for their findings.

However, it seems obvious to me that at least one of the most likely reasons is that Levothyroxine (T4) often does not result in the same level of FT3 and FT4 that healthy people with a working thyroid gland enjoy. All too frequently, T4 medication results in lower FT3 and higher FT4 than the patient had when they were well. In some cases, this may be due to their T4 dosage never being raised to a high enough level because the patient's doctor thought TSH was too low (see the articles in Chapter 6 on the flawed use of TSH). In other cases, various issues may have compromised the ability of the patient to convert T4 to T3 as efficiently as they used to (the loss of thyroid tissue can do this, as well as other factors).

Hence, in my view, some of these thyroid patients would be a lot healthier on a mix of T4 and T3 medications, rather than Levothyroxine only. So, a combination of synthetic T4 & T3 or natural desiccated thyroid (NDT) would be healthier for many thyroid patients. The reliance on TSH as the main indicator of thyroid hormone adequacy during treatment, also needs to be revised.

As I mentioned in the introduction, this does not mean that all thyroid patients on Levothyroxine have an increased risk of cancer. Some thyroid patients are extremely good converters of T4 to T3 and they will, of course, have sufficiently good levels of T3 to have no increased risk at all. Those thyroid patients on Levothyroxine who feel really healthy, are also likely to have sufficient T3 and be completely fine. So, this is not a blanket issue for all thyroid patients on Levothyroxine.

This research simply points out the risk to some thyroid patients on Levothyroxine. I would think that the people in the higher risk category are those with high levels of FT4, low levels of FT3 and/or high levels of reverse T3 (due to poor conversion from T4 to T3), and those that have remaining symptoms of hypothyroidism.

This research provides even more evidence that there is far too much reliance on T4 monotherapy. The faith of doctors and endocrinologists in the effectiveness of Levothyroxine is seriously flawed. Something has to change!

Here is the information on the study:

Chieh-Chen Wu, Mohaimenul Islam, Phung Anh Alex Nguyen, Tahmina Nasrin Poly, Ching-Huan Wang, Usman Iqbal, Yu-Chuan Jack Li, Hsuan-Chia Yang. April 2021. Risk of Cancer in Long-Term Levothyroxine Users: Retrospective Population-based Study. Cancer Sci. doi: 10.1111/cas.14908.
Abstract: https://pubmed.ncbi.nlm.nih.gov/33793038/
Full text: https://onlinelibrary.wiley.com/doi/10.1111/cas.14908

My belief that the increased cancer risk is likely to be connected to the lower levels of T3 generated by Levothyroxine, has further support.

We know from research that dendritic cells play a central role in fighting cancer. These dendritic cells are highly dependent on T3. Research using mice with cancer concluded that T4 therapy showed no increase in the activity of the dendritic cells. However, when the mice were given T3, it helped to destroy the cancers: https://pubmed.ncbi.nlm.nih.gov/31214123/

Experience of working with thyroid patients also suggests that T4/T3 and T3-Only treatments tend to cause patients to get far fewer colds, sinus infections, etc. This is anecdotal evidence but it fits well with the idea of Levothyroxine treatment often providing inadequate immune system support.

I hope you found this article interesting and important.

16. LIOTHYRONINE (T3) USE IS BENEFICIAL IN ISCHEMIC HEART DISEASE

Here is another research study that concludes that T3 replacement therapy is 'Safe'.

Note: ischemic heart disease is also known as coronary heart disease. It is where the heart muscle does not receive enough blood and oxygen. It is the most common type of heart disease.

This research goes completely against the negative views of many medical professionals that T3 causes heart attacks etc.

Here is the article:

"The impact of thyroid hormone dysfunction on ischemic heart disease" Madalena von Hafe et al. May 2019, Endocrine Connections 8 (5).
Full scholarly article: https://www.ncbi.nlm.nih.gov/pmc/articles/PMC6499922/
The PDF version of the article for printing is here:
https://www.ncbi.nlm.nih.gov/pmc/articles/PMC6499922/pdf/EC-19-0096.pdf

Key points in the research article related to thyroid patients and T3 use:

1. There has been over-emphasis on hyperthyroidism and thyrotoxicosis by many doctors who believe that only excess FT3 and FT4 are bad for the heart. This article shows that the real thyroid hormone issue with respect to the heart is actually hypothyroidism (too little FT3, possibly due to too little FT4, but sometimes poor conversion of T4 to T3). Note: We have known for decades that hypothyroidism, and low FT3 in particular, leads to a rise in bad cholesterol: https://pmc.ncbi.nlm.nih.gov/articles/PMC3473203/

2. The article discusses T3 use extensively, and even goes into the ways in which T3 therapy can reduce cardiovascular risk and promote healing.

3. The article also states that the use of levothyroxine requires the preservation of peripheral deiodinase activity to convert FT4 into the active hormone FT3. It states that administration of T3 may be a better option (than T4) in patients with impaired conversion. The doctors openly acknowledge that impaired FT4 to FT3 conversion is actually a genuine issue with potentially serious consequences - cardiac issues and death in some cases.

4. The article discusses the improved health of patients treated with T3 thyroid hormone. These patients had severe heart issues (St-elevated myocardial infarction and non-thyroidal illness syndrome in acute coronary syndrome). The results of the study showed that T3 is safe and improved the health of these patients with no side effects.

5. The authors discuss the importance of the T3 thyroid hormone, as it is the biologically active thyroid hormone. It highlights how important a good conversion rate from FT4 to FT3 is.

6. The authors also make it very clear that T3 is the most important thyroid hormone and that it is 20 times more potent than T4. My books discuss the potency of the T3 thyroid hormone and the fact that it binds far more readily to thyroid receptors than T4.

7. The article acknowledges that not all T4 is destined to become T3. FT4 converts to some FT3, but also to other thyroid hormones including reverse T3 (rT3). The authors do not talk about rT3 very much, but there is research that shows that rT3 is a T3-blocker, i.e., rT3 actively slows metabolism when it goes too high. Although the article does not refer to this, I felt I had to state it.

8. The article makes it clear that it is T3 that is the thyroid hormone that is responsible for the major necessary effects on the myocardium (muscular tissue of the heart).

9. The article makes it clear that T3 does many useful things. It stimulates nearly all of the transporters and ion channels involved in calcium myocardial fluxes. It enhances calcium uptake and release. It stimulates both diastolic myocardial relaxation and systolic myocardial contraction. It upregulates α-MHC and downregulates β-MHC (heart muscle-specific proteins). It increases resting heart rate, cardiac contractility, and venous tone almost immediately, increasing cardiac preload and cardiac output. It increases myocardial sensitivity to the adrenergic system by increasing the number of adrenergic membrane receptors and other necessary effects.

10. The authors state that hypothyroidism (low FT3 and FT4 thyroid hormones) reverses or blocks the long list of good things from happening in the cardiovascular system. The hypothyroid state results in lower heart rate and decreased myocardial contraction and relaxation, with prolonged systolic and early diastolic time intervals, culminating in advanced stages of heart failure. It is hypothyroidism, not T3 use, that cause heart failure.

11. This article finally admits that a low T3 syndrome IS a form of hypothyroidism. How could a syndrome characterized by a low thyroid hormone (T3) not be hypothyroidism? Just because TSH is not elevated and patients exhibit no 'clinical signs' of hypothyroidism, it is still possible to suffer an FT3 deficit. Decades of endocrinology have seen Low T3 syndrome as not hypothyroidism. This article corrects that error.

12. Another revolutionary factor in this article's discussion is that they discuss how other bad conditions take time to develop in the presence of hypothyroidism, e.g., insulin resistance and atherosclerosis.

13. The authors also admit that deiodinase Type 3 (D3), destroys thyroid hormone and leaves in its wake reverse T3 (rT3) hormone and that this can be pathological. Yes,

they actually use the word pathological. Recent studies show that expression of D3 is increased in some pathological contexts in a cell-specific manner, which are cancer, cardiac hypertrophy, myocardial infarction, chronic inflammation or critical illness. They talk about the process by which this pathological overexpression of D3 and chronic inflammation and hypoxia lead to local cardiac hypothyroidism – in which the heart has even less FT3 than you can measure in the bloodstream. In low T3 syndrome, by definition, blood FT3 is already lower than the body needs it to be, and this article says FT3 is even lower in the heart muscle itself.

14. The article makes it clear that a significant percentage of patients with acute coronary syndrome have NTIS [Non-thyroidal Illness Syndrome, a.k.a. Low T3 syndrome]. It also states that patients with ST-elevation myocardial infarction (STEMI) and alterations in thyroid function have almost a 3.5-fold increased risk of major adverse cardiac events, including cardiogenic shock and death, compared with patients with STEMI and no thyroid disorder.

15. Low FT3 levels and/or high Reverse T3 at the time of the acute myocardial infarction (heart attack), has long-term effects on recovery 6 months later. The 1-year mortality increases.

16. They are so concerned with the risk of low levels of FT3 and making heart surgery more successful that studies are looking into pre-treatment with T3 before going into surgery. The interest in the role of thyroid hormones cardio-protection is increasing.

17. Later sections in the article discuss thyroid hormone treatments. They are clear that all thyroid hormones are on the table, from levothyroxine to T3 to other thyro-mimetic compounds that target thyroid hormone receptors. This is music to my ears as I have been saying this for years and this is stated over and over again in my books and other articles.

18. The pros and cons of Levothyroxine and T3 therapy are discussed. The negative side of levothyroxine, again, is that the body needs to convert it to T3, which is less likely to happen in patients with poor FT4 to FT3 conversion, which is common in heart failure and other heart conditions. The negative side of using T3, of course, relates the risk of overdose, i.e., a bad dosing protocol (which I protect against in my safe and careful protocol in the Recovering with T3 book). T3's potency, its ability to heal, is its Achilles heel IF the dosing is not managed with care (which it can be if a sensible protocol is followed).

19. Far, far more is written here about the studies that show T3's benefits, alone or in combination with T4, both in human trials and in animal studies. Even children — yes children! — are the objects of studies of T3 pre-treatment for cardiac surgery.

20. In another research study they review, even a low daily dose of T3, a mere 1.2 micrograms per 100g in rats, confers benefits to their healing from a heart attack, and the practical applications to humans are profound: Low-dose T3 might offer a suitable

treatment option after myocardial infarction in patients who are intolerant to aerobic exercise training.

21. The authors also make it clear that tiny changes in thyroid hormone levels within the reference range, or not noticed in blood, are significant! Yes, symptoms and signs show the effect of thyroid hormone effect - not necessarily the lab results! They state that "Evidence suggests that the hypothyroid tissue state may be present independent of normal circulating levels of thyroid hormones. Therefore, it is important to identify a good biomarker of tissue hypothyroid-like state in order to treat patients effectively." What matters more than the reference range boundary is whether or not tissues like the heart muscle and blood vessels are getting enough T3. Even tiny doses can help.

22. Overall, the research article makes it very clear that they see immense value in treating lower than needed FT3 (even if it is within the reference range already). T3's benefits to the heart and the protection and healing it offers during the crises of acute coronary events is too important to ignore. The authors write, "The results are promising so far; experimental and clinical studies demonstrate that thyroid hormones can limit ischemic injury, attenuate cardiac remodelling, and improve hemodynamics." When they use the term 'thyroid hormones' the authors mean ensuring that the patients have enough FT3.

23. Their final brief paragraph trumpets the declarations doctors need to hear. First of all: Low thyroid hormone levels are the main issue when it comes to cardiovascular tissue. It is not about TSH-based definitions of hypothyroidism, nor is it about a certain magic number. 'Low' thyroid hormone means 'low' from the perspective of the body, not from the perspective of some arbitrary statistical population reference range boundary. They state: "It is now recognized that even subtle changes in thyroid hormone levels can lead to adverse effects in the cardiovascular system. Experimental and clinical evidence suggests a close link between low thyroid hormone levels and poor prognosis in ischemic heart disease. This condition should, therefore, be regarded as a cardiovascular risk factor." Notice this - Low thyroid hormone levels, not necessarily high TSH, "should, therefore, be regarded as a cardiovascular risk factor."

I will end with this quotation from the conclusion:

"Accordingly, thyroid hormone replacement therapy may yield improvements in lipid profiles, potentially reversing myocardial dysfunction and preventing the progression to heart failure. TH replacement treatment exhibits anti-ischemic and cardio-protective effects, acting as a promising target for ischemic heart disease. Moreover, subclinical hypothyroidism treatment and nonthyroidal illness syndrome constitute topics garnering increased interest; recent studies suggest that therapy with physiological doses of T3 is safe and provides beneficial effects on ischemic heart disease."

Evidence is mounting but it needs more to convince those sceptics who are controlling thyroid treatment guidelines.

Another piece of evidence is present in this research that supports the use of T3 for patients with atrial fibrillation after heart surgery (as low FT3 is linked to Afib):

"Free triiodothyronine: a novel predictor of postoperative atrial fibrillation" Alfredo Giuseppe Cerillo, Stefano Bevilacqua, Simona Storti, Massimiliano Mariani, Enkel Kallushi, Andrea Ripoli, Aldo Clerico, Mattia Glauber. European Journal of Cardio-Thoracic Surgery, Volume 24, Issue 4, October 2003, Pages 487–492. https://doi.org/10.1016/S1010-7940(03)00396-8

17. LIOTHYRONINE (T3) USE REDUCES THE RISK OF DEMENTIA AND MORTALITY

Here is a recent research study that provides more evidence on the benefits of including T3 in thyroid replacement therapy. One of the authors is a previous president of the American Thyroid Association, Professor Antonio Bianco.

Professor Bianco's statement on the research study is: "These results were obtained through the analysis of 1.26 million patients with hypothyroidism, seen in 126 health organizations across 17 countries. Over a 20-year follow-up, patients receiving combination therapy (LT4+LT3 or DTE) had 27% lower risk of dementia and 31% lower risk of mortality. These results should reset the approach to the treatment of hypothyroidism".

It will be interesting to see whether the endocrinology community pay any attention. I can imagine that many of them will choose to dismiss the findings. However, as time goes on, the evidence for many thyroid patients benefitting from T3, is mounting.

Here is the article:

"Treatment of Hypothyroidism that Contains Liothyronine is Associated with Reduced Risk of Dementia and Mortality"
Fabyan Esberard de Lima Beltrao, Antonio Bianco et al.
June 2025, The Journal of Clinical Endocrinology & Metabolism, dgaf367.
https://doi.org/10.1210/clinem/dgaf367

Chapter 10

Other Issues Related To Hypothyroidism

1. COULD ATROPHIC THYROIDITIS BE YOUR PROBLEM?

This article is based on a website post by another thyroid patient advocate, Dr Tania S. Smith. As I had Atrophic Thyroiditis myself, as well as Hashimoto's, I can also add my own experience here. Please see the reference to the website link by the author at the end of this article.

Atrophic Thyroiditis is defined generally as a thyroid gland volume of 5.0 mL (millilitres) or less (5.0 mL = 5000 cubic mms (millimetres).

This shrinkage is NOT caused by Hashimoto's TPOAb antibody, nor is it caused by ageing.

In Hashimoto's, the thyroid tissue is destroyed but the gland itself does not shrink. The vast majority of Hashi's patients keep their normal adult thyroid volume during their entire adult lives, including into old age, even if they began with Hashimoto's at a very young age.

In Atrophic Thyroiditis, you do not need the TPO antibody to be raised. You can have Atrophic Thyroiditis with or without the presence of Hashimoto's (detected by elevated TPOAb or TGAb autoantibodies) or Graves' Disease (often detected by testing for TSAb or TSI and TRAb autoantibodies).

Atrophic Thyroiditis is caused by an antibody called the 'TSH receptor blocking antibody' or TBAb. The antibody blocks TSH from stimulating the thyroid gland (instead of overstimulating as it does in Graves' disease). A severe flare of TBAb can block more than 98% of TSH receptors, so that TSH cannot reach the gland, no matter how much TSH you have in circulation.

A small percentage (10%) of Hashi's patients also have this antibody, when researchers have taken a random sampling of patients with elevated TPO levels and clinically diagnosed hypothyroidism.

The raised TBAb antibody can flare up and then go away again. Therefore, the TBAb antibody need not be constantly raised. As a result, it can be extremely difficult to detect.

Atrophic Thyroiditis caused by the TBAb antibody is another type of autoimmune thyroid disease that can occur with or without the presence of Hashimoto's.

Atrophy can happen before Hashi's, or during Hashi's, or in a person who never has had Hashimoto's (i.e., they have never had an elevated TPO). Most Hashi's patients do not experience severe thyroid atrophy.

But Atrophic Thyroiditis is not Hashi's because it is not caused by the TPO antibody.

Gland atrophy does not always happen when the TBAb flares up, and if it happens, it does not always happen at the same rate in all people. Here are the conditions:

The stimulating antibody TSAb will prevent the death of thyroid cells. Therefore, if you have TSAb (thyroid stimulating antibody), in circulation at the same time as TBAb (which is common), they counteract each other, then atrophy will not occur.

If you only have TBAb in circulation, your gland is vulnerable to atrophy.

As mentioned above, there are significant issues with testing for Atrophic Thyroiditis and so it is better to diagnose it in other ways.

Few labs have the ability to test the TBAb autoantibody, and the antibody is not always present. You would have to know you are in the middle of a TBAb antibody flare while testing so you can c'atch it in the act'!

TBAb blocking antibodies also disappear in half or more people who have them. They can completely disappear after doing their damage (atrophy), and then they can flare up again years later when someone is on therapy and they can wreak havoc with thyroid levels.

A bad flare of this TBAb blocking antibody can steal more FT4 to FT3 conversion from you than DIO1 or DIO2 genetic polymorphisms can. As a result, your FT3 may be low, even without any rT3 elevation.

A flare can also cause significantly raised TSH, as the receptors for TSH are blocked and the pituitary attempts to achieve more of a response from the thyroid gland.

The biggest clue of all though, is the presence of less than 5.0 mL gland volume. This is indicative of TBAb action, i.e., Atrophic Thyroiditis.

One very important thing to keep in mind is that during flares of Atrophic Thyroiditis, the effect of the antibody can significantly affect the conversion rate of FT4 to FT3. In a person without Atrophic Thyroiditis, the D2 deiodinase enzyme activity is normally upregulated by TSH i.e., the body makes more D2 enzymes when TSH rises, in order to convert more FT4 to FT3. So, in a healthy person, the cells will convert more of the FT4 to FT3, so the FT3 level will rise.

However, in a person with Atrophic Thyroiditis, the TSH signalling throughout the body can be blocked by high levels of the TBAb antibody. This prevents the FT4 to FT3 conversion rate from being up-regulated and at the level it should be. In fact, FT3 levels can remain far too low, when TBAb levels rise during a flare. So, those on T4 medication may find it very difficult to remain stable. During an Atrophic Thyroiditis flare the FT4 (from any remaining thyroid tissue or from T4 medication) will not get converted to as much FT3, but when the flare is over the conversion rate will improve and FT3 levels rise. It can be a highly unstable situation for the Atrophic Thyroiditis sufferer. This is especially true if they are using T4-based thyroid medication, e.g., Levothyroxine or NDT.

Once the thyroid gland is destroyed, the variation in the effect of TSH, due to flares in TBAb (which can continue even once the gland has atrophied), can still continue to affect the conversion rate of FT4 to FT3 in those patients on T4-based thyroid medication.

Therefore, some thyroid patients who suffer from this condition may find that they do significantly better on T3 medication once most of their thyroid gland has been destroyed by Atrophic Thyroiditis. This is because T3 is already biologically active and is NOT affected in the same way as T4 by the TBAb antibody. Any changes in TSH, and up-regulation or down-regulation of FT4 to FT3 conversion, is irrelevant to those thyroid patients who only use T3 therapy.

Note: things are made worse by the fact that the loss of the thyroid gland itself will already have significantly worsened the individual's FT4 to FT3 conversion ability, as the thyroid gland is the most important converter of FT4 to FT3 in the body (with usually at least a 25% contribution of the body's ability to convert T4). Again, this adds more evidence that thyroid patients with Atrophic Thyroiditis usually do far better on T3-Only monotherapy.

Here is the website post that I referred to at the start. There is a detailed section in the article on Atrophic Thyroiditis:
https://thyroidpatients.ca/2020/04/12/the-spectrum-of-thyroid-autoimmunity/

2. B12 – CRITICALLY IMPORTANT BUT OFTEN NOT DIAGNOSED OR TREATED PROPERLY

Vitamin B12, also known as Cobalamin, is a critical and very complex essential vitamin within the human body. As we cannot manufacture B12 in our bodies, it must be ingested either in food, a supplement or in an injection.

I became interested in B12, as low B12 seems to affect many thyroid patients. This might be due to the fact that low B12 makes T4 to T3 conversion worse. However, low thyroid hormone is also likely to make the absorption of B12 from food or supplements less effective.

Moreover, thyroid disease is often caused by autoimmune disease (Hashimoto's thyroiditis). We know that where there is one autoimmune disease, others can be present. Low B12 can be caused due to an autoimmune condition in some people.

Anyway, let me discuss B12 in more detail, and why it is so important to investigate it properly.

B12 is used in the process of making good-quality red blood cells. If B12 is too low, we cannot make the quality of red blood cells needed to carry oxygen around in the body. Sometimes, low B12 affects the number of red blood cells produced and it can cause the ones that are made to die off early. Red blood cells are cycled within the body every 3-4 months, but they can die off and be recycled far sooner if B12 is low.

B12 is also critical in the maintenance of nerve cells, including in the brain. B12 helps to maintain our DNA, energy levels, spinal cord, hair, and skin. B12 is also involved in glucose metabolism and adenosine triphosphate (ATP) production which provides cellular energy and helps both cortisol and T3 to work properly. It is critical in many of our systems.

Low B12 often results in a condition known as anaemia.

Anaemia is the most common disorder of the blood. It is caused by either a low, or below-average number of red blood cells in the blood or less than the normal amount of haemoglobin in the blood. If a patient has a normal number of red blood cells, but they have lower than normal haemoglobin, the patient is usually diagnosed as having iron deficiency anaemia, as iron is used to make haemoglobin. Low iron can therefore impact the ability to carry oxygen around because the oxygen is carried in haemoglobin. Iron deficiency anaemia is often detected by low haemoglobin in a Full Blood Count (FBC).

As mentioned above, low B12 can impact the quality and the number of red blood cells, as it is needed to make them in the bone marrow. Low B12 may be present with, or without Pernicious Anaemia, which is an autoimmune condition where the body attacks itself, and cannot make enough Intrinsic Factor in the stomach. Intrinsic Factor is essential in order for the B12 to be absorbed in the small intestine (in the ileum – the last stage of the small intestine).

There are at least two types of autoantibodies that can cause Pernicious Anaemia. One type, Anti-Intrinsic Factor Antibodies, attacks the intrinsic factor itself. The other type, Parietal Cell Antibodies, attack the parietal cells in the stomach that make the intrinsic factor (and parietal cells also make our stomach acid). Anything that disrupts the parietal cells can also reduce the level of Intrinsic Factor, e.g., Helicobacter Pylori bacteria.

When B12 deficiency is severe, it can reduce the number of red blood cells in the body, resulting in low red blood cell count (RBC). Very low B12 can also cause red blood cells to enlarge and be less effective in carrying oxygen. This can be measured by the mean corpuscular volume (MCV). Both RBC and MCV are also present in an FBC, but there are problems with detecting low B12 that I will discuss later in this article.

I have just been reading Martyn Hooper's excellent book: What you Need to Know About Pernicious Anaemia and Vitamin B12 Deficiency. I was prompted to write this, as I have just read that research has shown that there is an approximately 40% prevalence of B12 deficiency in hypothyroid patients! This is staggeringly high! Whether this is because many hypothyroid patients have the autoimmune condition Hashimoto's thyroiditis, and pernicious anaemia is another autoimmune condition, I do not know.

The information above appears to suggest that diagnosing and treating B12 ought to be straightforward.

However, the diagnosis and treatment of low B12 in all its forms is far from straightforward.

Let me give a brief summary of some of the numerous symptoms, and some signs, of B12 deficiency:

- Tiredness / Fatigue
- Shortness of breath.
- Inability to do exercise like you once did.
- Low cortisol symptoms, and/or low cortisol test results.
- Brain fog/confusion/memory problems.
- Headaches & migraines. Can be severe and very prolonged, whilst B12 is low.
- Heart palpitations, high heart rate.
- Pins & needles/numbness (esp. legs/feet) / nerve damage (can be permanent).
- Muscle & joint pain.
- Worst case with pernicious anaemia and very low B12 – spinal cord damage, brain lesions and serious nerve damage.
- Balance/coordination/changes in the way you move / clumsiness.
- Hair loss.
- Mood changes/irritability.
- Sore mouth/ sore tongue/mouth ulcers.
- Tinnitus.
- Depression.
- Diarrhoea.
- Nausea.
- Loss of appetite/weight loss.
- Almost any neurological problem from anxiety, and panic to depression because low B12 affects the red blood cells and the nervous system.
- Elevated homocysteine which can cause elevated blood pressure.
- …and more.

Low B12 might be detected by Total Serum B12 or possibly Active B12 (if you can get the test). However, both tests have severe drawbacks. One particular one to be aware of is that any supplement that contains B12 must be stopped for 4-6 MONTHS prior to testing B12. Even a multi-vitamin can compromise the test results as B12 can continue to circulate in the bloodstream for many months and simply not enter the cells.

'Total Serum B12' tests what the name implies, i.e., all circulating B12. This includes a large portion of B12, which is bound to protein and unavailable to the cells. There is a new test called the Holotranscobalamin test (the Active B12 test), that still measures B12 in the blood, and still does not show whether the B12 is truly adequate within the cells.

In the UK, the reference range for Total Serum B12 is typically about 180 – 1000 pg/ml (or ng/L) With results below 180 pg/ml considered low, 180-350 pg/ml is considered borderline, and more than 350 pg/ml is considered normal. Note: in the UK the NICE guidance (Draft for Consultation, July 2023) on Vitamin B12 deficiency in over 16s now proposes 350 pg/ml (or ng/L) as the low end of the range for either further testing or a trial of B12 injections.

However, there is huge controversy over this. In other countries, the low end of the range is higher. In Japan, for instance, a patient would be put on routine B12 injections if their levels were below 500 pg/ml. Many B12 medical researchers and doctors who focus on the B12 issue consider that 550 pg/ml should be the low-end cut-off point.

Note: it is also possible for some patients to have faults in their cell receptors and have high B12 results, but still, be clinically B12 deficient. There are pressure groups & charities working at present to get the low threshold of the B12 reference range, raised to at least 300 pg/ml and hopefully higher.

The Active B12 test has its own issues and researchers and doctors are still not entirely sure whether it is going to give a more reliable diagnosis than the Total Serum B12 test. This test still measures a blood level of B12 – it does not reflect B12 that is actually active within the cells (as the name might imply to some readers).

Methyl Malonic Acid (MMA) is one of the better tests for B12 (a urine MMA test or a serum MMA are good). MMA is elevated in 90-98% of cases of low B12. MMA is an expensive test though. Sometimes, MMA is not available. Homocysteine can also be used and is often elevated with low B12 – but it is not as reliable as MMA. Homocysteine can be high with folate deficiency, or low with methionine deficiency (common in vegans).

However, please be aware, that neither the MMA nor Homocysteine tests have had any thorough investigation in the case of people taking B12 supplementation. These tests are also thought to provide invalid results (false negative results) when any B12 supplementation has been used within 4 months of the test. This view was given to me directly by Martyn Hooper (the previous chairman of the Pernicious Anaemia Society and author of two books on low B12). As Martyn Hooper points out, there is so much B12 fortification in foods these days that all the tests for low B12 may be severely compromised.

Pernicious Anaemia (PA) is severe anaemia brought about by the inability to produce enough Intrinsic Factor needed to absorb the B12 in the gut. PA has additional tests that can be done. These are the Parietal Cell Antibody test and the Intrinsic Factor Blocking Antibody test. But there are issues with these tests too. People with PA caused by either destruction of the Parietal Cells (which produce intrinsic factor and stomach acid), or destruction of Intrinsic Factor, invariably need B12 intramuscular injections to maintain their B12 levels. The frequency of these needs to be determined based on symptoms. Unfortunately, some countries have poor guidelines for how frequently the injections to be done. The UK is currently one of these. Many low B12 patients require self-administered B12 injections multiple times per week, in order to maintain their health.

Note: in some countries like Germany, B12 is considered an entirely safe supplement and important to maintain at good levels. So, in Germany, B12 ampoules of all types of B12 may be purchased in pharmacies, with syringes and needles, for home injection, by anyone who feels that they require them. When regular injections are required, it is far more convenient for people to do their own at home, as they are very easy to do. Of course, one injection should always be done first by a pharmacy, or nurse to ensure that the person has no adverse response to them (which is rare).

Two important research papers appeared in the New England Journal of Medicine in 2012.

One research paper clearly showed that the presence of Intrinsic Factor Antibodies causes false-positive levels of B12 in the blood. This causes clinicians to rule out B12 deficiency.

A second paper in the same journal showed that the current machines that are used to test for B12, yield false-positive results in up to 35% of patients – again causing misdiagnosis. It is also known that Intrinsic Factor Antibodies only show positive in 40-60% of cases, and often have false-negative results!

On top of all of this, any test of blood-based B12 does not necessarily show how well the B12 is being effective within the cells. No such test is possible yet. The tests for Intrinsic Factor Antibodies and Parietal Cell Antibodies are known to be unreliable and misleading.

The British Society for Haematology have guidelines on Intrinsic Factor Ab testing: "Patients negative for intrinsic factor antibody with no other causes of deficiency may still have pernicious anaemia, and should be treated as anti-intrinsic factor antibody-negative pernicious anaemia. Lifelong therapy should be continued in the presence of an objective clinical response".

Furthermore, it is now known from research that:

1. Low B12 levels can be present in the absence of enlarged red cells in over 60% of cases, and
2. Neuro-psychiatric abnormalities due to low B12 can be present in a significant number of patients with normal haemoglobin and normal red blood cell count.

If low B12 is present, and you have a balanced diet, it is likely that you require proper treatment. Proper treatment probably means B12 injections.

To complicate things further, low folic acid can also have an impact; if it is low, you also cannot produce enough healthy red blood cells. So, testing Serum Folate is also important.

All in all, the current diagnosis methods for low B12 are flawed. The campaigners and doctors who specialise in B12 are aware of this and are pushing for major changes.

So, all the various tests may show that everything looks completely fine with respect to B12. However, the person might still have low B12 and be struggling with the myriad of symptoms that can come from it, e.g., depression, fatigue, headaches, shortness of breath, diarrhoea, pins and needles, other neurological issues including paranoia and even psychosis, to name but a few. Testing of B12 is currently inconclusive even if the test result shows no issue.

Left untreated, low B12 can result in permanent nerve damage! Permanent!

What if you have been on B12 supplements and then test B12?

If someone has been on any form of a supplement containing B12, it can leave the serum levels of B12 elevated for a long time afterwards. To get a true assessment of B12 level, the individual needs to have stopped any form of B12 supplement for 4-6 MONTHS! Many of the other tests for low B12 can also be compromised if supplementation has occurred during this time.

If someone has been taking a B12 supplement, or even a multivitamin, this will artificially make the blood levels of B12 remain high. This is the case even though cellular levels of B12 can be desperately low and cause nerve damage!

This latter point makes the testing of B12 in the blood relatively futile once any treatment is started and is, therefore, not likely to result in any clear diagnosis.

If someone has been supplementing with B12 tablets or patches or sublingual tablets, their blood level of B12 is likely to be high, yet they may have inadequate cellular levels of B12. In many cases, the B12 taken this way is bound to protein and just continues to circulate in the bloodstream, i.e., it does not get cleaved from protein and very little of it reaches the cells where it is needed. Hence, for someone with symptoms of low B12, it would be better to do the testing before any supplemental B12 is ever used. I have highlighted this last point as thyroid patients often take a lot of supplements in an attempt to ensure that they 'have enough of everything'. For most of the other things, they might want to test, taking supplements will not cause much of an issue if the supplement is stopped for a week or two prior to the testing. However, for B12 it makes a massive difference.

I cannot stress the last point enough, so please read this paragraph. If you have not had a B12 test prior to taking any supplement containing B12, you will probably not have true serum B12 results (with all of its faults). If you are on some form of B12, your results are likely to be high. The B12 test result is useless! Taking more oral B12 supplements (even sub-lingual) is likely not to help in many cases!

Please be aware that if you have been on oral supplementation of B12, and your results now look good or high, the B12 could still be dangerously low in the cells. So, supplementation ought to be avoided for many months if you plan to test B12. You have to be off ALL B12 supplements for 4-6 months to get a valid B12 test result.

Oral B12 supplements just end up circulating around the body in some individuals. This B12 may not ever arrive within the cells. In some patients, the B12 can just remain bound to protein and never be released for use within the cells. Some patients have been known to appear to have good B12 levels due to supplementation. However, because their cells were starved of B12, they suffered permanent neurological damage.

See the following document by the Dutch Research group, an official government group, the only one specifically mandated to research B12 in the world: https://b12-institute.nl/caution-note-about-oral-supps/

Once on B12 injections, serum levels remain high, which is needed to repair neurological damage, and there is no toxicity, as stated by the World Health Organisation. The injections are a very high dosage, and they bypass the stage where it attaches to one protein and is blocked there. It does get cleaved. When you take a tablet, the gut attaches a protein that needs to be cleaved along the way, and it does not happen if the circuit is broken somewhere. Additionally, there is a 1% passive absorption in all forms of B12, but nowhere enough to repair the damage.

What does this all imply?

This means it is a very complex situation, and it can be extremely difficult to get a clear diagnosis of B12 deficiency or Pernicious Anaemia.

Some people have methylation issues which affect their ability to convert some forms of B12 to the active form (methyl B12). Hydroxy or cyanocobalamin products can be less efficient for these people, and they may do better with methyl-cobalamin. This issue might possibly be detected by some of the genetic tests that can be done through companies like Ancestry.com or 23andMe.com. However, interpretation of the results can be difficult.

Please be aware that if someone has methylation issues and is on the incorrect type of B12 for them, this will result in B12 lab test results that appear excellent. However, they can still have many symptoms of low B12. I have had thyroid patients who have been on hydroxy cobalamin injections, but have had many symptoms still. In some cases, knowing that they have MTHFR issues, has allowed me to suggest switching to methyl B12 injections, with the correct co-factors. The results can sometimes be spectacular, with symptoms just vanishing, including low cortisol. Methylation issues can work both ways - sometimes the patient can only handle inactive B12 injections, e.g., hydroxy cobalamin.

I worry that a lot of thyroid patients who are not responding to thyroid treatment may well have undiagnosed B12 issues.

Even if someone is diagnosed with low B12, they often fail to get the treatment that they need to keep the effects of low B12 at bay, i.e., the required frequency of intramuscular B12 injections. Many of them find that within a few weeks of a B12 injection, their symptoms are starting to return.

For these people, far more frequent injections are required. This is hard to get in some countries unless the patient has a good haematologist or doctor.

Some of the most affected PA patients need much more frequent injections e.g., every other day or twice per week. In these cases, being able to self-inject is a good option. B12 is very easy, and painless, to administer this way. Sometimes, even regular intravenous B12 is required.

In many cases of low B12, frequent loading doses of B12 are needed for several weeks, and possibly months, in order to get the levels up quickly. Often this means 2-3 times per week, and in rare cases, even once a day. After this, the frequency of the B12 injections could be reduced to the level for the individual that keeps symptoms at bay. However, some low B12 patients continue to need frequent injections – often for life. B12 blood tests cannot be used to monitor for a good result. As explained already, the B12 in the blood can be extremely high after any supplementation and this does not mean that cellular levels are good. Note: when a patient requires regular B12 injections, it does make sense for them to be able to do them themselves at home.

All in all, the entire situation is a bit of a shambles.

The Pernicious Anaemia Society charity in the UK, chaired by Martyn Hooper, is trying to work with the medical profession and other groups to create awareness and bring about change. There is still a long way to go.

If someone has symptoms that fit extremely well with B12 deficiency, or PA, and there is any doubt about the blood tests at all, it is worth seeking a referral to a good Haematologist. They ought to know that the clinical presentation is the most important thing

Sometimes a therapeutic trial of B12 injections is the only valid diagnostic test.

Doing a proper trial and assessment of the person's response to regular B12 injections might be the only way to reach a correct diagnosis.

In addition to all the above, there are numerous co-factors that may be needed to enable B12 to function correctly within the cells.

If Methyl-Cobalamin (methyl B12) is the chosen form of B12, then a supplement called Adenosyl-Cobalamin should be taken each day.

B12 and Folate (B9) work together. One cannot work without the other. It is best to keep folate in the 3rd or 4th quartile of the reference range. Stop the folate for a week and test serum folate. With infrequent or monthly injections of B12, some people manage adequate folate with only 400 mcg per day of folic acid or folinic acid. Those on two injections per week may need 1 or 2 mg per day to keep folate levels up, and I know of some patients on daily or twice daily B12 injections that need 5 mg of folate per day, but that is more unusual. Getting feedback via testing folate after taking no supplement of it for a week, is the best way to judge the right amount to supplement with. Note: some people may need one of the active folates like Methyl Folate or Folinic Acid if they have genetic issues (MTHFR) processing Folic Acid. If Methyl Folate does not work well, this does not mean that Folinic Acid will also not work, and vice versa. Sometimes, the non-active form, Folic Acid, actually works better. Frequently, the person does not know what particular type of folate is going to work best for them, until they try.

Also, look into Iron, Vitamin D and Magnesium levels as these can be deficient also, (this is common when the person has Parietal Cell Antibodies but these nutrients can be low, even when this is not the case).

Beyond the above, it is essential to have functional B2 for B12 to cycle correctly. So, for ideal B12 usage, the person requires the following supplements: at least 5 mg/day B2 (via B2 or a B complex). B6 is also helpful as it is used alongside B12 and Methyl Folate to make red blood cells. Sometimes the B6 needs to be in the active form also − Methyl-B6 (also known as Pyridoxine-5-phosphate or P-5-P). Note: Low B6, or methylation cycle problems leading to low methyl B6, can also cause high homocysteine. You can over-dose on B6. So, taking 25 mg of B6 is safe for a very short time, but 10 mg of B6 per day is far safer if you intend to take it daily for the long-term.

Also, some other supplements may be helpful: 150 mcg/day Iodide, 55 mcg/day of Sodium Selenite (in some Selenium supplements), 100 mcg/day of Sodium Molybdate (in some Molybdenum supplements).

Further Reading.

I recommend reading these excellent books by Martyn Hooper: What you Need to Know About Pernicious Anaemia and Vitamin B12 Deficiency, and Pernicious Anaemia: The Forgotten Disease. Both books cover both B12 deficiency and Pernicious Anaemia (the autoimmune version of low B12).

A less easy, but also excellent read is 'Could it be B12?' by Pacholok and Stuart.

See also:

http://www.vitaminb12deficiency.net.au/VB12Hypothyroidism.htm
and:
https://www.facebook.com/groups/946944078825502/

For more information, please see the link to the 2014 guidelines on B12 and folate treatment from the British Society of Haematologists, and the summary of that from the Pernicious Anaemia Society (PAS), which is a little more digestible.

Summary for the diagnosis and treatment of cobalamin and folate disorders (from the British Society of Haematologists – for medical professionals) See: https://onlinelibrary.wiley.com/doi/full/10.1111/bjh.12959

Here is the summary of this report from Martyn Hooper of the Pernicious Anaemia Society:

In June 2014 the British Committee for Standards in Haematology issued new; revised Guidelines on Vitamin B12 and Folate. The new guidelines acknowledge the failings of the current assay used to determine B12 status in patients. Below are the main recommendations of the committee:

1. The clinical picture is the most important factor in assessing the significance of test results assessing cobalamin status because there is no 'gold standard' test to define deficiency.

2. Definitive cut-off points to define clinical and subclinical deficiency states are not possible, given the variety of methodologies used and technical issues.

3. In the presence of discordance between the test result and strong clinical features of deficiency, treatment should not be delayed to avoid neurological impairment.

4. The absence of a raised MCV cannot be used to exclude the need for cobalamin testing because neurological impairment occurs with a normal MCV in 25% of cases.

5. Some assays may give false normal results in blood serum that contains high titre anti-intrinsic factor antibodies.

6. It is not entirely clear what should be regarded as a clinically normal serum cobalamin level.

7. It is even less clear what levels of serum cobalamin represent 'subclinical' deficiency.

8. Neurological symptoms due to cobalamin deficiency may occur in the presence of a normal MCV.

9. IFAB is positive in only 40-60% of cases, i.e., low sensitivity, and the finding of a negative IFAB assay does not therefore rule out pernicious anaemia (hereafter referred to as AbNegPA).

10. Standard initial therapy for patients without neurological involvement is 1000ug intramuscularly ['i.m.'] three times a week for 2 weeks. The BNF advises that patients presenting with neurological symptoms should receive 1000ug i.m. on alternate days until there is no further improvement.

11. Care must be taken if low dose supplements are prescribed, as such an approach risks the suboptimal treatment of latent and emerging pernicious anaemia with possible inadequate treatment of neurological features.

12. There are arguments against the use of oral cobalamin in initiation of cobalamin therapy in severely deficient individuals who have poor absorption, especially due to pernicious anaemia.

13. Patients with pernicious anaemia need treatment for life regardless of serum cobalamin levels.

3. POSSIBLE CAUSES OF HAIR LOSS IN SOME THYROID PATIENTS

Unfortunately, some thyroid patients suffer from hair loss. This is obviously very distressing for those with this problem and often it can be extremely difficult to discover what is causing it. It might be connected with their hypothyroidism, or it might not be.

Over the years I have been asked the question of what could be causing hair loss. I have usually answered that hair loss is not a symptom that I focus on very much. This is not because I do not care, it is just because it is not a symptom that I know a great deal about.

Sometimes, the thyroid patient associates some change in their thyroid medication to a worsening of the condition. However, I believe that this is often because a change in thyroid medication has further exposed some other underlying issue.

Whilst, I am no expert in hair loss causes, I have managed to accumulate some suggestions of issues that can contribute to hair loss.

Here are just some of the possible causes of hair loss:
- Low iron (testing for serum iron, ferritin, TIBC and transferrin saturation % is a good idea).
- Heavy metals in excess.
- Hypothyroidism (esp. low T3).
- High testosterone, DHEA or DHT.
- Polycystic ovary syndrome (PCOS).
- Insulin resistance.
- Low blood sugar or low blood pressure − both can limit the nutrients getting to the scalp.
- Cortisol imbalances − high cortisol and low cortisol can both cause hair loss.
- Hormonal changes in menopause. Esp. low oestrogen or progesterone.
- Micronutrient deficiencies (vitamin B12, biotin, iron, zinc, silica, and essential fatty acids especially).
- Immune system dysfunction (e.g., alopecia and lichen planopilaris).

- Environmental (skin mites).
- Drug side effect (such as those used for cancer, arthritis, depression, heart problems, gout and high blood pressure).
- A stressful event or shock.
- Some hair treatments.

Note: a few thyroid patients who are on T3-Only have told me that sometimes adding a little T4 medication can help to avoid the hair loss. Even as little as 10 to 25 mcg has helped some to overcome this issue. But clearly this is not going to help everyone. However, the vast majority of patients on T3-Only do not have any hair loss at all.

As I said earlier, I am definitely no expert in this area. However, the above may help some of you to begin your own investigations into the cause and solution for this distressing problem

4. IS THERE A CONNECTION BETWEEN THYROID HORMONES AND DEPRESSION

Far too many anti-depressants are prescribed these days when the real issue is some underlying cause.

I know of many cases where anti-depressants were prescribed by a doctor to a patient whose actual problem ended up being improperly treated hypothyroidism or low vitamin B12 and, in a few situations, sex hormone imbalances.

This short article will focus on the link between thyroid dysfunction and depression. I was prompted to write it by a thyroid patient who showed me an article that Dr Kent Holtorf, M.D. wrote a few years ago.

I will provide the link to Dr Holtorf's article shortly, but his thesis is simple: there are large studies that show that the majority of patients being treated with anti-depressants fail to respond to them, or have side effects that are severe enough to discontinue them. The research showed that T3 was far more effective than anti-depressants, with fewer side effects.

Dr Holtorf believes that many depressed or bipolar patients actually have undiagnosed or improperly treated thyroid hormone dysfunction and that T3 therapy is actually more appropriate than anti-depressants.

It is very clear that hardly any doctors focus on the Free T3 (FT3) test result and assess whether the patient's T3 levels are possibly too low before writing a prescription for anti-depressants. Even in the case of a patient with diagnosed hypothyroidism, FT3 is rarely the focus − but it should be. Equally, other issues like low B12 are often simply not looked for before the anti-depressant is offered.

Many of us know from friends, family members and possibly personal experience that anti-depressants frequently do not work and can have undesirable side-effects. They can also be difficult to withdraw from. So, investigating these other possible causes before prescribing anti-depressants would be preferable.

Let me be clear. I am not trying to imply that all cases of depression or bipolar disorder or other mental health issues have a root cause in hypothyroidism or low B12 etc. That would be a very silly position to take. However, it is extremely likely that a subset of those patients with depression actually does have an underlying root cause such as hypothyroidism and that this root cause remains untreated.

Here is the link to Dr Holtorf's short but important article:

https://holtorfmed.com/articles/mental-health/thyroid-dysfunction-as-cause-of-depression

Here are just a few additional links to research papers and writings on the subject. There is too much out there on the Internet to ignore the connection between thyroid dysfunction and mental health issues:

https://www.ncbi.nlm.nih.gov/pmc/articles/PMC3246784/

https://psychcentral.com/blog/is-thyroid-dysfunction-driving-your-depression/

https://www.ncbi.nlm.nih.gov/pmc/articles/PMC3968440/

https://pubmed.ncbi.nlm.nih.gov/29331701/

https://psycheducation.org/treatment/thyroid-and-bipolar-disorder/

I recommend that if you are interested in this important subject area that you do your own research, as there is a lot of information out there.

5. THYROID BLOOD TESTS – CONDITIONS LIKE CFS, ME AND FIBROMYALGIA

There are conditions like chronic fatigue syndrome (CFS), myalgic encephalopathy (ME) and fibromyalgia for which our current treatments are inadequate.

Patients with these conditions often never get full restoration of health.

The symptoms associated with all three of these conditions overlap hugely with those of hypothyroidism.

Some people with apparently perfectly normal-looking thyroid blood test results after treatment with T4 or T4/T3 can still continue with severe symptoms of hypothyroidism.

A proportion of these thyroid patients often continue to fail to respond to T4 or T4/T3 thyroid hormone replacement. For these thyroid patients T3-Only replacement therapy frequently fully restores their health. I have seen thousands of cases like these, of thyroid patients with good looking thyroid blood test results when on T4, T4/T3 or NDT, who still cannot get well until T3-Only is used.

It does not take much imagination to see that it is possible for someone who has never had an obviously underactive thyroid, potentially to have a similar issue, i.e., an undiagnosed thyroid hormone issue. This undiagnosed issue could have its origins within the cells and not be subject to diagnosis through a standard set of thyroid laboratory tests.

I believe that it is very likely that some percentage of CFS, ME, or fibromyalgia patients have some form of thyroid hormone issue underlying their symptoms.

Many thyroid patients who eventually recover using NDT, T4/T3, or T3-Only had a CFS, ME, or fibromyalgia diagnosis at one time. One of my own endocrinologists and my own family doctor both said I had ME or CFS.

Consequently, the questions I would like to leave readers with is:

How many of the ME, CFS or Fibromyalgia sufferers, who have been tested for thyroid disease, and have been told their "lab test results were normal", actually have thyroid hormone issues at the cellular level. Might some of these respond to a trial of NDT, T4/T3 or T3-Only replacement therapy?

We know there are serious dangers in mechanically using thyroid reference ranges.

It is also important to be aware that when patients develop thyroid problems, their thyroid hormone levels can adjust from their individual healthy levels to different, unhealthy levels for them. These new, unhealthy levels may still be well within the large population ranges, and so they may never be diagnosed with thyroid problems. An endocrinologist or doctor may just tell them that there is nothing wrong with their thyroid or thyroid hormones.

If there were laboratory tests that could measure how well our cells were being regulated by thyroid hormone, I would expect some proportion of the sufferers of these types of conditions to have problems with thyroid hormones at the cellular level. I do believe this to be true.

The worrying thought is that people in this category may never have this found out because no existing laboratory test can show the actual level of regulation of cell function by thyroid hormone.

The late Dr. John C. Lowe discovered, from his own research over many years, that treatment with T3-Only was absolutely necessary to relieve many patients of the symptoms of fibromyalgia.

I believe that T3 treatment may also help some patients who have been given diagnoses of conditions like chronic fatigue syndrome (CFS) and ME.

However, we desperately need more research to be done to provide adequate laboratory tests that show the actual level of cell regulation by thyroid hormone.

We need medical research to make some big breakthroughs for thyroid patients. These breakthroughs need to happen in the field of diagnostic tests for actual regulation of cell function at the nuclei and mitochondria by thyroid hormone.

Only with these types of tests can a proper indication of thyroid hormone activity be seen. These tests would be the laboratory test equivalent of going beyond the old basal metabolic rate (BMR) test.

Advances in science will enable this research to occur at some point, and the lives of thyroid patients and some sufferers of other related conditions like CFS, ME and fibromyalgia will improve dramatically.

6. TESTOSTERONE AND MEN

Note: some aspects of this article are relevant to women also.

Testosterone levels are often low for men with thyroid problems.

This is no real surprise as all systems of the body are impacted when thyroid hormones are low or are not working effectively.

Low testosterone often causes significant symptoms in its own right. Two of the most common symptoms are depression and low libido. Muscle loss and lower energy levels can also result. You can look up more information on symptoms quite easily on the Internet.

I will assume in this article that all the basics of low iron, B12, other nutrients, low cortisol and blood sugar issues have been addressed and are not relevant.

When looking at testosterone levels it is important to test:

- Total Testosterone. Note: total testosterone on its own tells us very little.
- Sex Hormone Binding Globulin (SHBG). SHBG binds most of the testosterone. Albumin also has a weak binding effect on testosterone. High SHBG may be limiting how much free testosterone there is.
- Free Testosterone (although this can be estimated using total testosterone and SHBG).
- In some cases where aromatisation is a concern, estradiol should also be checked.
- In addition, checking prolactin may also be important as raised prolactin can suppress testosterone levels.

Free Androgen Index (FAI) is sometimes used to estimate Free Testosterone if all you have is Total Testosterone and SHBG. FAI = Total Testosterone x 100/SHBG

There are Free and Bio-Available Testosterone Calculators on the Internet. These require Albumin, as well as SHBG and Total Testosterone, and are a more accurate estimate of Free Testosterone than FAI.

Here is a good link with which to begin your own research in relation to thyroid hormone, the deiodinase enzymes and testosterone:

http://nahypothyroidism.org/deiodinases/

For a man with low cortisol not caused by Addison's disease, or hypopituitarism, the Circadian T3 Method (CT3M) can be a real blessing.

CT3M can often raise testosterone levels in men. Male thyroid patients have often seen 30% increases in total testosterone levels when using CT3M.

Whether you can use the CT3M depends on whether you have low cortisol or not. If you do not have low cortisol, then CT3M will not help you, and in fact, could cause issues by raising cortisol to too high a level. But for those men that need to address low cortisol, CT3M may work well to raise testosterone levels.

Let me briefly discuss sex hormone-binding globulin (SHBG).

In both men and women, SHBG is the main protein that carries the sex hormones testosterone and oestrogen. Albumin also carries some of the testosterone and oestrogen but the sex hormones are only weakly bound to albumin. Only the testosterone and oestrogen that is not bound to SHBG (and albumin to a lesser extent), is biologically active.

If testosterone levels stay the same and SHBG rises, there is less biologically active testosterone and a guy can feel very unwell. So, when a man (or a woman) has testosterone checked, they should have SHBG checked at the same time.

For those thyroid patients who have to use T3 replacement, this sometimes drives up SHBG. Multi-dosing, using the dosage management process in the Recovering with T3 book, helps because the process arrives at an effective T3 dosage with low individual T3 doses.

If SHBG is still an issue then there are multiple approaches.

Some patients have said that the use of milk thistle can sometimes bring SHBG down.

Stinging nettle root extract (it has to be the root) in capsules can also help to **lower SHBG.** Stinging nettle root comes in 250 mg and 500 mg capsules and the dosing typically is done 2-3 times per day over the course of the day.

There is also a drug called Danazol that can be used in low doses to reduce SHBG (50-200 mg every other day is typical). Danazol supposedly cuts SHBG in half within 6-8 weeks. Note: Danazol is a prescription drug and its use to reduce SHBG is an 'off label' application. Danazol should only be considered under the supervision of a knowledgeable physician. There are other medications that might also work. Male thyroid patients should do their own research on this.

Some doctors prefer to provide transdermal, or injected testosterone to a high enough level to overcome any SHBG, as testosterone will ultimately suppress SHBG, although this can lead to other problems e.g., higher estrogen levels (aromatisation). Sometimes total testosterone needs to be over range in order for free testosterone to be at a healthy level.

There are many connections that men should be aware of:

- It is free testosterone that is active and has an effect, not total testosterone.
- Low thyroid hormone often results in low testosterone levels.
- Low testosterone in men will result in a lowering of the D1 deiodinase enzyme activity (resulting in worse conversion of FT4 to FT3, and increased rT3).
- Low thyroid hormone levels may lead to lower growth hormone levels and this, in turn, may reduce FT4 to FT3 conversion and increase reverse T3 (growth hormone supplementation is known to increase FT4 to FT3 conversion and reduce reverse T3).
- Increased free testosterone can lower thyroid binding globulin (TBG) which increases free T4 (FT4) and free T3 (FT4). Lowering free testosterone increases TBG, lowering FT4 and FT3.
- Increased free testosterone can displace cortisol from cortisol binding globulin (CBG), which increases free cortisol. Lowering free testosterone can cause more cortisol to be bound to CBG, resulting in lower free cortisol.

If low testosterone is an issue, it should be discussed with a knowledgeable doctor or specialist. Testosterone replacement can be challenging. Often more than just testosterone itself needs to be provided to ensure the treatment works. Plus, one type of testosterone replacement may not suit everyone. See Article 5 in Chapter 8 for connections to Free T3 and cortisol.

7. ESTROGEN DOMINANCE, THE USE OF PROGESTERONE AND DEALING WITH HIGH ADRENALINE

I never intended to write about sex hormones but over the last few years, it has become increasingly clear that there is a connection between sex hormones and thyroid hormones and that some women never get full relief from symptoms until both have been adequately treated. However, I have found that a few women appear to react poorly to the introduction of progesterone, and it leads them to give up too soon. This is why I wrote this article.

The parts of this article that discuss dealing with high adrenaline may also be relevant to men.

Please note that in all cases where I discuss treatment with progesterone, I mean bio-identical progesterone of some kind. Bio-identical progesterone is the only safe form of progesterone that women should ever consider using, as synthetic progesterone is linked with cancer.

It is also worth mentioning that in some countries (including the UK), many doctors simply do not believe that replacement with progesterone is needed in any other than a small dosage to protect the lining of the womb. Certainly, in the UK, the NHS doctors believe that estrogen is the only hormone that will resolve post-menopausal symptoms, and that the idea of 'estrogen dominance' is nonsense. Women often need to find a functional medicine doctor or a specialist in bio-identical hormone replacement (if they cannot resolve their issues on their own). I fully intend to use the term 'estrogen dominance' as I know for a fact that it is a very real issue for many post-menopausal women.

Please see the sex hormone chapter in my book, The Thyroid Patient's Manual, for specific details on testing progesterone and estrogen in post-menopausal women. Estrogen dominance occurs when the woman's progesterone level is not high enough to balance the amount of estrogen. The book should be really helpful in assessing this. It would take too much space int this article to cover it. You can use this calculator to assess your estrogen to progesterone ratio. This ratio for post-menopausal women is usually best at 200:1 or 300:1: https://www.omnicalculator.com/health/pg-e2-ratio.

In recent years, I have tried to help some post-menopausal thyroid patients who have estrogen dominance. Estrogen dominance brings with it its own set of symptoms including weight gain, fatigue, mood issues and breast tenderness. It is difficult to treat thyroid problems when estrogen dominance is also present. Estrogen dominance, or high estrogen, also increases thyroid binding globulin which lowers the free levels of thyroid hormone.

Treating estrogen dominance through added progesterone, usually works well. However, in some cases, the progesterone appears to produce a bad reaction. The reaction is similar to having high adrenaline with tension, anxiety and elevated heart rate. I have never really understood this, as surely adding the progesterone would help?

Recently, from talking to several practitioners and reading Dr Michael E. Platt's book 'Adrenaline Dominance', I think I may now understand why this can happen, and what to do about it.

Through working with patients over many years, Dr Platt is convinced that many of them are dealing with excess adrenaline. This can be true for both men and women. Adrenaline is produced when the person is under either physical or emotional stress. Adrenaline and cortisol can also be elevated when the brain is not getting enough blood sugar. They both raise blood sugar through a process called gluconeogenesis, which I have discussed many times in my writings. The net result of the raised blood sugar can be raised insulin, which unfortunately, can cause fat around the stomach, elevated blood pressure, ageing, and very likely, type 2 diabetes. The raised insulin also lowers blood sugar, causing insulin-induced hypoglycaemia. In turn, the hypoglycaemia causes more adrenaline. It is a vicious circle. Adrenaline, is implicated in many negative conditions, including anxiety, depression, insomnia, diabetes, IBS, weight gain, early ageing, headaches, addictions and possibly fibromyalgia. Excess adrenaline is great to get you out of danger but otherwise is it not good news!

However, there is good news! Progesterone has an important role in controlling adrenaline. Dr Platt believes that progesterone can prevent the action of insulin at insulin receptor sites and stop the hypoglycaemia. Plus, progesterone appears to directly block the effect of adrenaline. Progesterone might also have an effect on the pancreas cells themselves and prevent excess insulin production.

Dr Platt, through his years of practice, is convinced of the effect of progesterone on hypoglycaemia, excess adrenaline, and high insulin levels. Unfortunately, there are no studies on this as it is not an area that has elicited much interest from researchers.

Note: progesterone has no single dosage that is usable by everyone. It has to be adjusted to suit the patient. Also, treating the patient based on symptoms and signs is far superior to using lab test results. If transdermal bio-identical progesterone cream is used, then it is best used on the inner forearms, upper chest, back of the neck or face – where the skin is thin and there is a good blood supply. Often these transdermal creams need to be applied two-three times per day, as the half-life is fairly short. However, there are other forms of progesterone and different methods of use for their absorption (micronised progesterone capsules, buccal lozenges, suppositories, even sublingual drops like Progest-E/Pro-E which is very pure/additive free). One type/use of progesterone may suit some patients but not others patients. The different forms of progesterone, methods of use and dosages are beyond the scope of this article to cover.

Returning to the thyroid patients with estrogen dominance that seem to be intolerant of progesterone.

There are at least two aspects to this:

1. Firstly, there is a concept discussed amongst bio-identical hormone practitioners called "estrogen kickback", or "estrogen breakthrough", where the female patient uses too low a dosage of progesterone and the progesterone stimulates the estrogen receptors. The kickback effect is thought to be due to the estrogen receptors being sensitised, or becoming more active, in the presence of progesterone. This is also referred to as 'estrogen receptor stimulation' and 'estrogen receptor antagonization' in quite a number of research articles. If there is not enough progesterone to balance this estrogen effect, then estrogen dominance occurs with all the symptoms it brings. However, the main question is, how much estrogen is there to be balanced and how much progesterone will be needed. Some bio-identical hormone replacement practitioners believe that there is far more estrogen in the body than what is measured in the blood, and essentially estrogen is stored in tissues and is also constantly supplied

by our estrogenic environment/foods etc. That is why there might be the need for far more progesterone to balance estrogen than mainstream doctors believe.

The estrogen kickback effect can cause far more of a response to the already dominant estrogen effect than any current estrogen dominance issue is already giving the patient. The symptoms can be varied: mood swings, irritability, fatigue, depression, headaches, weight gain, bloating, and breast tenderness, elevated heart rate, hot flashes and anxiety. Plus, the response can be very strong and quite alarming. This may sound contradictory but I have heard this view expressed by many experienced practitioners. However, many patients simply give up attempting to use the progesterone at this stage because they think it is not going to work for them.

2. Secondly, patients that do have an adrenaline issue, often need MORE progesterone. Success usually comes when the progesterone dosage is increased, step by step, until the symptoms subside. However, many patients just baulk at using progesterone, once they have had any bad symptoms appearing after starting it.

The bottom line, for both the cases above, is that many women simply need to stick with the progesterone they are taking and wait for the symptoms to subside OR that they actually require a much higher dosage of progesterone in order to overcome the issue. Sometimes it is necessary to try different types of progesterone OR different absorption methods (transdermal creams, oral bio-identical progesterone, suppositories etc. are all options these days for bio-identical hormone replacement).

Therefore, when there is estrogen dominance, the presence of adrenaline and estrogen kickback should always be a consideration when dosing progesterone. Progesterone is the only known hormone to actually deal with both estrogen dominance and high adrenaline. Therefore, sometimes, persisting with its use, or even increasing the dosage, is often the only way to actually get rid of the horrible symptoms and effects of estrogen dominance and high adrenaline.

It is also worth noting a couple of other important things:

• For progesterone therapy to work properly, other issues may well need to be addressed. I am not going to list all of these but low iron, low ferritin and low B12 are just examples.

• Also, sex hormones can have an impact on thyroid hormones. So be on the lookout for this and be prepared to adjust thyroid hormone dosage if you think it appropriate.

Finally, progesterone has been largely neglected by mainstream medicine. Despite this, a large and growing number of women are finding that it can often help them. But, just like T3 (which is also a natural hormone), it may not always work for everyone. Both T3 and progesterone are natural substances and should work for everyone. However, sometimes, there are people who struggle to use them without symptoms that are too difficult to cope with. This is much more likely to be due to other issues, or conditions, that the person has, or to as yet unknown factors, given how scant the research is in this area. What should be done if there is no relief of symptoms on higher doses of progesterone, despite changing delivery methods and addressing other issues? Or what if the symptoms of intolerance are far too difficult to cope with? In these situations, it is recommended to stop the progesterone, or wean it down, as clearly things are not working.

I have five articles that cover the various relationships of thyroid hormone, cortisol and sex hormones. They include Article 3, 4, 5 and 6 in Chapter 8, along with Article 7 (this article), in Chapter 10. They have helped me to assist many thyroid patients.

Thank you to Chemaine Linnie for directing me to Dr Platt's book. Thanks also to Keith Littlewood for emailing with me on this topic. Also, many thanks to Aldona Z. Coldicott for her very helpful input.

8. THE IMPORTANCE OF IRON TO THYROID PATIENTS AND LINKS TO GUT HEALTH

Many thyroid patients struggle to keep their iron levels up to a healthy level, as a result of the effect of prolonged hypothyroidism.

The four main tests to use to determine if iron is adequate within the body are:

- Serum iron.
- Serum Ferritin.
- Total Iron Binding Capacity (TIBC).
- Transferrin Saturation %.

From patient experience, thyroid patients usually feel better if:

- Serum iron is over 90 ug/dL and ideally closer to 100-110 ug/dL. This is based on a lab range of 65-176 ug/dL for men and 50-170 ug/dL for women.
- Serum ferritin is at least in the range 80-100 ng/mL for women (men do well with similar results or even a little higher). This is based on a lab range of 22-320 ng/mL for men/post-menopausal women and 10-290 ng/mL for pre-menopausal women.
- If iron supplementation is being considered, TIBC should be at or above the lower quartile. This is so that it is clear there is capacity to supplement with iron.
- Transferrin saturation % in the 35-45% range.

This article is not about iron itself, or about supplementing it to achieve healthy levels. It is about the digestive system, and its role in absorbing iron, and the implications of this.

The absorption of the majority of nutrients takes place in the jejunum (the middle section of the small intestine), with the following notable exceptions:

- Iron is absorbed in the duodenum and first part of the jejunum.
- Vitamin B12 is absorbed in the terminal ileum (the last part of the small intestine).
- Water and lipids are absorbed throughout the small intestine.
- Sodium bicarbonate, glucose, fructose and amino acids are also absorbed in the small intestine.

The mechanism of iron transport from the gut into the blood stream remains a mystery, despite intensive investigation.

However, the physical state of iron entering the duodenum greatly influences its absorption.

Gastric acid lowers the pH in the duodenum (makes it more acidic), enhancing the solubility and uptake of iron. When gastric acid production is impaired (for instance by acid pump inhibitors, such as the drugs Prilosec or Omeprazole), iron absorption is greatly reduced.

Heme is the name of a number of naturally occurring organic molecules that contain iron. Heme is found in meat. Interestingly, heme is absorbed by machinery completely different to that of inorganic iron. The process is more efficient and is independent of duodenal PH.

Consequently, meats are excellent nutrient sources of iron. Meat is the best form of food from which to obtain iron, as even when stomach acid is reduced, (which it often is in hypothyroid patients), the natural form of organic iron is still absorbed extremely well. Heme iron may also be provided in supplement form.

Many people discuss the benefits of eating vegetables like spinach, but this form of iron is not as well absorbed as the heme in meat (red meat, liver and kidneys especially). The shortage of meats in the diets of many of the people in the world adds to the burden of iron deficiency.

A number of dietary factors influence iron absorption. Vitamin C can often increase iron uptake, in part by acting as weak chelators to help to make the iron more soluble in the duodenum. However, it is better to take this as Whole Food Vitamin C, as sometimes the standard type can lower ferritin. So, if iron is supplemented then vitamin C is often taken with the iron supplement. Supplements include iron bis-glycinate and heme iron which can be found in capsule form. Sometimes both the bis-glycinate, and the heme iron may be required to get serum iron and ferritin to improve.

Iron absorption is inhibited by plant phytates and tannins. These compounds also chelate iron, but prevent its uptake by the absorption machinery. Phytates are prominent in wheat and some other cereals, while tannins are prevalent in (non-herbal) teas.

So, the health of the digestive system is critical to the raising, and maintenance, of good iron levels, as it is the duodenum that absorbs iron.

Low stomach acid may also affect the absorption of iron.

It is also important to note that all iron is not equal. Iron in meat is very effectively absorbed. In addition to this, for someone with a gut that is already compromised in some way, then they often have a group of pathogenic bacteria growing in their gut. These pathogens are iron-loving bacteria, and they consume much of any inorganic iron supplements that are taken, which in turn feeds the population and creates further imbalances in the gut flora. These bacteria include: Actinomyces spp., Mycobacterium spp., strains of E.coli, Cornybacterium spp., and others.

Consequently, for someone with a compromised gut, taking iron supplements may make this situation worse, and particular attention may need to be given to healing the gut.

If someone has a compromised gut then they may continue to struggle to raise iron levels, and, as a consequence, they may struggle to have effective thyroid hormone action and adrenal health. However, a compromised gut does not always mean that the individual has obvious digestive system symptoms.

Sometimes, the overall health of the person, their response to thyroid hormone, laboratory test results of nutrient levels, their diet and past history (antibiotic use etc) may need to be assessed to get some idea that the gut is involved. Healing a compromised gut can, in some cases, be the most important action that a thyroid patient can take in order to get well.

For people who struggle to raise their iron storage, infusions or injections may be needed from their doctor.

The bottom line is that iron is critical to the function of many of our systems, including thyroid hormone action. Good iron levels are essential, but we must not ignore the digestive system. Improving the health of a thyroid patient's digestive system may be critical to the absorption of iron and other nutrients, as well as limiting the entry of other toxins into the bloodstream.

9. CALMING THE AUTOANTIBODY ATTACK IN HASHIMOTO'S THYROIDITIS

Some people believe that it is possible to calm the immune system and stop Hashimoto's Thyroiditis.

This article provides a starting point for those that want to find out more about reducing the TPO and Tg autoantibodies that are raised in Hashimoto's thyroiditis.

Strategies believed to calm the immune system in Hashimoto's Thyroiditis:

- For a thyroid gland that is under attack (evidenced by raised TPO and Tg autoantibodies), ensuring that the right thyroid treatment is in place and the patient is not hypothyroid in terms of FT3 and symptoms/signs is a good starting place.

- The right thyroid hormone treatment will not be effective if cortisol levels are low. Consequently, it is important to test cortisol with a 24-hour adrenal saliva test and an 8:00 am morning blood cortisol test, and then correct any low cortisol issue found.

- Many of my articles, and parts of the Recovering with T3 book, are concerned with the need for the healthy adrenal output of cortisol and, when necessary, the use of the Circadian T3 Method (CT3M), so I will say no more about this subject here.

- Vitamin D3 supplementation has been shown to be helpful in reducing the autoimmune attack in Hashimoto's thyroiditis. Vitamin D levels can be tested with a 25-hydroxy vitamin D test. Supplementation with vitamin D3 is essential if vitamin D is low. Supplementation with 5000 IUs of vitamin D3 may make sense, even if vitamin D levels are within range. Some doctors recommend higher doses of vitamin D3, but it is important to take medical advice on vitamin D3 supplementation (especially if a patient has kidney issues as vitamin D can cause further kidney damage).

- If iron levels are low this will put stress on the processing of thyroid hormones, so iron should be properly tested and supplemented if it is not at a healthy level.

- Vitamin B12 and folate should also be tested as, if these are low, this will also create stress on the body and impair thyroid hormone action.

- Selenium 200 mcg per day is also known to be effective in lowering autoantibodies.

- Gluten is known to be a factor in the development of Hashimoto's thyroiditis. This is a massive topic in itself. One of the strategies that many thyroid patients adopt is to go gluten-free. This, and many other relevant topics, may be found in Datis Kharrazian's book "Why do I still have symptoms when my lab tests are normal?"

- Low dose naltexone (LDN) is a drug that is known to modulate the immune system. Many thyroid patients have had good results using LDN and have seen their TPO and Tg autoantibodies reduce significantly.

- Finally, Izabella Wentz has an excellent book entitled Hashimoto's Thyroiditis. She appears to be one of the leading advocates for diet and supplementation to deal with Hashimoto's.

This article is just a menu of potential options that thyroid patients may wish to investigate further themselves.

However, I hope the above may provide some readers with a starting point for their own investigations.

10. COULD LOW DOSE NALTREXONE (LDN) BE HELPFUL IN HASHIMOTO'S

Could Low Dose Naltrexone (LDN) help some thyroid patients to calm down the immune system, and reduce thyroid destruction in Hashimoto's thyroiditis?

At high doses, naltrexone is an opioid antagonist that has been used and approved to treat opioid addiction and alcohol addiction.

When naltrexone is taken in low doses, it is known as low dose naltrexone or LDN. LDN has been shown by researchers to work in a different way to the doses of naltrexone used to treat opioid and alcohol addiction.

LDN stimulates the production of more endorphins, which can modulate the immune system and re-balance any excessive immune system responses.

LDN is usually used with a starting dose of 0.5-1 milligrams, rising to 4.5 milligrams at the most. Therapeutic doses can be anywhere in the middle of that range and frequently between 2 and 3.5 mg.

Taking too much LDN can cause side effects, so increases are usually by only 0.5 milligrams and only every 4-6 weeks. These side effects are minor but can include fatigue, sleep disturbances, diarrhoea, nausea and becoming more emotional.

Although extensive clinical trials have not been done specifically on LDN, there is information available on the safety of the much higher dosage Naltexone, which is an approved medication.

Low dose naltrexone (LDN) is currently being used to treat some autoimmune diseases including rheumatoid arthritis, multiple sclerosis and Crohn's disease. Other autoimmune conditions may also benefit from LDN treatment. Research teams are continuing to investigate the potentially very important benefits that LDN is alleged to bring.

I have communicated with many Hashimoto's thyroiditis patients who have told me that LDN has made their Hashimoto's autoantibodies drop to lower levels. They say it has relieved many of their symptoms including fibromyalgia.

Some claim that LDN has fixed their fibromyalgia or brain fog.

I have also spoken to patients with other autoimmune conditions who have told me that LDN has made a significant difference in their lives, and in many cases has eradicated their symptoms. However, I know some patients who have tried LDN without any benefit. So, it appears to be very individual and I do not think this is understood yet.

It is important to be absolutely clear that full clinical trials resulting in approval to use LDN for a wide range of autoimmune thyroid conditions have not been done yet. Campaigners are in the process of trying to get approval for these trials.

There is a reasonable amount of information on LDN available on the Internet and via patient-based forums.

I do not know if LDN will turn out to be widely used by Hashimoto's thyroiditis patients but at least for some, it appears to help.

Here are some resources for thyroid patients who want to find out more about LDN:

The main website for low dose naltrexone: http://www.lowdosenaltrexone.org/

The LDN Research Trust website: http://www.ldnresearchtrust.org

11. AUTOIMMUNE PROTOCOLS MAY NOT BE RIGHT FOR EVERY THYROID PATIENT

These days, there is a lot of focus on diet and supplements as a solution to autoimmune thyroid problems. The basic idea behind these approaches is to reduce, and ideally stop, any autoimmune response that may be damaging to the thyroid gland. These all fall under the umbrella description of Autoimmune Protocols. However, in some special cases, this may not always be the right approach.

In most countries, thyroid levels are only tested once a person has become symptomatic. It is rare for routine health screening to contain a complete thyroid hormone assessment, including the most common autoantibodies TPOAb and TgAb (those associated with Hashimoto's thyroiditis). However, if one is performed and a patient is told that they have raised autoantibodies, they may well want to find out what can be done to stop this response before it does any serious damage to the thyroid gland.

Therefore, if someone discovers that they have Hashimoto's thyroiditis in its early stages before the thyroid gland is damaged, then reducing the autoimmune response using an Autoimmune Protocol (AIP) can be extremely helpful indeed.

However, by the time some people find out they have Hashi's, their thyroid gland is often already very damaged. Because the thyroid gland is the most important organ for converting T4 to T3, the loss of thyroid tissue greatly reduces the patient's ability to convert. Once most of the thyroid gland is destroyed, a thyroid patient typically loses around 25% of their total T4 to T3 conversion capability. Furthermore, the loss of T3 can be far more than this, because for some people, the T3 contribution of their thyroid gland through conversion of T4 and through direct production of T3, can be very large. I explain this in more detail in my book, The Thyroid Patient's Manual.

Losing a significant amount of production and conversion capability can be a huge problem. It can, in some cases, make using an AIP problematic. Let me discuss my own history first, before talking more generally about this.

Paul Robinson's own history of Hashimoto's and losing a lot of T4 to T3 conversion capability.

I was diagnosed with Hashimoto's thyroiditis around the age of thirty. My symptoms were already quite extreme when I went to see my family doctor: severe fatigue, weight gain, dry skin, dry hair, memory issues, slow thinking etc. Surprisingly, she ran a full thyroid panel and found that my TSH was around 70 and my FT4 and FT3 levels were below the bottom of the reference ranges. Hashimoto's was already advanced. During the previous year or two, I had probably had some more minor symptoms, but my thyroid gland had compensated a great deal, even though it was being severely damaged. Thyroid tissue does not recover from this attack and it simply becomes dead non-functional tissue.

Over the last few years, I have tested DIO1 and DIO2 and found that both my parents gave me a copy of the defect in each gene. Hence, I am homozygous for both DIO1 and DIO2. When this is the case and the gene defects have manifested, which I believe mine did when I was in my late twenties, the effect is to have more of the bioavailable FT4 in the blood be converted to Reverse T3 (rT3) and to have less FT4 converted to FT3 (the active thyroid hormone). So, when this happens, the person is much more likely to be symptomatic with thyroid hormone issues, even when they are on Levothyroxine (T4) treatment. I will give you a link at the end to more information about these gene defects and how to test for them.

So, because Hashimoto's had destroyed a lot of my thyroid gland, I would already have lost a great deal of my ability to convert from T4 to T3. The DIO1 and DIO2 gene defects would also have been likely to further impair this conversion ability.

It is no surprise that Levothyroxine (T4) medication never worked for me at all and left me with all the symptoms that I had when I was first diagnosed. Even T4/T3 combination therapy failed to resolve my symptoms. T3-Only (T3-monotherapy) did help a great deal. However, for the first few years on T3-Only therapy, I found it hard to get my T3 daily dosage over 35-40 mcg. I felt much better on the T3, but not completely optimal. This was true even though I had created a way of using T3 to correct my low cortisol (the Circadian T3 Method – or CT3M).

The reason that I could not become optimal on the T3 at the beginning was that I still had some thyroid function left. It was impossible for me to shut this production off by taking enough T3 to completely suppress the thyroid gland without becoming hyperthyroid. So, I had some T4 left in my system. It may well have been at the very low end of the reference range (or just below it) but it was there and measurable on blood tests. Reverse T3 (rT3) could not be tested back then, but I imagine that a lot of the T4 my remaining thyroid tissue was making, was converting to rT3. This is because my TSH was very low due to T3-Only therapy. We know that low TSH tends to increase the conversion to rT3, because low TSH downregulates the production of the deiodinase enzymes that convert T4 to T3. My autoantibodies were also still present, albeit at a lower level than when first diagnosed.

Over a period of a few years, the ongoing autoimmune attack gradually destroyed my thyroid gland completely. As my thyroid was destroyed, my autoantibodies got lower and my FT4 got closer to zero. I was gradually able to increase my T3 dosing and as it approached 50 mcg per day, my health, energy and wellness began to return to normal.

After a few years, I was able to get my T3 dosage to 60 mcg per day. This slow process of increasing the T3 was not anything about me slowly getting adjusted to it. It was that, whilst my thyroid gland was producing T4, I was simply unable to get the T3 dosing up. Any T4 produced by my thyroid would have given me some small amount of extra FT3 but also enough rT3 that I simply could not cope with.

When I was at 60 mcg of T3, I felt extremely well. I could function as well as I could before I had become ill. At that point, I had no thyroid tissue left at all.

What is the point of my story? Well, here is the important bit.

I did try a number of autoimmune protocols e.g., using selenium supplements and adopting a gluten-free and dairy-free diet for over two years. They failed to make any difference to me. However, if these approaches had been successful in stopping the autoantibodies earlier on, the consequence would have been to PERMANENTLY LEAVE ME WITH ILL HEALTH! I will explain why this would have been the case.

I had a major T4 to T3 conversion issue that had nothing to do with the ongoing autoimmune response. It was everything to do with the gene defects and the loss of thyroid gland tissue. Basically, I had lost too much T4 to T3 conversion ability already. I actually NEEDED to get my T4 totally out of my system. The only way I could do that effectively was to have the Hashimoto's run its course and destroy my thyroid gland completely. Once my thyroid could no longer make T4, I could get my T3 higher and feel well. The fact that my autoantibodies, fell to zero had little or no benefit – that was just a side effect of having no more thyroid tissue.

I did try several times to raise my T3 beyond 50 mcg when I had some thyroid tissue left because I wanted to get the T3 dose up and to shut down my thyroid, but it just made me feel hyper and ill. I was simply unable to completely shut the thyroid gland down, whilst I still had some thyroid tissue left.

The above is also backed up by the fact that, even today, I am unable to add even 5 mcg of T4 medication per day without feeling ill within a week. I just cannot cope with the T4 and the rT3 it produces.

I now consider myself lucky that my Hashi's ran to completion and destroyed my thyroid gland utterly. When I was first diagnosed it was already too late to ever regain decent T4 to T3 conversion – the thyroid tissue loss combined with the gene defects had already made it impossible for me to deal with T4 properly.

I never wrote about this aspect of my own health issue in my book, Recovering with T3, as I felt it was far too complex and would have made the book too long. I also did not know when I first wrote it, that I had the DIO1 and DIO2 gene defects.

What are the implications for other Hashimoto's patients considering using an AIP?

The dietary and supplement approaches that are currently popular in terms of reducing and stopping the thyroid autoimmune response are excellent if the person finds out they have Hashimoto's thyroiditis early in the process. There is no doubt of this. I think these approaches are excellent early on, before there is significant thyroid tissue damage.

However, they do suffer from a couple of problems:

1. Often, it is too late to avoid thyroid tissue damage and the lost conversion ability that comes with it. The diagnosis of Hashimoto's frequently comes at the point when much of the thyroid gland has already been destroyed.

2. There are often many other problems that cause T4 to T3 conversion issues that no amount of working with diet or supplements is going to help, e.g., DIO2, DIO1 gene defects do not go away, lost thyroid tissue does not come back etc.

Let me be very clear, if the autoimmune issue is found early enough, before very much thyroid damage is caused, and if the autoimmune response can quickly be stopped in its tracks, then this is extremely helpful. In addition, if the thyroid patient is unlikely to lose a significant amount of their conversion ability, then an AIP can also help. AIP can avoid years of problems and the need to go on lifelong thyroid medication.

However, for those with a severe T4 to T3 conversion issue caused by either lost thyroid tissue or gene defects or both, AIP could be a total and utter disaster. For these people, stopping the autoimmune response could prevent them from ever getting on the right level of T3 that resolves all their symptoms. Thyroid patients in this category could be left with no autoimmune reaction, a partially working thyroid gland but very poor conversion. They would then potentially find it difficult to take the right balance of T4 and T3 hormones to make them feel well.

For some people, it may be better to let the autoimmune attack run its course and do what it needs to do! I suspect that you have not heard anyone say that before – but in some circumstances, it can be true.

Those that have a severe T4 to T3 conversion issue (through lost thyroid tissue, gene defects or both) need to be careful what they wish for regarding stopping any autoimmune response using an autoimmune protocol (via diet or supplements).

I also believe that the most important thing with thyroid problems, especially if they are not caught early, is to get people on the right balance of thyroid hormones for them. People need to get well fast. This is the single best approach to avoid all the other dreadful consequences to jobs, relationships etc. Life is too short to spend years trying other approaches out. The kind of collateral damage that can come with being unwell for a prolonged period of time, really needs to be avoided.

Trying to fix Hashimoto's with dietary or supplement approaches can be effective if the issue is caught very early on, before significant thyroid damage occurs and if the person responds well to the AIP approach. However, if the thyroid patient already has serious conversion issues, the AIP approach needs careful consideration.

To find out more about AIP you can visit Dr Westin Child's website, one of his links is here:
https://www.restartmed.com/root-causes-of-hashimotos/#more-88438

Izabella Wentz also has some very good books on the subject of AIPs.

I hope this quite complex article has been informative and helpful to you.

12. BREAST IMPLANTS AND HYPOTHYROIDISM SYMPTOMS

A while ago, I spoke to a patient, Melissa. I determined that I could not find any evidence of a genuine thyroid problem. I do not find thyroid problems in everyone I talk to. On occasion, I even recommend that people stop taking thyroid medication because it is not actually needed. In some cases, a different condition is causing the patient's symptoms.

In Melissa's case, there did not seem to be a thyroid problem at all. However, there were definite low iron issues (from labs and symptoms), and I suggested some iron supplementation and some other basic nutrients to cover the bases.

Later, Melissa got back to me and told me that she had been diagnosed with Breast Implant Illness (BII).

The idea to consider this had not arisen during our communications. I do not even think she told me that she had implants. Why would she? It would not have seemed relevant.

Melissa is a good, kind woman and wants to let others know about this issue, so she has asked me to write something about it.

The best way to do this is to use her own words, which she has given me permission to use, so here they are:

"Hello Paul!

I hope you are doing well!

I am not sure if you remember me, I had a discussion with you about two months ago and we went over my labs and we were trying to figure out if I had hypothyroidism. To recap my main symptoms, I went through major hair loss, brain fog, and low energy. We figured out that the main culprit was low iron and probably stress, but not my thyroid.

Since our talk, I have started on the recommended supplements and hormones, and have completely changed how I eat. I would love to say that everything got 100% better but they have not, because the real culprit is something I never thought of....my breast implants. I am emailing you to try and get the word out to as many people as I can.

After doing much research, I have found the sickness due to breast implants is called Breast Implant Illness (BII) and women are developing autoimmune diseases, Lymphoma, hypothyroidism, hormone imbalance, early menopause, miscarriages, Lupus, and the list goes on and on.

I am not sure if all my symptoms are due to my breast implants, but I believe many of them are due to the fact that they are "foreign bodies" inside of me. I have found a surgeon who specializes in "explant" and taking the entire "capsule" out when taking out the implant. A woman's body naturally builds a barrier (capsule) around the implants to protect the rest of the body from this foreign body and I am finding out how important it is to have these capsules removed, along with the implants.

The very sad and upsetting thing about all of this is that seven years ago, when I had the implants put in, I along with millions of other women were never told of the health risks. In fact, I was told that they were safe and that if they leaked, the saline would naturally be absorbed by the body......they forgot to mention that the outer shell is made of silicone and contains different metals and other materials that are toxic to the human body.

In September 2018, one of the largest ever studies published shows breast implants ARE associated with rare diseases. The article is "US FDA Breast Implant Postapproval Studies". Here is also a link to the US FDA Q&A on the subject: https://www.fda.gov/medicaldevices/productsandmedicalprocedures/implantsandprosth etics/breastimplants/ucm241086.htm

There is also a chemist in Canada that has examined and studied implants after they have been removed and what he has found is astonishing: mould, fungus and bacteria, all inside the implants!

What is the view where you are at, in the UK? Are women returning to the surgery table to get these "toxic bags" removed, or is this surgery still the top plastic surgery performed every year like it is in the US? I believe in 10 or 20 years from now, they will be banned and the women from 1960 until when they are banned, will have become the guinea pigs. Thank you for the help you provided two months ago!"

I asked Melissa if I could use her exact words and this was her reply:

"Absolutely! I am more than happy for you to use any information you need from me to get this information out. I do not mind if you use all the details you need about my personal situation. You can even use my name and let people know that I can be reached through Facebook as I am contemplating starting a blog about my journey to get this information out there.

To give you a little more history, I got my implants in March of 2012. Life moved on without any health issues until July 2018. I am finding that between 6-10 years is when many women start seeing health problems associated with their implants. However, some women start having health issues right away. Let me know if there is any other specific information you might need from me.

Thank you so much for writing about this! Information is essential for others to know what might be going on in their own bodies!
Truly grateful,
Melissa"

If anyone wants to contact Melissa, they can message her on Facebook. Her Facebook ID is: https://www.facebook.com/melissa.ourbiijourney.5
Melissa also provided me with another document that discusses this:
https://www.fda.gov/medicaldevices/productsandmedicalprocedures/implantsandprosth etics/breastimplants/ucm239995.htm

I know the above will only apply to a small percentage of women, but if this article helps just a handful of women, it would be a good result. As a postscript to this, I have also worked with another thyroid patient who I suspected might have the same issues. She did. She had an explant procedure and her health improved rapidly afterwards.

13. T3 TREATMENT AND CT3M – RELEVANCE IN MANY CONDITIONS

I know from personal experience and from dealing with thousands of thyroid patients over a period of more than 15 years, that T4/T3 combination therapy (including the use of natural desiccated thyroid) is often required. Some thyroid patients need T3-Only therapy. All the treatment options need to be available for every doctor to choose from when dealing with individual patients. In some cases, the Circadian T3 Method (CT3M) is also required in order to raise cortisol levels.

Every thyroid patient is different. We are not all the same in the way our systems work and do not work. Some thyroid patients have lost thyroid tissue (through thyroidectomy or Hashimoto's) – this loses around 25% of their T3, mostly through the loss of T4 to T3 conversion capability. Other thyroid patients have poor conversion ability due to deiodinase enzyme production defects in their genetic makeup (DIO1 and DIO2 gene defects).

T3 stimulates every tissue and organ to ensure they can perform their function well. It is critical for energy production in every organ. This includes the hypothalamic-pituitary (HP) system. Low thyroid effect in the HP system reduces all hormones. This is why hypothyroidism should always be considered in cases of testosterone deficiency, amenorrhea (loss of menstrual cycles), growth hormone deficiency, and hypocortisolism.

T3 in T4/T3 combination therapy and especially in T3-Only therapy often manages to raise cortisol from a low level to a normal level. This sometimes requires the use of my Circadian T3 Method (CT3M) protocol (defined in my book, Recovering with T3, and in The CT3M Handbook). I have seen this many times in thyroid patients being treated with T3. Research studies make it clear that the pituitary is known to have the highest concentration of T3 within its cells compared to other tissue in the body. The pituitary produces its own D2 deiodinase enzymes and is a prolific converter of T4 to T3. So, in a healthy person with good conversion, the pituitary basically runs on T3, as its fuel.

In my book, Recovering with T3, I describe what I did to raise my own cortisol level from dreadfully low to normal using CT3M. I discovered that taking T3 several hours before people get up in the morning helps the pituitary to produce the high early morning levels of ACTH and get morning cortisol back up to normal.

This is why I think that T3 use could be instrumental, not only for thyroid patients who remain with severe symptoms of hypothyroidism when on T4-monotherapy, but also for patients suffering from conditions like fibromyalgia, chronic fatigue syndrome (CFS) and ME. I believe in many of those conditions, the problem is the hypothalamic-pituitary (HP) system that is no longer ensuring the end hormones are produced at a good enough level. This is especially true if patients with these conditions have low cortisol.

The T4 hormone does virtually nothing. It has effects only if it is converted to T3 (in healthy people who are good converters of T4 to T3). If T4 monotherapy does not work well and results in lower levels of T3 production than in a healthy person, then T3 needs to be used either in combination therapy or on its own in T3-Only treatment.

I believe that T3 ought to be one of the options available when treating conditions like CFS, ME, and fibromyalgia (where end hormones like cortisol and T3 are often lower than ideal).

Higher T3 levels stimulate ACTH and cortisol production, and other end-hormones modulated by the HP system. In hypothyroidism, ACTH and cortisol production are often significantly reduced, even to the point to suggest there is a pituitary problem.

In summary, T3 therapy, and CT3M, should be an option for thyroid patients who do not respond well to other treatments. These treatments also should be an option for CFS, ME, and Fibromyalgia patients who need to have their hypothalamic-pituitary system given a boost. T3 is about the easiest way to help the HP system.

Here are some relevant research references:

- Sánchez-Franco F, Fernández L, Fernández G, Cacicedo L. – Thyroid hormone action on ACTH secretion. Horm Metab Res. 1989;21(10):550-552. The Abstract is here: https://www.ncbi.nlm.nih.gov/pubmed/2553572 This paper clearly provides actual research backing for why the Circadian T3 Method (CT3M) works so well. By providing the hypothalamic-pituitary system with enough T3 when it needs to drive ACTH high, CT3M helps to raise morning cortisol to normal levels.
- Lizcano F, Rodríguez JS. Thyroid hormone therapy modulates hypothalamo-pituitary-adrenal axis. Endocr J. 2011;58(2):137-142. The abstract may be found here: https://www.ncbi.nlm.nih.gov/pubmed/21263198
- Bigos ST, Ridgway EC, Kourides IA, Maloof F. Spectrum of pituitary alterations with mild and severe thyroid impairment. J Clin Endocrinol Metab. 1978;46(2):317-325. The abstract may be found here: https://academic.oup.com/jcem/article-abstract/46/2/317/2677356?redirectedFrom=fulltext
- Tunbridge WM, Marshall JC, Burke CW. Primary hypothyroidism presenting as pituitary failure. Br Med J. 1973;1(5846):153-154. The abstract and full text are available here: https://www.ncbi.nlm.nih.gov/pmc/articles/PMC1588401/
- Paula Bargi-Souza · Rodrigo Antonio Peliciari-Garcia · Maria Tereza Nunes. Disruption of the Pituitary Circadian Clock Induced by Hypothyroidism and Hyperthyroidism: Consequences on Daily Pituitary Hormone Expression Profiles. Thyroid. 2019 Apr;29(4):502-512. doi: 10.1089/thy.2018.0578. Epub 2019 Mar ·13. The abstract is: https://www.ncbi.nlm.nih.gov/pubmed/30747

www.ingramcontent.com/pod-product-compliance
Lightning Source LLC
Chambersburg PA
CBHW082351270326
41935CB00013B/1584